Reduced Dose Mammography

edited by

Wende Westinghouse Logan, M.D.
Consultant, Roswell Park Memorial Institute
Buffalo, New York

E. Phillip Muntz, Ph.D.
Professor of Aerospace Engineering and
Diagnostic Radiology
University of Southern California
Los Angeles, California

 MASSON Publishing USA, Inc.
New York · Paris · Barcelona ·
Milan · Mexico City · Rio de Janeiro

Proceedings of the Second Reduced Dose Mammography Meeting, Roswell Park
Institute, Buffalo, New York, October 4–6, 1978

Acknowledgments

This symposium was funded by the Bureau of Radiological Health, FDA (Contract No. FDA 223-78-6012), and held on October 4–6th, 1978, in cooperation with the Roswell Park Memorial Institute, New York State Department of Health, Buffalo, New York.

Preface

Because of public and professional interest in questions concerning the benefits and risks to be associated with mammography, there have been widespread efforts over the past few years to reduce the dose required for mammography examinations. Reduced dose mammography is now universally practiced in the United States and is being accepted in many other countries.

Sensitive detector systems and numerous equipment modifications, as well as revised breast positioning and other technique changes, have resulted in images that are not only obtained at low doses, but which appear to permit simultaneously improved diagnostic performances. For example, in the Breast Cancer Detection Demonstration Project, the ability of mammography as the sole method of detection of breast carcinomas in asymptomatic women under the age of 50, when compared with the ability to detect carcinomas in the same women solely by physical examination, has increased 18-fold relative to the original HIP screening study in the mid-1960s.

Rationalizing the apparently improved performance of modern mammography systems, as well as discussing ways to continue improving these systems, were two major objectives of this symposium. At the symposium the status of reduced dose mammography was reviewed in a coherent, carefully chosen program. The central issues associated with reduced dose mammography—radiation effects, proper indices for risk, diagnostic and clinical performances, and risk-benefit analyses—were discussed. In addition, the technical and diagnostic basis for the continuing optimization of mammography was examined.

We hope that the material presented here will provide a scientific focus that will encourage further developments in technology, technique, and diagnosis. A review of the material in this volume suggests that further mammography dose reductions are possible without degradations in image quality; or alternatively, there can be important image quality improvements without concomitant dose increases.

We would like to thank the contributors to this volume for their cooperation in permitting as much editing as possible within the constraints of the photo-ready format. (Our secretaries, Sandy Lantieri, Gayle Callaghan, Alyce Norder, and Julie Syverson-Routly have been a great solace during the past six months.) The format was chosen primarily because it permits timely publication at a reasonable cost. The value of this symposium was greatly enhanced by the financial and academic support of the Bureau of Radiological

Health, for which we are very grateful. We also wish to thank the staff (Kevin Craig *et al.*) of the Roswell Park Memorial Institute for their valuable assistance in coordinating and holding the meeting.

Wende Logan
Phillip Muntz

Contributors

Erik Åkerlund   Department of Surgery, Central Hospital, Falun, Sweden

Lars Baldetorp   Institute of Surgery, University of Linköping, Sweden

Gary T. Barnes   Department of Diagnostic Radiology, University of Alabama School of Medicine, The University of Alabama in Birmingham, Birmingham, Alabama 35233

Lloyd M. Bates   AAPM-CRP Coordination Office, Suite 307, 6900 Wisconsin Avenue, Chevy Chase, Maryland 20015

Eugene V. Benton   Professor of Physics, University of San Francisco, San Francisco, California

Martin Braun   Radiologic Sciences Inc., 2920 Coronado Drive, Santa Clara, California 95051

Phillip C. Bunch   Eastman Kodak Company, Rochester, New York 14650

John R. Cameron   Department of Radiology, University of Wisconsin, Madison, Wisconsin 53706

C. H. Joseph Chang   Department of Diagnostic Radiology, University of Kansas Medical Center, Kansas City, Kansas 66103

Richard P. Chiacchierini   Epidemiological Studies Branch, Division of Biological Effects, Bureau of Radiological Health, FDA, Rockville, Maryland 20857

Andrzej J. Demidecki   AAPM-CRP Coordination Office, Suite 307, 6900 Wisconsin Avenue, Chevy Chase, Maryland 20015

Larry A. DeWerd   Department of Radiology, University of Wisconsin, Madison, Wisconsin 53706

Gerald D. Dodd   Departments of Diagnostic Radiology and Physics, Section of Experimental Diagnostic Radiology, The University of Texas System Cancer Center, M.D. Anderson Hospital and Tumor Institute, Houston, Texas 77030

Kunio Doi   Kurt Rossman Laboratories for Radiologic Image Research, Department of Radiology, The University of Chicago, and The Franklin McLean Memorial Research Institute, Chicago, Illinois 60637

Robert L. Egan   Chief, Mammography Section and Professor of Radiology, Emory University, Atlanta, Georgia 30322

Gunnar Fagerberg   Institute of Radiology, University of Linköping, Sweden

Panos P. Fatouros   Medical College of Virginia, Radiation Physics Division, Box 72, Richmond, Virginia 23298

Stephen A. Feig   Department of Radiology, Thomas Jefferson University, Philadelphia, Pennsylvania 19107

Bertil Fors   Department of Pathology, Central Hospital, Falun, Sweden

Michael Friedrich   Klinikum Steglitz, Klinik für Radiologie und Nuklearmedizin, Institut für klinische Physiologie, Freie Universität Berlin, Berlin, Federal Republic of Germany

Adel Gad Department of Pathology, Central Hospital, Falun, Sweden

B. M. Galkin Department of Radiology, Thomas Jefferson University, Philadelphia, Pennsylvania 19107

John J. Gisvold Consultant, Department of Diagnostic Radiology, Mayo Clinic and Mayo Foundation, Rochester, Minnesota

Richard H. Gold Professor of Radiological Sciences, Chief, Diagnostic Division, Department of Radiological Sciences, UCLA Center for Health Sciences, Los Angeles, California 90024

R. O. Gorson Department of Radiology, Thomas Jefferson University, Philadelphia, Pennsylvania

Otto Gröntoft Institute of Medical Microbiology and Pathology, University of Linköping, Sweden

John F. Hamilton, Jr. Eastman Kodak Company, Rochester, New York 14650

G. Richard Hammerstein* Northeast Center for Radiological Physics, Memorial Sloan-Kettering Cancer Center, New York, New York 10021

Arthur G. Haus Departments of Diagnostic Radiology and Physics, Section of Experimental Diagnostic Radiology, The University of Texas System Cancer Center, M.D. Anderson Hospital and Tumor Institute, Houston, Texas 77030

Robert L. Hirschfeld Greater Baltimore Medical Center, Baltimore, Maryland

Gunnila Holje Kurt Rossmann Laboratories for Radiological Image Research, Department of Radiology, The University of Chicago, and The Franklin McLean Memorial Research Institute, Chicago, Illinois 60637

Ronald G. Jans Bureau of Radiological Health, Food and Drug Administration, U.S. Department of Health, Education, and Welfare, 5600 Fishers Lane, Rockville, Maryland 20857

Robert Jennings Medical Physics Branch, Division of Electronic Products, Bureau of Radiological Health, FDA, Rockville, Maryland 20857

Gerhard Jost Philips-Mueller, Medical Systems Division, 200 Hamburg 1, Germany

Emil Kaegi Xonics Inc., Van Nuys, California 91406

Lester Kalisher Saint Barnabas Medical Center, Department of Radiology, Livingston, New Jersey 07039

Michael A. King Department of Diagnostic Radiology, University of Alabama School of Medicine, University of Alabama in Birmingham, Birmingham, Alabama 35233

Lars-Olof Lamke Institute of Surgery, University of Linköping, Sweden

M. Lassen Department of Radiology, Thomas Jefferson University, Philadelphia, Pennsylvania

Richard G. Lester Professor and Chairman, Department of Radiology, The University of Texas Medical School at Houston, Houston, Texas 77030

John Lewis Xonics, Inc., 6849 Hayvenhurst, Van Nuys, California 91406

Wende W. Logan Consultant, Roswell Park Memorial Institute, 1351 Mt. Hope Avenue, Rochester, New York 14620

Frank E. Lundin Epidemiological Studies Branch, Division of Biological Effects, Bureau of Radiological Health, FDA, Rockville, Maryland 20857

Mary E. Masterson Memorial Hospital, 1275 York Ave., New York, New York 10021

* Deceased

Daniel W. Miller Memorial Hospital, 1275 York Ave., New York, New York 10021

Myron Moskowitz Professor of Radiology, University of Cincinnati Medical Center, Cincinnati General Hospital, Cincinnati, Ohio

E. Phillip Muntz Departments of Aerospace Engineering and Radiology, University of Southern California, Los Angeles, California 90007

Rudolph Nerlinger Department of Radiology, Thomas Jefferson University, Philadelphia, Pennsylvania

Ann Westinghouse Norlund 1351 Mt. Hope Ave., Rochester, New York 14620

Patricia A. O'Brien Chief Mammography Technologist, Emory University, Atlanta, Georgia 30322

Thomas R. Ohlhaber Bureau of Radiological Health, Food and Drug Administration, U.S. Department of Health, Education, and Welfare, 5600 Fishers Lane, Rockville, Maryland 20857

Arthur S. Patchefsky Department of Radiology, Thomas Jefferson University, Philadelphia, Pennsylvania 19107

David D. Paulus Departments of Diagnostic Radiology and Physics, Section of Experimental Diagnostic Radiology, The University of Texas System Cancer Center, M.D. Anderson Hospital and Tumor Institute, Houston, Texas 77030

Saar A. Porrath Department of Radiology, Santa Monica Hospital Medical Center, Santa Monica, California

Gopala U. V. Rao Medical College of Virginia, Radiation Physics Division, Box 72, Richmond, Virginia 23298

Bernard Roth Eastman Kodak Company, Rochester, New York 14650

Gordon F. Schwartz Department of Radiology, Thomas Jefferson University, Philadelphia, Pennsylvania 19107

Gary S. Shaber Department of Radiology, Thomas Jefferson University, Philadelphia, Pennsylvania 19107

Melvin P. Sieband Department of Radiology, University of Wisconsin, Madison, Wisconsin 53706

Ruth E. Snyder Attending Radiologist, Memorial Sloan-Kettering Cancer Center, New York, New York 10021

Perry Sprawls Professor and Director, Division of Physics and Engineering, Department of Radiology, Emory University, Atlanta, Georgia 30322

Leonard Stanton Department of Radiation Therapy and Nuclear Medicine, Hahnemann Medical College and Hospital, Philadelphia, Pennsylvania 19102

Alfred M. Strash Radiation Physics Division, Medical College of Virginia, Richmond, Virginia 23298

László Tabar Department of Mammography, Central Hospital, Falun, Sweden

Cornelius A. Tobias Professor of Medical Physics, Radiation Biophysics Group Leader, Lawrence Berkeley Laboratory, Berkeley, California

Edward A. Sickles Department of Radiology, University of California School of Medicine, San Francisco, California 94143

Robert F. Wagner Medical Physics Branch, Division of Electronic Products, Bureau of Radiological Health, FDA, Rockville, Maryland 20857

Robert E. Wayrynen E. I. du Pont de Nemours & Co., Inc., Wilmington, Delaware 19898

Edward W. Webster Division of Radiological Sciences, Massachusetts General Hospital, Boston, Massachusetts 02114

Peter Weskamp Klinikum Steglitz, Klinik für Radiologie und Nuklearmedizin, Institut für klinische Physiologie, Freie Universität Berlin, Berlin, Federal Republic of Germany

John F. Wochos Department of Radiology, University of Wisconsin, Madison, Wisconsin 53706

Kay H. Woodruff Consulting Pathologist, Lawrence Berkeley Laboratory, Berkeley, California

Michael V. Yester Department of Diagnostic Radiology, University of Alabama School of Medicine, University of Alabama in Birmingham, Birmingham, Alabama 35233

Contents

Part II: TECHNICAL CONSIDERATIONS

This book is dedicated to G. Richard Hammerstein (1942–1978) in recognition of his work in mammography dosimetry

PART I

BENEFIT AND RISK

A SYSTEMS ANALYSIS OF MAMMOGRAPHY: AN OUTLINE OF AN INTEGRATED APPROACH TO REDUCED DOSE MAMMOGRAPHY

by

E.P. Muntz, Ph.D.
University of Southern California

INTRODUCTION

A system analysis is like a good business plan. You do not expect it to be absolutely correct, particularly when dealing with the behavior of a complicated system. But you do expect it to provide a baseline that can be used to keep track of departures from expected behavior, or to indicate the way to possible improvements. In the case of mammography, we can use analysis to indicate directions for further study as well as to identify potential improvements in present systems.

The purpose of this paper is not to pretend to describe in precise detail all aspects of an examination and diagnosis. It is an attempt to provide a framework of understanding that permits one to begin to address, in a system- atic manner, the really central issues confronting the practice of mammography, viz, for what techniques and for what levels of tissue dose is there an optimum benefit compared to the associated risks? It must, of course, be noted that the conditions leading to an optimum will likely depend on the patient population's risk level; that is, depend on whether one is dealing with a screening population or a referral population.

In the past few years there have been numerous pressures and subsequent responses associated with mammography. The pressures have appeared in the form of a semi-scientific debate in the lay and scientific press over the benefits and risks to be properly associated with mammography. The responses, at least in North America, have included: reduced patient cooperation; a limiting of certain classes of screening-type examinations; increased efforts to establish the efficacy of the examination, particularly in younger women; and rather dramatic reductions in dose by means of technique and hardware changes, with some accompanying alteration of image quality.

Two major purposes of this symposium were; to investigate and document the image quality changes that can be associated with the reduced doses, and to study the diagnostic and clinical implications of such changes. There are really three fundamental questions associated with these aspects of mammography.

First, what equipment characteristics and technique parameters provide the greatest amount of basic (technical) information content per unit of carcinogenic effect?

Then, for diagnostic purposes, what is the best way to display this information content? And a corollary, what is a meaningful way to describe the connection between the technical information and the displayed diagnostic information?

3

Finally, we must ask how the amount of displayed diagnostic information varies with the carcinogenic effect of the examination and how much and what kind of diagnostic information is really required to achieve specified clinical results?

To answer the first question, it is necessary to understand in a quantitative way the interrelationships of the elements in a mammography examination and to determine appropriate technical measures for information content and carcinogenic effect

After this, the display of the technical information must be understood in terms of diagnostically significant measures. One possible but not necessarily always good example of such a measure is an appropriate signal to noise ratio.

For the third question, the displayed diagnostic information characteristics and carcinogenic effects of the newer techniques and the older ones should be compared to their corresponding clinical performances, in order to relate diagnostic information and carcinogenic effects to clinical results. In addition, different configurations and techniques should be sought that provide the same diagnostic information as accepted existing systems, but with less carcinogenic effect.

DISCUSSION

The basic questions associated with mammography and an outline of the information needed to answer these questions has been presented above. In what follows is a brief sketch of some attempts at being more specific with particular reference to the subjects dealt with by the many excellent papers in this volume. Together, these papers provide a significant advance towards providing the information that is required to formulate specific answers to the questions that have been asked.

It is useful to outline what is understood about attempting to answer at least the first question mentioned above. A list of the several elements of a mammography examination that interact to provide an image can be written. It is the simultaneous interaction of these elements that must be considered in order to optimize a mammographic examination to provide a specified image quality for the least possible carcinogenic effect.

A list of these elements along with an indication of where in this volume the subject, or a related subject, is discussed (indicated by senior author's name in parentheses) is:

- focal spot size (Braun, Haus)
- photon spectrum (Jennings, Siedband)
- source detector distance (Barnes, Haus)
- patient size distribution (Jost, Logan)
- targets to be detected including their surround (panel discussions: Cameron, Egan, Friedrich, Gold, Haus, Kalisher, Moskowitz, Miller, Sickles, Snyder, Stanton
- air gap (Barnes, Haus, Jost, Logan, Sickles, Stanton)
- scatter suppression devices (Barnes, Jost, Logan, Stanton)
- effective detector quantum efficiency (Doi,Friedrich,Lewis,Roth,Wagner)
- detector resolution (Doi, Fatouros, Friedrich, Haus, Wagner)
- detector sensitivity (Doi, Fatouros, Friedrich, Haus, Kaegi, Lewis, Roth, Wagner, Wayrynen)
- exposure time and tube output (Braun, Logan, Siedband)

- carcinogenic effects (Chiaccierini, Feig, Hammerstein, Lester, Moskowitz, Muntz, Webster)
- technical indicators of image quality (Doi, Fatouros, Friedrich, Wagner; panel - Cameron, Egan, Friedrich, Miller)

A careful look at any one of these items will usually result in a fairly clear outline of what important unsolved problems remain. For example, consider the case of carcinogenic effects. If a linear dose effects relationship is assumed, an average dose for the glandular tissue is appropriate as an indicator of carcinogenic effect (Ref. 1) -- assuming, of course, that all of the glandular tissue is equally sensitive. In order to obtain an estimate of carcinogenic effect, we then need to know: age specific spatial distribution of glandular tissue, age specific breast thicknesses during examination, depth dose information, and the assumed linear dose-effects relationship. We now have adequate depth dose information (Ref. 2 and Hammerstein); we do not have very quantitative information on the age specific distribution of sensitive tissue nor age specific breast thickness distributions during mammography. While obtaining this information represents a certain amount of effort, it is not difficult to imagine creating a well defined and reasonably limited program to do so.

Although there is not sufficient space here to go into each item on the preceding list, the results of such an inquiry show that there are only two major points other than the two indicated above, where there is not enough information. One relates to the question of patient motion and exposure time, and in particular how long an exposure is possible without the motion problem becoming unacceptable; the other to target specification, particularly soft tissue targets. For the remaining items there is sufficient information to begin an analysis of how the various elements in a mammography examination simultaneously interact with each other. Indeed, the limited number of places where more information is needed can be avoided to some extent by simply using in the analysis several possibilities, such as several maximum exposure times.

How important is the interrelationship between the elements of a mammography system? I will consider two examples for illustrative purposes. The first is photon energy control and the second is an analysis of magnification mammography. I will have to be brief; for more details on these subjects, related articles in this volume should be consulted, as well as the original work which appears in references 3 and 4.

As an illustration of the effects of photon energy control (also refer to article by Jennings in this volume) the exposure of a Stanton mammography phantom, using a Min-R detector, has been studied (Ref. 3). For this phantom, the performance of the Min-R system was examined by theoretically determining the exposure multipliers associated with hypothetical systems, each having one of the individual performance degrading characteristics of the Min-R system. It has been shown (Ref. 3 and Jennings) that for the detection of calcifications in mammography there are optimum photon energies that depend on phantom thickness, composition, etc. The results of the study described in reference 3 indicate that energy de-tuning (too low) in the Min-R exposure accounts for an exposure multiplier of 3.3; quantum efficiency effects account for a factor of 2.5 and system blur a factor of 2.1. The beam energy in film screen mammography is low because of contrast requirements. Thus, the analysis indicates that if detectors with greater contrast could be found and used along with suitable generators (see Braun's and Siedband's articles in this volume), there could be significant savings in exposure for a given image quality (see also Jennings in this volume).

Now consider the more complicated situation of an analysis of magnification mammography including; scattered radiation, focal spot and detector blurring, and assuming various generator outputs and focal spot sizes. Such an analysis has been done (Ref. 4) by referencing the magnification situation to contact exposures, assuming a constant sensitivity detector and equal exposure times for all the exposures. Among the conclusions of the study was that focal spot size and tube outputs interact in a complicated way with the scattering reduction due to an air gap such that, for reduced dose mammography systems, somewhat better performance may be realized for a given exposure increase using tubes with intermediate size ($\approx$300 μm) focal spots. The analysis also indicates that if say 4 sec. exposure times could be tolerated, tubes with focal spots around 150 μm would be preferred.

In both of the examples given above, it is the interaction between the properties of a few or larger number of the elements of the system I want to emphasize. In fact, when these types of studies are examined in detail, it becomes clear that in terms of optimizing a mammography examination, the interaction of the elements of the examination is at least as important as the detailed characteristics of each individual element. Note also that all the elements of the examination are important, not simply the traditional ones of detector resolution and speed and focal spot size.

So far, only the first question mentioned in the introduction of this article has been addressed. The second and third questions are more difficult, although the work reported by Chiacchierini, Moskowitz, Feig and Tabar in this volume make a significant contribution towards reaching an answer to the third one. In the case of the second question, more work needs to be done, for the most part connected with the radiographic clutter produced by normal tissue. This is primarily of importance when attempting to decide on gross optimum characteristics of the display modulation transfer function (e.g., between high edge effect or none). If, on the other hand, one is satisfied with a compromise that compares various possible systems with similarly shaped modulation transfer functions (as in different film screen systems), question two is not quite so terrifying. Indeed, it then seems reasonable to rely on signal to noise ratios and contrast for various sized targets as satisfactory indicators (see, for instance, the article by Friedrich in this volume).

SUMMARY

Based on the brief sketch given above as well as more detailed work reported elsewhere, it is my opinion that with the help of the new information presented in this volume, we are approaching an ability to be able to answer, at least to a first approximation, the fundamental questions affecting reduced dose mammography. It is important to remember that the simultaneous interrelationship of all the elements in a mammography examination must be considered in order to achieve as low a carcinogenic effect as possible for some required clinical performance.

A list of information that is still needed to in fact reach the goal of a satisfactory absolute optimization is:

- exposure time (how long a time can be tolerated before serious motion problems are encountered)
- quantitative age specific distribution of glandular tissue
- age specific patient size distributions
- additional target specification and characterizations

- connection between technical information content and displayed diagnostic information (particularly for dissimilar modulation transfer functions).
- information on the relationship between displayed diagnostic information content and, say, person-years saved.

It is to be hoped that over a period of a few years most of this information can be obtained. In the interim it is quite reasonable to do restricted optimization based say on the most dose effective way to achieve present levels of diagnostic information content. It is my opinion that such restricted optimizations are possible with the amount of information that is presently in hand.

On a more practical note, combining the results given by Chiacchierini in this volume with those of Moskowitz and Tabar, also in this volume, it is possible to sketch an answer to the global question of what benefit for what risk. This, of course, does not represent other than a possibly accidental optimization, but it is a starting point. The more detailed information requirements discussed here are necessary to proceed beyond such an input output result in order to optimize the mammographic breast cancer detection system.

References

1. E.P. Muntz: "On the Relative Carcinogenic Effects of Different Mammography Techniques". To be published, Medical Physics, 1979.

2. D.W. Miller, G.R. Hammerstein, D.R. White, M.E. Masterson, and J.W. Laughlin: "Radiation Absorbed Dose in Mammography." Presented to AAPM, Cincinnati, Ohio, August 1-4, 1977.

3. E.P. Muntz, M. Welkowsky, E. Kaegi, L. Morsell, E. Wilkinson, G. Jacobson: "Optimization of Electrostatic Imaging Systems for Minimum Patient Dose or Minimum Exposure in Mammography." Radiology, 127(2):517, 1978.

4. E.P. Muntz: "On the Significance of Scattered Radiation in Reduced Dose Mammography Including: Magnification Effects, Scatter Suppression, Focal Spot and Detector Blurring." To be published, Medical Physics, March/April 1979.

EPIDEMIOLOGY OF RADIATION RELATED BREAST CANCER

Stephen A. Feig, M.D.

Department of Radiology, Thomas Jefferson University Hospital, Phila.,Pa.

This paper will examine the assumptions of radiation risk which would enter a benefit risk equation for mammography. Data for this evaluation will be obtained from several groups of women who, after exposure to high doses of ionizing radiation, exhibited an excess breast cancer incidence when compared to similar populations of non-irradiated women. These groups were comprised of:

1. Japanese women exposed to gamma and neutron radiation from atomic bombings at Hiroshima and Nagasaki (13).
2. Women from Rochester, N.Y. treated with radiotherapy for postpartum mastitis (18).
3. Swedish women treated with radiotherapy for fibroadenomatosis and other benign breast conditions (1).
4. Women who received multiple chest fluoroscopies during artificial pneumothorax treatment for pulmonary tuberculosis. Two groups of women were evaluated in separate studies. These were from sanatoria in
   A. Nova Scotia (12, 14, 15)
   B. Massachusetts (3)

The risk of radiation carcinogenesis in humans is generally expressed in terms of absolute risk such as excess cases / 10^6 exposed persons / year / rad. For breast cancer, this would mean that if one million women each were to receive one rad tissue dose to the breast, there would be for each yearly period an excess of observed minus expected breast cancers. This yearly excess would not occur until after a latent period of a given number of years and it would persist for a duration of another given number of years.

It remains a paradoxical necessity that risk estimates for possible breast cancer induction in humans have only been derived from populations exposed to relatively high doses of radiation. The reason for this is simply that the induction rates are extremely low (possibly 3.5-7.5 cases/10^6 women/ year/rad)(21). As dose decreases, the incidence of radiation induced breast cancer becomes harder and harder to separate from the background noise of the natural breast cancer incidence. For U.S. women the age adjusted annual incidence of breast cancer is 720 cases/10^6 women (2). To derive statistically adequate risk estimates directly from women receiving doses of one rad or less would require an exposed population of several million women.

To circumvent this problem, workers in the field of radiation protection have adopted the linear hypothesis. This states that risk per rad remains constant regardless of dose or dose rate and can be extrapolated downward as a straight line from high doses to low doses. This represents a conservative estimate of the upper limits of risk. In terms of radiation protection, it is a simplifying assumption which has never proven a problem in terms of protective shielding. Nor has it hampered the performance of most radiographic procedures which are meant to solve an immediate clinical problem (rather than screen an asymptomatic population for breast cancer). In the former situation, benefit and risk do not lend themselves to a quantitative balance.

Nevertheless, it must be realized that estimates of risk derived from high doses of radiation may represent significant overstatements of risk for patients.

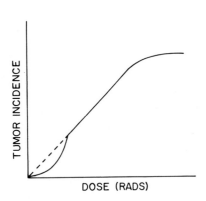

Figure 1.   Dose - response curve for
     radiation carcinogenesis in animals.

exposed to low doses. Most animal experiments show a curvilinear dose - response relationship where risk decreases exponentially at low doses (Figure 1) (20). One possible exception may be mammary carcinoma in Sprague - Dawley rats where expressed as the proportion of animals with mammary carcinoma, the risk may be a linear or curvilinear function of dose at low doses (17). In terms of mammary tumors per animal however, Kellerer and Rossi have demonstrated a clearly curvilinear relationship (16).

The ICRP cautioned in its 1977 report that "linearity may lead to an overstatement of radiation risk which in turn could result in the choice of alternative practices that are more hazardous than a practice involving radiation exposure" (9). This statement should be kept in mind as risk estimates for breast cancer induction derived from human populations are reviewed.

LATENT PERIOD AND DURATION

The minimal latent period refers to the time between exposure and appearance of an excess of observed cancers in the irradiated group compared to those expected from the control group. Graphic portrayal of latent period for the Rochester mastitis series is seen in figure 2. Data from this series as well as from the New England fluoroscopy study would suggest a minimal latent period of 15-17 years.

However, a considerably shorter latent period of 5-9 years is suggested for the Japanese A bomb survivors.There are three possible explanations for this disagreement. First, the Japanese population had a mean age of 34 years in contrast to a mean age of 27 years for the two groups of western women. Secondly,Japanese women were exposed to nearly instantaneous dose of mixed gamma and neutron radiation. Lastly,a larger number of breast cancers were studied in the two North American series.

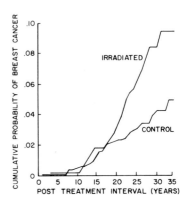

Figure 2.   Determination of latent period for excess breast cancer incidence in Rochester, N.Y. women treated by radiotherapy for postpartum mastitis. (Modified from ref. 18).

The duration of carcinogenic effect is unknown, but data from all studies would indicate that it has persisted until at least the thirtieth post exposure year. It is not known what length of follow-up will be necessary to measure the entire cancer risk.

DOSE RESPONSE RELATIONSHIP

The dose-response curves produced in animal experiments consist of three components as seen in figure 1. The midportion of the curve is a rising straight line where incidence is directly proportional to the first power of dose. Above this, at higher doses, the curve flattens as radiation produces cell killing and degeneration as well as carcinogenesis. The low dose portion (below 50 or 100 rads) is usually concave upwards as incidence varies as an exponential function of dose. Effect per rad here is less than at medium or high doses.

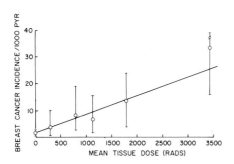

Figure 3. Relationship of breast cancer incidence to estimated breast tissue dose from fluoroscopy of Nova Scotia sanatoria patients. (Modified from ref. 2).

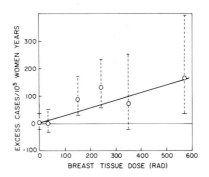

Figure 4. Relationship of breast cancer incidence to estimated breast tissue dose from fluoroscopy of Massachusetts sanatoria patients. (Modified from ref. 3).

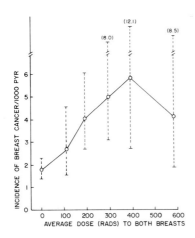

Figure 5. Relationship of breast cancer incidence to breast tissue dose in Rochester, N.Y. women treated by radiotherapy for postpartum mastitis. (Modified from ref. 18).

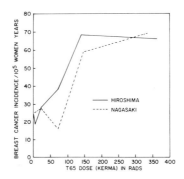

Figure 6. Relationship of breast cancer incidence to estimated dose in atomic bomb survivors. (Modified from ref. 13).

In several respects, the curves for radiation related breast cancers in humans resemble those produced in animal experiments. Those for the Nova Scotia and New England fluoroscopy series, Rochester mastitis study, and Japanese A bomb survivors are shown in figures 3,4,5,6 respectively. All contain a linear portion which rises at doses above 100 rads. Three of the studies (New England, Rochester, and Japan) suggest a flattened or decreasing response at higher doses.

For low doses, however, the curves provide little information to permit a choice between a linear or curvilinear response. The lowest tissue doses recorded on the Nova Scotia and Rochester graphs are 261 rads and 112 rads respectively. Actually, if the Rochester data is analyzed on the basis of rads per breast rather than the average rads to both breasts (only 1/3 of patients received treatments to both breasts), the lowest mean dose per breast would be 150 rads. In this category, two cancers were observed and 1.47 expected.

A dose category ranging from 1-99 rads (mean = 35 rads) can be seen on the New England graph. For this subgroup of 469 women, 10 breast cancers were observed and 9.6 expected. At first glance, failure to demonstrate an excess breast cancer incidence in this group of women might seem to indicate that either risk is absent or effect per rad considerably diminished at this dose level. However, the product of women years at risk and rads absorbed is not of sufficient magnitude to statistically exclude a breast cancer risk of 6 cases/10^6 women/year/rad seen at higher dose levels in the Massachusetts study.

The same may be said of the failure to demonstrate an excess breast cancer incidence in 269 Toronto sanatoria patients who received an average depth dose of 17 rads (5). Similarly, Kitabatke followed 568 Japanese women who also received PA fluoroscopy during pneumothorax treatments. No deaths resulted from breast cancer although 0.4 were expected based on Japanese national statistics (11). PA fluoroscopy results in considerably lower breast tissue doses than does the AP technique used for the Nova Scotia patients.

Analysis of the Japanese data is complicated by the fact that both gamma and neutron radiation were emitted. Though, at Nagasaki, neutrons accounted for less than 2% of the total dose in rads, at Hiroshima they amounted to 25%. Because of the relatively dense ionization track produced by neutrons (high LET) they result in a significantly higher relative biological efficiency (RBE) than do gamma rays. For acute effects such as epilation and bleeding and for leukemia as a delayed effect, neutrons are considered 5 times as effective as gamma rays (20).

Most animal experiments reveal that dose-response curves for neutron induced carcinogenesis remain linear even at low doses while the curves for the same effect produced by gamma rays becomes curvilinear. Thus, divergence of neutron and gamma ray curves for the production of the same biological effect would suggest that gamma rays are less effective per rad as dosage declines (16).

At nearly all dose levels, breast cancer incidence is consistently higher for Hiroshima women exposed to both gamma and neutron radiation than for Nagasaki survivors exposed to gamma radiation alone. This difference is most marked at 50-99 rads. Between 10 and 49 rads, the cancer incidence is very small and therefore the two curves appear to approach each other again. Thus, one could infer that below 100 rads the Nagasaki graph may be curvilinear while the Hiroshima graph retains a linear shape.

Nevertheless, the relatively smaller number of Nagasaki survivors compared to the larger Hiroshima population does result in some statistical variability. Moreover, the shape one interprets for the curves at low doses does depend on what one sets as the base line of expected breast cancer incidence. For each city, one of three possible base lines may be used: women not in the city at time of bomb, those in the city but exposed to 0 rads, and those exposed to 1-9 rads. As can be appreciated from table I, the data are consistent with a variety of dose-response curves.

Table I   Breast Cancer Incidence* Rates for Hiroshima and Nagasaki Women Exposed to Low Doses of Radiation and For Those Not Exposed   (From ref. 13)

City	\multicolumn{5}{c}{Dose (Rads)**}
	0***	0****	1-9	10-49	50-99
Hiroshima	188	245	179	283	384
Nagasaki	157	123	255	279	159

*   Age adjusted incidence per 10^6 person years for all survivors older than 10 years of age

**   T-65 dose = total tissue Kerma in free air at a point corresponding to the center of the body

*** Not in city at time of bomb

****In city at time of bomb

RISK ESTIMATES

Strictly speaking, risk estimates should be applied only to groups of women similar in all factors which might affect radiation sensitivity to the population from which the risk estimate is derived. Factors which may influence breast sensitivity would include: patient age (over 35 years), race (largely caucasian), pregnancy status (neither pregnant nor postpartum). Type of radiation (gamma or neutron) should be the same. Exposure doses and absorbed doses should be accurately known. Extrapolation of risk between populations is valid only if the risk per rad remains constant between the doses and dose rates incurred. The study population should be sufficiently large so that valid conclusions for each age group and dose group can be made. Although the populations which have been most thoroughly studied do not fulfill many of these criteria, risk estimates derived from them are provided in table II.

Based on radiotherapy records, exact exposure doses are known for Rochester N.Y. and Swedish women and,from these, tissue doses can be estimated. The postpartum breast, however, is characterized by an enormous proliferation of glandular and ductal tissue as well as a high state of physiological activity related to lactation. If radiation sensitivity is increased in the postpartum period or by postpartum mastitis, then risk estimates derived from these women would be too high.

There is much uncertainty concerning dosage estimates for the Nova Scotia sanatoria patients. Much depends on the recollection by physicians as to the average duration of fluoroscopic examination. Technical settings of kV and mA as well as presence or absence of aluminum filtration for individual studies must be assumed in retrospect. Dosage estimates for Massachusetts sanatoria patients have been derived by means of a more thorough methodology and probably represent more reliable retrospective measurements (4).

Table II Estimates of Absolute Breast Cancer Risk in Exposed Populations

Population	Reference	Type of Radiation	Period After Irradiation Upon Which Risk Estimates Based (Years)	Tissue Dose (Rads) Range	Tissue Dose (Rads) Mean	Mean Age at Exposure	Absolute Risk (Cases/ 10^{6}Women/ Yr/Rad)
Rochester Mastitis	18	gamma	10-34	40-1500	377	27	8.3
Swedish Radiotherapy	1	gamma	1-42	130-4249	713	38	5.6
Nova Scotia Fluoroscopy	2,12, 14	gamma	10-30	260-4000	1215	26	8.4
Massachusetts Fluoroscopy	3	gamma	10-45	1-1027	150	25	6.2
Japan A-bomb	13	gamma + neutron	5-25	10-600	81	34	1.9

Risk estimates for Japanese A bomb survivors may not be directly applicable to mammographic exposure of western women for several reasons. First, the natural breast cancer incidence in Japan is only 20% of that in the U.S.(10) and therefore sensitivity to radiation may also differ. Secondly, three fourths of the exposed women were from Hiroshima where neutrons comprised 25% of the exposure dose in rads and probably a much greater proportion of the total dose expressed in rems. Since all women received total body radiation, associated hormonal or immunologic effects might have altered the response to direct breast irradiation.

As can be seen in figure 7, women over 35 years of age account for more than 97% of the natural breast cancer incidence. In terms of benefit, this is considered a suitable age to begin mammographic screening of asymptomatic patients. In assessing possible risks from screening, it would be valuable to have a risk estimate appropriate to this age group. It is apparent, however, from table II that estimates on western women have been derived either for those less than 30 years of age and/or from breasts which, because of pregnancy, resemble those of younger women. However, when these populations are analyzed by age groups, a considerable dependence of sensitivity on age at exposure is evident.

Both Hiroshima and Nagasaki data show an absolute breast cancer induction risk that strongly depends on age at time of exposure (Table III). For combined cities, women exposed at 35 years of age or above were only 1/3 to 1/2 as sensitive to radiation as those below 35 years of age. Since Nagasaki survivors were exposed to gamma radiation only, they approximate a population exposed to diagnostic xrays more than do Hiroshima survivors who received mixed gamma and neutron radiation. For Nagasaki, breast cancer induction in the 35-49 age and 50+ age group are approximately 30% and 20% respectively of that found in the 20-34 age group.

14

Table III Absolute Breast Cancer Risk as a
Function of Age at Time of Bomb
for Japanese A-bomb Survivors

Absolute Risk*

| Age ATB | Beir Type | Regression Type | |
(Years)	Both Cities	Hiroshima	Nagasaki
10-19	4.0	2.9	2.2
20-34	1.2	1.7	2.5
35-49	0.9	0.5	0.9
50+	1.3	1.6	0.5

* Excess Cases/10^6 Patient Years/Rad
(From ref. 13)

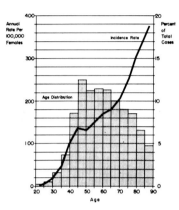

Figure 7. Natural breast cancer
incidence rates and distribution of cases by age.
(From ref. 19).

Table IV Relation of Relative
Breast Cancer Risk*
to Radiation Dose
and Age at Exposure
for A-Bomb Survivors
(Modified from ref 13)

| Age at Time | Dose (Rads) | |
of Bomb	10-99	100+
10-99	5.6*	8.7**
20-34	0.8	3.1**
35-49	1.1	1.9**
50+	1.0	3.0***

* Relative risks compared to
0-9 rad group
** $p < 0.05$
*** $p < 0.01$

It should be emphasized that the 10-19 age group at time of bomb is the only one to later show an elevated risk for 10-99 rads vs. 0-9 rads (Table IV).

Nova Scotia sanatoria patients also demonstrated a striking dependence of radiation sensitivity on age at time of exposure (Table V). If the control incidence of 1% is subtracted for each age interval, then the rate of cancer induction in women over 30 years of age is less than 20% of that seen in younger women.

Among Massachusetts sanatoria patients 35 years of age or older at time of first treatment, there were fewer cancers than expected. For women 30-35 years of age at onset of treatment, there was a statistically insignificant increment (Table VI). Combining these two groups, it can be seen that no excess breast cancers were detected in women 30 years of age or older at time of first exposure.

Swedish radiotherapy patients also showed a higher risk of developing breast cancer when breasts were irradiated at lower ages although this may be partly due to variation of exposure dose with age at exposure. Nevertheless, breast cancer induction in women over 30 years of age at exposure was only 20% of that observed in women below 30 years of age (Table VII).

Table V   Relationship of Breast Cancer Incidence to Age at Exposure for Nova
           Scotia Sanatoria Patients (From refs 14, 15, 16)

Sanatoria Patients	Age at Exposure	Number of Patients	Breast Cancers	Percent Incidence
Fluoroscoped	0-19	59	6	10
	20-29	181	23	13
	30-60+	86	3	3
Control	0-60+	535	7	1

Table VI   Relationship of Breast Cancer Incidence to Age at Exposure for
            Massachusetts Sanatoria Patients (From ref 3)

	Age at Exposure						
	0-15	15-19	20-24	25-29	30-34	35-39	40+
Number of Women	99	242	263	200	105	75	63
Breast Cancers Observed	2	13	9	9	4	2	2
Breast Cancers Expected	0.9	3.4	5.4	5.5	3.2	2.5	2.2
Observed per Expected	2.1	3.8	1.7	1.6	1.2	0.8	0.9
Observed Minus Expected Per 10^6 Women Years	4.4	13.3	4.6	6.2	3.0	-3.2	-3.7

Only in one group of women, Rochester, N.Y. patients treated for postpartum mastitis, was there no variation in radiation sensitivity with age. Adjusted absolute risk estimates for women below and above age 30 were 7.9 and 9.2 cases/ 10^6 women/year/rad respectively. The most plausible explanation for this finding would be that as far as radiation carcinogenesis is concerned, full term pregnancy returns the breast to an earlier, more sensitive physiologic state. Most likely, pregnancy negates an age-related resistance to radiation.

To determine the risk for western women irradiated after age 35, the National Cancer Institute has first estimated the absolute breast cancer risk for Japanese women exposed below and above age 35 as 2.8 and 1.25 cases/10^6 women/year/rad respectively. The NCI has then applied an adjustment of 1.25/ 2.8=0.45 to the average absolute risk of 7.5 cases/10^6 women/year/rad obtained from the Nova Scotia and Massachusetts fluoroscopy series and Rochester mastitis series. These calculations yield a risk of 3.5 cases/10^6 women/year/rad for women age 35 or over at time of exposure (21). Examination of the Nova Scotia, Massachusetts, and Swedish studies, however, would suggest that this may be an overly conservative estimate and that considerably greater adjustment for age dependent sensitivity might be justified.

Table VII   Relationship of Breast Cancer Incidence per Rad per 10^6 Breasts to Age at Exposure in Swedish Women Treated with Radiotherapy for Benign Breast Conditions (From ref 1)

Age at Irradiation	Number of Breasts	Breast Cancers Observed	Breast Cancers Expected	Average Mean Breast Dose(Rads)	Excess Rate/Rad/ 10^6 Breasts
10-19	28	2	0.25	285	219
20-29	205	31	3.4	437	308
30-39	333	28	8.3	667	89
40-49	311	20	8.9	886	40
50-	119	7	3.1	965	34
All	996	88	24.0	713	90

REFERENCES

1. Baral, E, Larsson, L-E, and Mattson, B: Breast cancer following irradition of the breast. Cancer 40: 2905-2910, 1977

2. Beir Report. The effects on populations of exposure to low levels of ionizing radiation. National Academy of Sciences, National Research Council, Washington DC, 1972

3. Boice, J D, and Monson, R B: Breast Cancer following repeated fluoroscopic examinations of the chest. J Natl Cancer Inst 59: 823-832, 1977

4. Boice, J D, Rosenstein, M, and Trout, E D: Estimation of breast doses and breast cancer risk associated with repeated fluoroscopic chest examinations of women with tuberculosis. Radiat Res 73: 373-390, 1978

5. Delarue, N C, Gale, G, and Ronald, A: Multiple fluoroscopy of the chest: carcinogenicity for the female breast and implications for breast cancer screening programs. Can Med Assoc J 112: 1405-1411, 1975

6. Dodd,G D: Present status of thermography, ultrasound, and mammography in breast cancer detection. Cancer 39: 2796-2805, 1977

7. Feig, S A: Can breast cancer be radiation induced? p 5-14 in Breast Carcinoma The Radiologist's Expanded Role, ed by Logan, W W. New York, John Wiley and Sons, 1977

8. Feig, S A: Ionizing radiation and human breast cancer. Crit Revs in Diag Imaging, in press, 1978

9. International Commission on Radiological Protection: Recommendations of the International Commission on Radiological Protection. Annals of the I C R P 1: 1-53, 1977

10. International Union Against Cancer: Cancer Incidence in Five Continents. New York, Springer-Verlag, 1970, p 205

11. Kitabatake, T, Kurokawa, S, Yamasaki, M, et al: A prospective study on the incidence of chest malignancies after repeated fluoroscopy during artificial pneumothorax therapy for pulmonary tuberculosis. Nippon Acta Radiologica 35: 895-899, 1975

12. MacKenzie, I: Breast cancer following multiple fluoroscopies. Brit J of Cancer 19: 1-8, 1965

13. McGregor, D H, Land, C E, Choi, K, et al: Breast cancer incidence among atomic bomb survivors, Hiroshima and Nagasaki, 1950-1969. J Natl Cancer Inst 59: 799-811, 1977

14. Myrden, J A, and Hiltz, J E: Breast cancer following multiple fluoroscopies during artificial pneumothorax treatment of pulmonary tuberculosis. Can Med Assoc J 100: 1032-1034, 1969

15. Myrden, J A, and Quinlan, J J: Breast carcinoma following multiple fluoroscopies with pneumothorax treatment of pulmonary tuberculosis. Ann R Coll Physicians Can 7: 45, 1974

16. Rossi, H, and Kellerer, A: Radiation carcinogenesis at low doses. Science 175: 200-202, 1972

17. Shellabarger, C J, Bond, V P, Cronkite, E P, et al: Relationship of dose of total body ^{60}Co radiation to incidence of mammary neoplasia in female rats. in Radiation-Induced Cancer, IAEA-SM-118/9, Vienna, 1969, p 161-172

18. Shore, R E, Hempelmann, L H, Kowaluk, E, et al: Breast neoplasms in women treated with x-rays for acute postpartum mastitis. J Natl Cancer Inst 59: 813-822, 1977

19. Seidman, H: Cancer of the Breast, Statistical and Epidemiological Data. New York, American Cancer Society, 1972, p 28

20. United Nations Scientific Committee on the Effects of Atomic Radiation: Sources and Effects of Atomic Radiation, 1977 Report to the General Assembly, with annexes. New York: United Nations, 1977

21. Upton, A C, Beebe, G W, Brown, J M, et al: Report of the NCI Ad Hoc Working Group on the Risks Associated with Mammography in Mass Screening for the Detection of Breast Cancer. J Natl Cancer Inst 59: 481-493, 1977

ANATOMIC AND PATHOLOGIC BASIS OF RADIATION RELATED HUMAN BREAST CANCERS

Stephen A. Feig, M.D.

Department of Radiology, Thomas Jefferson University Hospital, Phila., Pa.

The purpose of this chapter is to review those aspects of breast anatomy, histology, physiology, and pathology which are pertinent to radiation carcinogensis. Epidemiologic studies indicate that breast sensitivity to radiation strongly depends on age at time of exposure (1, 2, 6, 7, 18, 19). However, this observation can best be understood in terms of breast structure and cellular composition which vary with age as well as parity. Data on location and cell type of radiation induced breast cancers could prove useful in dosimetric calculations. Similarly, knowledge of the comparative clinical course of radiation induced and naturally occurring breast cancers could assist in benefit-risk analysis.

BREAST ANATOMY

The gross and microscopic structure of the breast is illustrated in figure 1. The glandular portion of the breast is comprised of 15-20 lobes. The lobes cannot be defined by anatomical dissection, but rather refer to the collection of glandular units which are drained by a single major lactiferous duct. There are no connections between neighboring lobes or ducts. However, some of the major ducts may merge prior to their termination on the nipple so that the number of duct openings is less than the number of major ducts (3, 9, 10, 12).

The terminal units of each lobe are the blind ending sacs or acini. These are lined by a single layer of cuboidal epithelium. Lobules consist of groups of 10-100 acini. The number of lobules per breast varies enormously at various stages in a woman's life and among different women (10).

The breast ducts form a branching structure which convey milk from the acini to the nipple. The various sized ducts have been described on the basis of their location as interlobar, intralobar, interlobular, and intralobular. The major (interlobar) lactiferous ducts are lined by stratified squamous epithelium which gradually merges into the columnar epithelium of the smaller ducts. Their peripheral portions have low columnar cells that blend into the cuboidal epithelium of the lobules and acini (3).

The glandular and ductal elements consititute the parenchyma. The breast stroma refers to fatty and fibrotic tissue which both surrounds and extends into the lobules. Usually, the periductal fibrous tissue is considered parenchyma, whereas the supportive fibrous connective tissue is stroma. Both parenchyma and stroma are contained within a sac formed when the superficial pectoral fascia splits into anterior (superficial) and posterior (deep) layers. Cooper's ligaments are tentlike projections of the superficial layer of superficial fascia through the fatty subcutaneous tissue to the skin. These contain extensions of parenchyma. However, in a broader sense, Cooper's ligaments may refer to all of the supportive fibrous connective tissue which forms a kind of fibrous skeleton between the superficial and deep layers of superficial fascia (9, 10).

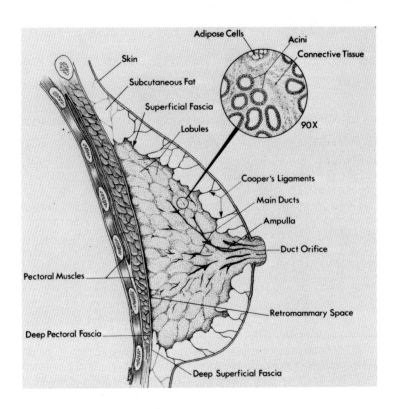

Figure 1. Anatomy of the normal human breast

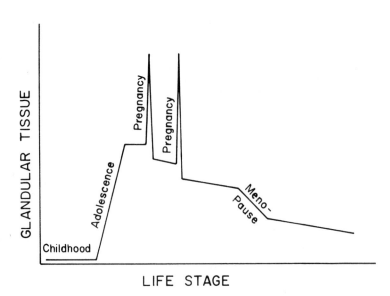

Figure 2. Relationship of breast glandularity to life stage in normal women.

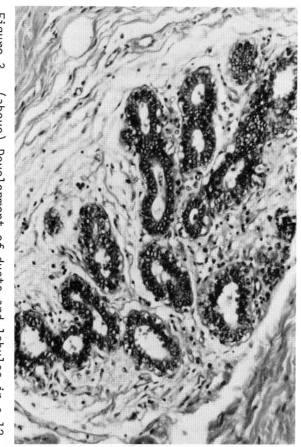

Figure 3. (above) Development of ducts and lobules in a 12 year old. (H & E x 190).

Figure 4. (right) Normal nulliparous breast in a 19 year old female is densely opaque on mammography due to the large amount of glandular and fibrotic tissue.

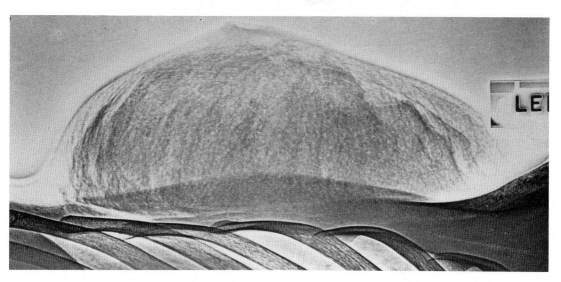

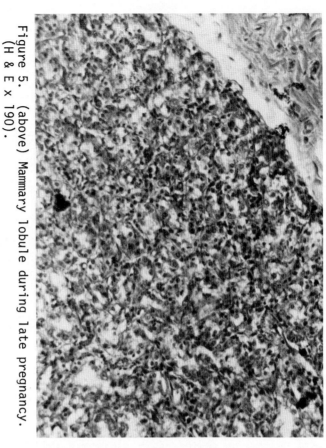

Figure 5. (above) Mammary lobule during late pregnancy. (H & E x 190).

Figure 6. (right) Negative mode xeromammogram during late stage of pregnancy shows further increase in size and opacity due to glandular proliferation.

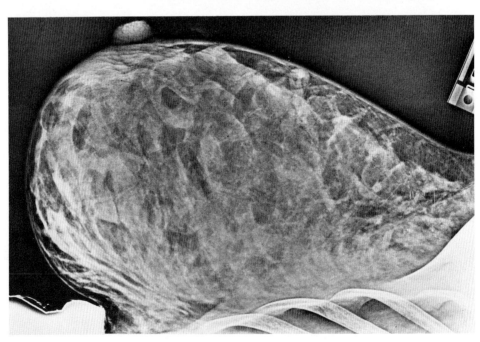

Similarly, there are also posterior projections of the deep layer superficial fascia which contain parenchyma and cross the retromammary space to fuse with the deep pectoral fascia which overlies the pectoralis muscles. These projections are known as the posterior suspensory ligaments.

AGE RELATED ANATOMY

Breast structure and composition vary considerably with age (Fig. 2) During adolescence, the breast undergoes both growth and differentiation. Ducts subdivide and penetrate further into the breast and there is marked budding of terminal ducts with lobule formation (Fig. 3). By late adolescence, the breast is a well developed glandular structure (Fig. 4).

With pregnancy, there is further increase in breast size. The number of acini are increased and there is proliferation of cells into duct lumens. By the end of pregnancy, the breast has been converted into an almost solid glandular structure (Figs. 5,6). If the mother breast feeds her child, these changes will persist into the period of lactation. Following pregnancy and/or lactation, there will be a marked decrease in the number of acini and the breast will be less glandular than it was prior to pregnancy (12).

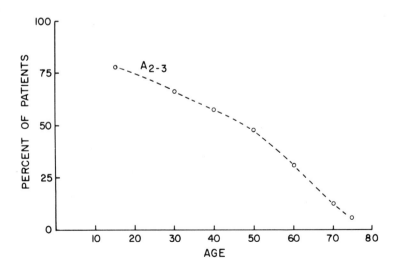

Figure 7. Relationship of alveolar patterns to patient age from mammograms of 2000 normal women. Alveoli (A) have been graded as 0: none, 1: strands, 2: Moderate, and 3: marked. (Modified from ref. 30).

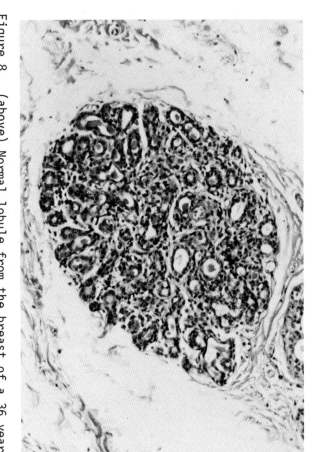

Figure 8. (above) Normal lobule from the breast of a 36 year old para 1 female is comprised of numerous acini (H & E x190).

Figure 9. (right) Breast of a 38 year old para 1 female shows intermediate density on xeromammography consistent with age and parity.

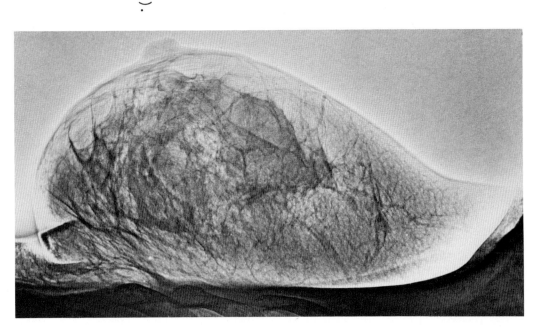

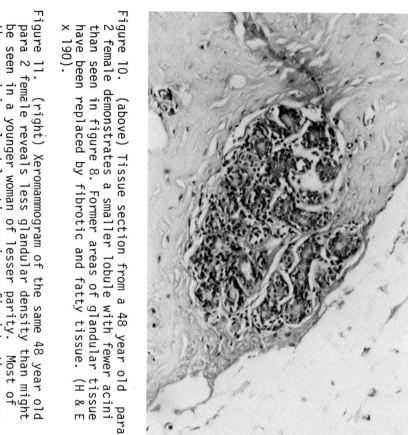

Figure 10. (above) Tissue section from a 48 year old para 2 female demonstrates a smaller lobule with fewer acini than seen in figure 8. Former areas of glandular tissue have been replaced by fibrotic and fatty tissue. (H & E x 190).

Figure 11. (right) Xeromammogram of the same 48 year old para 2 female reveals less glandular density than might be seen in a younger woman of lesser parity. Most of the remaining glandular tissue is confined to the upper-outer quadrant. The remainder of the breast is largely fatty.

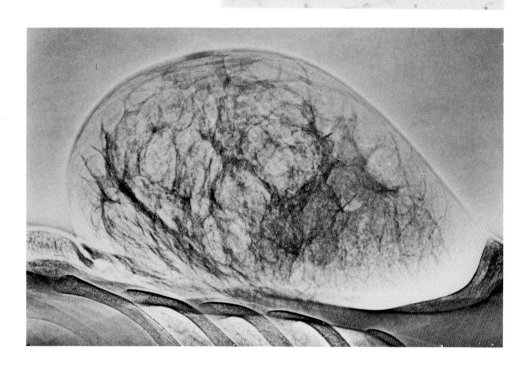

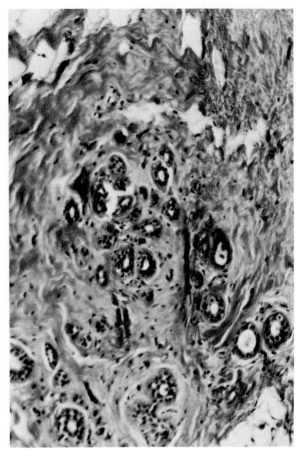

Figure 12. (above) Atrophic lobule from a 55 year old para 0 woman contains only a few acini. Surrounding tissue shows marked fibrotic replacement. (H & E x190).

Figure 13. (right) Breast of a 65 year old para 2 female shows virtually no residual glandularity. It is comprised almost entirely of fat.

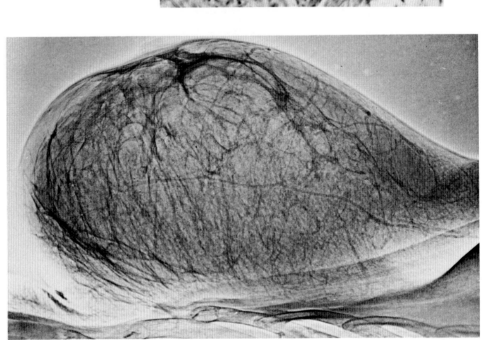

Mammographic studies would indicate that breast parenchymal atrophy begins in the early twenties or following the first pregnancy, whichever comes earlier. It continues with advancing age and accelerates at menopause (30) (Fig. 7). Coincident with this decrease in the number of lobules and acini, there is a relative increase in the proportion of fatty to glandular tissue. This is apparent on mammography (Figs. 8-13). Histologically, the ductal epithelium become atrophic but this change cannot be appreciated on mammography because the ducts are visualized on the basis of periductal collagenosis which neither increases nor decreases with age. On mammography, the ducts may show increased prominence with age which is more apparent than real and is due to regression of overlying alveolar elements (31).

BREAST CANCER HISTOLOGY

NATURALLY OCCURRING CANCERS

Nearly all naturally occurring breast cancers arise from the cuboidal and columnar epithelium of the breast ducts (17). Ductal lesions accounted for nearly 94% of all breast cancers diagnosed at our institution over the past 20 years. Lobular carcinoma which arises from the terminal alveoli of breast lobules was the primary histologic diagnosis in 5.5% of cases. Less than 1% of breast malignancies were of sarcomatous or other rare mesenchymal origin (26) (Fig. 14).

Ductal and lobular carcinomas may be further classified by stage of invasion. Non-infiltrative lesions are still confined to the ducts and acini. infiltrative lesions have broken through the basement membrane and invaded the breast stroma. Of those breast cancers encountered in clinical practice (non-screening situation) 95% are infiltrative and 5% are non-infiltrative (21).

RADIATION RELATED CANCERS

Several studies suggest that radiation induced breast cancer is histologically similar to other breast cancers. Wanebo et al report that the histologic type of breast cancer occurring in Japanese women exposed in Hiroshima and Nagasaki at over 60 rads were similar to those exposed at lower doses (29).

A more recent survey of A bomb survivors by Tokunaga (13) confirms the indication that types of breast cancers are induced in approximately the proportions in which they spontaneously occur in the Japanese population (Table I). It should be noted that Japanese women in general may have a higher proportion of intraductal to infiltrative ductal carcinoma than do western women (22).

Yoshizawa and Kusama surveyed a number of published sporadic case reports of radiation induced breast cancer and note that most such cases are of ductal origin(33).

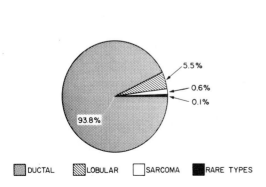

DUCTAL   LOBULAR   SARCOMA   RARE TYPES

Figure 14. Per cent distribution by histologic origin for 2888 breast cancers diagnosed at Thomas Jefferson University Hospital 1959-77 (From ref. 26).

Table I Breast Cancers Occurring in A-Bomb Survivors:
Per Cent Distribution by Histologic Types
(Source ref 13)

	Dose (Rads)		
	0	1-99	100+
Ductal Carcinomas			
Infiltrating	85	85	76
Intraductal	13	9	21
Other Types	2	6	3
Total Per Cent	100%	100%	100%
Total Number of Cancers	118	74	33

PROGNOSIS OF NATURALLY OCCURRING AND RADIATION RELATED BREAST CANCERS

Based on histologic types and proportion of invasive to non-invasive lesions, one would expect the prognosis of radiation related and naturally occurring breast cancers to be similar. This question can be more directly approached by comparison of breast cancer mortality to incidence. Analysis of data from McGregor et al (18) yields an identical mortality/incidence rate in 139 Hiroshima and Nagasaki women exposed to 0-9 rads and in 82 women exposed to 10-100+ rads. On data from the 1950-1969 period, the UNSCEAR Report has estimated mortality risk rates at 0.25x the incidence rates in the Japanese Life Span Study (27).

For Rochester, New York women who received radiotherapy for postpartum mastitis, 7 breast cancer deaths were reported for 37 breast cancer cases (mortality/incidence = 0.2) (25, 27).

Among Massachusetts sanatoria patients subjected to multiple fluoroscopic examinations, 23 breast cancer deaths occurred among 56 breast cancer cases (mortality/incidence = 0.41) (2, 27).

Thus, radiation related breast cancer would seem to be characterized by a rather slow course and high cure rate. When these figures are compared to the respective morbidity and mortality data for naturally occurring breast cancers in Japan and the United States, prognosis would seem to be no worse than that of naturally occurring breast cancers (4, 20, 23, 32).

BREAST CANCER LOCATION

NATURALLY OCCURRING CANCERS

As evident from clinical examination or mammography, the upper outer quadrant usually contains a greater bulk of glandular tissue than any other section of the breast. Probably for this reason, it accounts for a greater proportion of breast cancers than any other quadrant. Fully half of all breast cancers originate there. The next most common site is the retroareolar region (18%) on which ducts from the entire breast converge. Only 21% of breast cancers arise from the upper and lower inner quadrants (5,8, 11, 14) (Fig. 15).

RADIATION RELATED CANCERS

MacKenzie described a greater proportion of inner and central breast

Cancer in Nova Scotia women subjected to multiple fluoroscopies for pulmonary tuberculosis for 42 cancers occurring in women treated by pneumothorax, 26% (11/42) were in the outer breast, 41% (17/42) occurred centrally, and 33% (14/42) were in the inner breast (15). This finding can be explained by the fact that the xray beam tended to be focused more over the medial aspect of the chest wall on the side on which pneumothorax was induced.

POSSIBLE DETERMINANTS OF AGE RELATED RADIATION SENSITIVITY

The breasts of women 30 years of age and older are considerably less susceptible to radiation carcinogenesis than are those of younger women. This observation is now well established, having been confirmed in 4 major epidemiologic studies: Nova Scotia and Massachusetts sanatoria patients subjected to multiple chest fluoroscopies, Japanese A-bomb survivors, and Swedish women treated by radiotherapy for benign breast conditions (1, 2, 18, 19).

One explanation for this increased resistance to radiation might be a decrease in the amount of target tissue in older women. As seen on mammography, the amount of alveolar tissue does decline with age. Histologic evidence would suggest that the altered mammographic appearance is due to atrophy of both acini and terminal ductal epithelial from which most breast cancers arise (12).

Another possible explanation could be decreased sensitivity of target tissue in older women. At present, however, there is no known significant change in blood levels of estradiol, progesterone, FSH or LH between age 18 and 41. There is a significant decline in estradiol and rise in FSH beginning in the premenopausal period around age 46 (24, 28), but this hormonal change occurs too late in life to explain the earlier alteration in radiation sensitivity.

One reason for decreased radiation sensitivity could be the greater proportion of parous women in older age groups. The association between age at first birth and breast cancer risk is fully documented and represents one of the pillars of breast cancer epidemiology (Fig. 16) (16). It may be that completion of full term pregnancy prior to radiation exposure protects the breast from effects of radiation. Although this hypothesis could explain the marked decline in radiation sensitivity around age 30, it has not yet been subjected to epidemiologic investigation.

It is possible that the hypothetical risk from the low doses of radiation used in mammography may be greater in nulliparous than in parous women. Also, the postulated risks may be greater for women with benign dysplasias since their breasts contain a greater amount of glandular and ductal tissue than do the breasts of normal women of similar age group. However, since both nulliparous women and women with benign dysplasia are at a higher risk for naturally occurring breast cancer, the benefit/ risk ratio for mammographic screening would not be less than in other women.

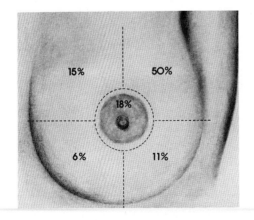

Figure 15. Per cent distribution by location of 3147 breast carcinomas (From refs. 5, 8, 11, 14).

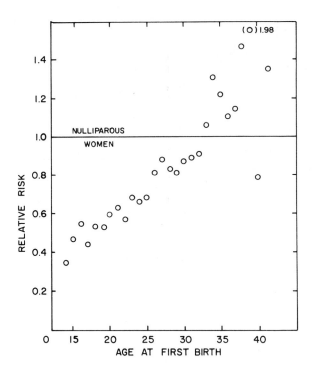

Figure 16. Breast cancer risk according to age at first birth.
Values are relative to a risk of 1.0 for nulliparous women
(From ref. 16).

CONCLUSION

Radiation induced breast cancers arise from the ductal epithelium and
alveoli. They do not differ in histologic appearance or degree of invasion
from the naturally occurring variety. Prognosis for radiation induced breast
cancers is no worse than for the naturally occurring type.

Most naturally occurring breast cancers are found in the outer breast and
subareolar region since these areas contain the bulk of ductal and glandular
tissue. Location of radiation related cancers may depend both on distribution
of sensitive tissue and distribution of absorbed radiation.

The risk of radiation carcinogenesis in the female breast has been found
to decrease with increasing age above 30 years of age. This may be due to the
progressive decline in the amount of glandular and ductal tissue after age 20
or to decreased sensitivity of breast tissue related to parity or undetermined
hormonal factors.

REFERENCES

1. Baral, E, Larsson, L-E, and Mattson, B: Breast cancer following irradiation of the breast. Cancer 40: 2905-2910, 1977

2. Boice,J D, and Monson, R B: Breast cancer following repeated fluoroscopic
examinations of the chest. J Natl Cancer Inst 59: 823-832, 1977

3. Cutler, M: Tumors of the Breast. Philadelphia, J B Lippincott, 1962.
Chap 1, Anatomy of the breast

4. Doll, R, Muir, C S, and Waterhouse, J A H (Eds.): Cancer Incidence in Five
Continents, vol II. New York: Springer-Verlag, 1970

5. Donegan, W L: Diagnosis of mammary cancer. In: Cancer of the Breast, ed
by Spratt, J S, and Donegan, W L. Philadelphia: W B Saunders Co, 1967 chap 3

6. Feig, S: Can breast cancer be radiation induced? In: Breast Carcinoma,
The Radiologist's Expanded Role, ed by Logan, W W. New York: John Wiley and
Sons, 1977, pp 5-14

7. Feig, S A: Ionizing radiation and human breast cancer. Crit Revs in Diag
Imaging, in press, 1978

8. Fisher, B, Slack, N H, Ausman, R K, et al: Location of breast carcinoma and
prognosis. Surg Gynecol Obstet 129: 705-716, 1969

9. Gray, H, and Goss, C M: Gray's Anatomy of the Human Body. Philadelphia:
Lea and Febiger, 1962, pp 1381-1385

10. Haagensen, C D: Diseases of the Breast. Philadelphia: W B Saunders, 1971,
Chap 1: Anatomy of the mammary gland

11. Haagensen, C D: Diseases of the Breast. Philadelphia: W B Saunders, 1971,
p 381

12. Ingelby, H, and Gershon-Cohen, J: Comparative Anatomy, Pathology, and
Roentgenology of the Breast. Philadelphia: University of Pennsylvania Press,
1960

13. Kato, H: Personal communication on work in preparation by Tokunaga, A,
Asano, M, Tokuoka, S, et al: Malignant breast tumors and their relation to
radiation, Hiroshima and Nagasaki, 1950-74

14. Leis, H P: Diagnosis and Treatment of Breast Lesions. London: H K Lewis
and Co, Ltd, 1970, p 126

15. MacKenzie, I: Breast cancer following multiple fluoroscopies. Brit J of
Cancer 19: 1-8, 1965

16. MacMahon, B, Cole, P, Lin, T M, et al: Age at first birth and breast
cancer risk. Bull Wld Hlth Org 43: 209-221, 1970

17. McDivitt, R W, Stewart, F W, and Berg, J W: Atlas of Tumor Pathology,Second
Series, Fascicle 2: Tumors of the Breast. Washington D C: Armed Forces
Institute of Pathology, 1968

18. McGregor, D H, Land, C E, Choi, K, et al: Breast cancer incidence among atomic bomb survivors, Hiroshima and Nagasaki, 1950-1967. J Natl Cancer Inst 59: 799-811, 1977

19. Myrden, J A, and Hiltz, J E: Breast cancer following multiple fluoroscopies during artificial pneumothorax treatment of pulmonary tuberculosis. Can Med Assoc J 100: 1032-1034, 1969

20. National Cancer Institute: Cancer Patient Survival Report Number 5, DHEW Publication (NIH) 77-992. Washington, D C: US Government Printing Office, 1976

21. National Cancer Institute: Prepublication data received from SEER Program. Biometry Branch, NCI.

22. Rosen, P P, Ashikari, R, Thaler, H, et al: A comparative study of some pathologic features of mammary carcinoma in Tokyo, Japan and New York, USA. Cancer 39: 429-434, 1977

23. Seidman, H: Cancer of the Breast, Statistical and Epidemiological Data. New York: American Cancer Society, 1972

24. Sherman, B M, and Korenman, S G: Hormonal characteristics of the human menstrual cycle throughout reproductive life. J Clin Invest 55: 699-706, 1975

25. Shore, R E, Hempelmann, L H, Kowaluk, E, et al: Breast neoplasms in women treated with x-rays for acute postpartum mastitis. J Natl Cancer Inst 59: 813-822, 1977

26. Thomas Jefferson University Hospital: Eighteenth Annual Report, Tumor Registry. Philadelphia, 1978

27. United Nations Scientific Committee on the Effects of Atomic Radiation: Sources and Effects of Ionizing Radiation, 1977 Report to the General Assembly with annexes. New York: United Nations, 1977

28. Vorherr, H, and Messer, R H: Breast cancer, potentially predisposing and protecting factors, role of pregnancy, lactation, and endocrine status. Am J Obstet Gynecol 130: 335-358, 1978

29. Wanebo, C K, Johnson, K G, Sato, K, et al: Breast cancer after exposure to atomic bombings of Hiroshima and Nagasaki. New Engl J Med 279: 667-671,1968

30. Wolfe, J N: A study of breast parenchyma by mammography in the normal woman and those with benign and malignant disease. Radiology 89: 201-205, 1967

31. Wolfe, J N: Breast parenchymal patterns and their changes with age. Radiology 121: 545-552, 1976

32. Wynder, E L, Kajitani, T, Kuno, J, et al: A comparison of survival rates between American and Japanese patients with breast cancer. Surg Gynecol Obstet 117: 196-200, 1963

33. Yoshizawa, Y, and Kusama, T: Search for the lowest irradiation dose from literatures on radiation induced breast cancer. Nippon Acta Radiologica 35: 1125-1130, 1975

MAMMARY CANCER INDUCTION BY LOW DOSES OF X RAYS

Edward W. Webster, Ph.D.
Division of Radiological Sciences
Massachusetts General Hospital
Boston, Massachusetts

The objective of this review is to provide some of the radio-biological background which underlies current intensive efforts to reduce the radiation dose to the breast in mammographic examinations. Its main conclusion is that the intensive effort to explore and implement low dose techniques is eminently justified by the present weight of radiobiological evidence. Nevertheless, it is of considerable significance to state at the outset that a discussion of radiobiological data at current mammographic dose levels (1 rad or less) would be exceedingly short--there are no data. Indeed, most workers in the radiobiological and epidemiologic fields confidently believe that we will never learn through any practical human or mammalian investigation the actual incidence of breast cancer following 1 rad of breast dose. This is because the sample sizes required for the exposed and control populations are too large for a feasible investigation. On the basis of a linear dose-effect relationship, the sample sizes increase in <u>inverse</u> proportion to the square of the excess number of cancer cases expected, and at an even faster rate if the relationship is less than linear. Thus, reducing dose from 100 rads to 1 rad would require 10,000 times (not 100 times) the sample size if the excess cancer rate is proportional to dose. Estimates of the breast cancer risk at low doses therefore depend on the trend of the incidence (or mortality) as a function of dose at levels considerably greater than 1 rad. The following discussion therefore depends heavily on the published literature concerning experience with both animal and human populations at those higher doses.

In the following brief review animal and human epidemiologic data will be presented in relation to: (a) the shape of the dose response curve particularly at low doses; (b) the dependence of sensitivity on subject age; and (c) the latent period after irradiation for manifestation of breast cancer.

DOSE RESPONSE RELATIONSHIPS

Many physicians interested in the medical applications of radiation are attracted to the <u>suggestion</u> that the incidence of late cancer produced by low LET radiation (x rays and gamma rays) is non-linear with dose. It has become apparent, particularly in mammalian experiments, that the rate of induction per rad of some kinds of cancer increases as the dose increases. The curvature of the response is attributed variously to the multihit nature of the primary lesion, or to the multicellular nature of the primary malignant lesion. There is some evidence of non-linearity between dose and carcinogenic effect in human populations for low LET radiation, such as bone cancer induction (1) and more recently leukemia induction (2). On the other hand some of the present evidence in animals and humans unquestionably support the linear hypothesis down to a few 10s of rads.

A non-linear dose/effect curve, particularly at low dose rates, should be associated with a time-dependent repair mechanism. Such an effect is illustrated in Figure 1 which shows the results of a recent study by Yuhas (3) of ovarian tumors in mice for gradually falling dose rates of x rays over a range of sixty. There is a marked reduction in incidence at the lower rates and also upward curvature of the dose/response relation at low dose rates.

A similar relation is suggested in a study by Upton (4) of myeloid leukemia in x-irradiated RF mice, the results of which are shown in Figure 2. The effectiveness of chronic irradiation is much smaller than that of acute radiation. In this case both responses are somewhat curvilinear at low doses. There is evident non-linearity of the leukemia response of the Japanese A-bomb survivors who received low doses in Nagasaki, where the radiation was almost entirely due to gamma rays. Figure 3 shows the mortality from leukemia over the years 1950 - 1972 as a function of absorbed dose to the bone marrow (2) and suggests that the linear response in Hiroshima is due to the fast neutron component (approximately 25%) in that city.

Most of the animal data on mammary cancer relates to the Sprague-Dawley rat and comes primarily from Brookhaven National Laboratory and the Argonne National Laboratory. This animal has a very high natural incidence of mammary cancer and the effect of radiation is to accelerate its appearance. Both adenocarcinoma and fibroadenomas appear. Figure 4 taken from the work of Shellabarger (5) shows very little reduction in the incidence of cancer as the dose is fractionated. The lowest curve is for thirty-two 15 R fractions and there are slight increases in effect for sixteen 31 R, eight 62 R, and four 125 R fractions, and for a single 500 R dose. The sparing for fractionated treatment was confined to the fibroadenomas (6). Figure 5 based on the work of several investigators (7) shows the counterpart to Figure 4, namely, an essentially linear dose response from about 25 rads upwards. However there is some suggestion of non-linearity (Fig.6) at lower doses in later work of Shellabarger and associates at Brookhaven National Laboratory (8). The linearity of the rat data, although suggestive, cannot be assumed to hold for breast cancer in the human female in which the natural incidence is far below 100%.

HUMAN EPIDEMIOLOGIC STUDIES OF BREAST CANCER

The 1972 BEIR Report of the U.S. National Academy of Sciences (9) reviewed breast cancer induction in several irradiated populations. Since then studies in the populations previously investigated have continued, particularly in the A-bomb survivors, and women receiving radiotherapy for post-partum mastitis. In addition, new populations have been investigated, especially young women who received multiple fluoroscopies in two Massachusetts TB sanitoria during pneumothorax therapy, and Swedish women who also received radiotherapy for benign breast conditions. This review is based on four papers published in 1977 concerning these populations.

Hiroshima and Nagasaki

The survey reported by McGregor et al. (10) covered the follow-up years from 1950 - 1969. Eighty-two cancers were discovered in women receiving between 10 and 600 rads and 144 cancers in those receiving smaller doses or zero. Despite the substantial fraction of neutron dose (13 - 30%) received in Hiroshima, the dose response relation is very similar to that in Nagasaki and it has seemed appropriate to pool these populations to improve the statistical validity of risk estimates.

The cancer incidence as a function of breast dose in rads is shown in Figure 7 for both cities. Both sets of data show best fits to a straight line rather than a curvilinear upward line. For Nagasaki only where there is minimal neutron dose, the statistics are given in Table 1 for the zero dose group and for those receiving less than 100 rads. In all age groups of women there is excess cancer in the irradiated population. For all age groups taken together the excess is significant at the 5% level. There is increased sensitivity in the age group 10 - 19 at the time of the bombing, but in the over-20 age group the excess cancer below 100 rads is significant at p = 0.07.

Taking both cities together, the actual observations at the lowest breast doses (2.7 rads, 16.7 rads, and 54.3 rads) in comparison with the group receiving zero exposure, strongly confirm the linearly increasing incidence with dose.

TABLE 1

BREAST CANCER IN A-BOMB SURVIVORS
AT NAGASAKI
1950-69

AGE-GROUP		10-19	20-34	35-49	> 50
Zero dose	Number/person-years	3/33842	6/27425	2/17357	1/6951
< 100 rad	Number/person-years	3/14882	11/29103	4/23736	5/10899

All ages: zero dose   12/85575   Signif. different
          < 100 rad   23/78620   p < .05

Over 20 yrs: zero dose 9/51733   Signif. different
         < 100 rad 20/63738   p = .07

(data from McGregor et al.)

The strength of the low dose excess cancer cases is strongly dependent upon the choice of the "control" population which is problematic in the Japanese studies. The options are the in-city zero-dose group, the in-city zero-9 rad group, the not-in-city at the time of the bombing group, and the Japanese national statistics age adjusted for the population at risk. In Nagasaki the incidence of all cancer in the zero dose group, including breast cancer, is considerably below that in the other three groups.

Thus, comparison with the Japanese national statistics will considerably diminish the excess cancer incidence observed for doses below 100 rads, such that although it remains positive, the excess is not significant. Indeed the choice of the zero dose group for control maximizes the apparent excess of cancer seen in Nagasaki at low doses.

Massachusetts Fluoroscopy Study

This study by Boice and Monson (11) concerns young women admitted to sanitoria for the treatment of tuberculosis and who received multiple chest fluoroscopies during pneumothorax therapy. The study covers breast doses ranging from 32 to more than 400 rads. Altogether 41 cancer cases were found in the exposed population of 1047 women compared with 15 found in 717 unexposed controls. Ten cancer cases were found in women receiving less than 100 rads compared with 9.6 cases expected. The average dose per fluoroscopy was 1.5 rads. In this study doses were much lower than those in the earlier Nova Scotia study (12), which was the first to associate breast cancer with multiple chest fluoroscopies. Although the dose effect relation is highly consistent with linearity, particularly after age standardization of the data, there is no significant difference between the control incidence and the incidence in patients receiving less than 100 rads. The increasing incidence with breast dose is shown in Figure 8 where the 80% confidence intervals for each dose point are included.

Table 2 provides data for the lowest dose point and shows that the observed excess at 32 rads breast dose is confined to the 15 - 29 year old age group.

TABLE 2
MASSACHUSETTS FLUOROSCOPY STUDY
Lowest Dose Data

Number of fluoroscopies   1 to 49
Dose range   1.5 to 75 rads
Mean dose   35 rads

Age Group	less than 15	15 to 29	over 30
Woman-years at risk	680	5949	2613
Expected ca.	0.2	4.3	3.6
Observed ca.	0	7	1

One of the weaknesses of this study, apart from the small number of cancer cases and the limited age range of the subjects, is the uncertainty regarding the doses which were actually received by the patients who later developed breast cancer. The dosimetry is based on an average exposure per exam based on the reported proportion of examinations given with the patient facing the x-ray tube and the proportion given while facing the physician. The dose differential between these two positions is very large: approximately 24 times greater when facing the tube. Thus a patient who faced the tube during all examinations would have received 3.5 times as much radiation as estimated in this study, while a person who always faced the physician would have received about 0.15 times the estimated dose. Unfortunately in the majority of patients the examination position was unknown.

New York Mastitis Study

An earlier study of this population has been extended by Shore et al.(13) and includes 571 exposed women of whom 36 developed breast cancers in comparison with 993 controls who developed 32 breast cancers. The dose range varied from 50 to over 600 rads with an average of 248 rads. The population contains relatively few persons receiving less than 100 rads: less than 10% of the women were in this group. Figure 9 shows the essentially linear trend of the data. However the lowest dose point is at 112 rads and at that level the incidence is not significantly different from that of the several control populations.

Irradiation of Benign Breast Disease in Sweden

In this study 1168 breasts were irradiated with doses in the range 200 - 1000 rads. A total of 115 cancers were observed compared with 28.7 expected based on the statistics of the Swedish population (14). In this study doses were very high and it is likely that the induced cancer incidence rate falls at these high dose levels due to cell killing. Moreover in this series there is a strong correlation between dose and patient age at the time of treatment. For women below age 40 where average doses were 400 to 800 rads, the risk is estimated at about 7 cases/million-year-rad.

AGE DEPENDENCE OF CANCER RISK

Attention has been given to the incidence of radiation induced cancer as a function of age in the above studies. It is clear that both in the Japanese and the Massachusetts fluoroscopy populations there is a considerably higher risk in the group aged 10 - 19 years at the time of irradiation. Table 3 shows the absolute risk for groups of increasing age. The risk falls in the 20 - 40 age group with a subsequent increase for older age groups. The relative risk (i.e., factor of increase over normal incidence) shows the same trend in Table 4, but the large values of relative risk for younger women stem partly from the low natural incidence of breast cancer in those women. The Massachusetts study shows the same trend. The raw data reproduced in Table 5 shows a maximum risk in the age group 15 - 19, with some reduction at older age groups. The data shows zero excess cancer for women over 35 years old but statistically the data is very thin since only about 10% of the total number of person-years at risk were in this older age group.

On the other hand the New York mastitis study shows no effect of age. In Table 6 the absolute risk in the age group 15 - 29 is essentially the same as that in the age group 30 - 45. It has been suggested that this may be attributed to the hormonal state of the breast during lactation (13), although increased cancer has not developed in lactating irradiated rats (15).

TABLE 3
ABSOLUTE CANCER RISK BY AGE GROUP
AT TIME OF BOMBING-HIROSHIMA AND NAGASAKI

AGE ATB	EXCESS RISK/ million-year-rad
0-9	0
10-19	4.0
20-34	1.2
35-49	0.9
50 +	1.3
average 10+	1.9

T-65 dose range 10 to 100+ rads
Years 1950-69

McGregor et al.(10)

TABLE 4
BREAST CANCER IN NAGASAKI
FOR DOSES LESS THAN 100 RAD
BY AGE AT TIME OF BOMBING

AGE GROUP	RELATIVE RISK*
10-19	7.7
20-34	1.1
35-49	0.4
50 +	1.4
average 10+	1.2

*Compared with incidence per 10^6 person-years
with 0-9 rad in same age group 1950-69

McGregor et al. (10)

TABLE 5
MASSACHUSETTS FLUOROSCOPY STUDY

Excess cancer by age at first
fluoroscopic exposure

Age group	<15	15-19	20-24	25-29	30-34	>35
# Women	99	242	263	200	105	138
Ca. observed	2	13	9	9	4	4
Ca. expected	0.9	3.4	5.4	5.5	3.3	4.8
O/E	2.1	3.8	1.7	1.6	1.2	0.8

TABLE 6
NEW YORK MASTITIS SERIES
EFFECT OF AGE AT IRRADIATION ON ABSOLUTE RISK

AGE AT IRRADIATION, years	15-29	30-45
ABSOLUTE RISK (ca/10^6P-Y-rad)	7.9	9.2

A good summary of this situation is provided in the Final
Report (16) of the NCI Ad Hoc Committee on Mammography Screening.
A lower limit for the absolute risk of Western women over 35 years
old was derived by modifying the average risk for all age groups
based on the Massachusetts fluoroscopy and the New York mastitis
studies (7.5 cases/million-year-rad) by a factor of 0.45 derived
from the Japanese age-dependence data (Table 3). As a result the
range of 3.5 - 7.5 excess cancers/million-year-rad was estimated,
the higher limit being prompted by the uncertainties in the estimates of age-specific risks for Western women.

LATENT PERIOD

The life-span studies of the Japanese A-bomb survivors suggest
an increase in breast cancer in exposed women starting well within
10 years after the bombing. However this onset time is age dependent and follows the time pattern of normal breast cancer development. Thus no cancer has been observed in women younger than 10
years in 1945. There is also no sign that the rate of appearance
of breast cancer is diminishing 24 years after irradiation.

In the Massachusetts fluoroscopy study excess breast cancer
incidence was discernible 15 years after exposure (as was also
the case in the New York study) and was continuing to appear 40
years after exposure. In the Swedish study the earliest time of
observation was about 8 years after irradiation and the median
latent period was about 24 years.

CONCLUSION

There appears to be no good evidence to presume that the risk
of induction of mammary cancer is non-linear with dose down to the
lowest levels. There also appears to be no reduction in the risk
as a result of the extensive fractionation in the fluoroscopy
studies compared to the relatively acute doses delivered in the
therapy studies. This fact suggests that the human breast cancer
primary lesion, as in the case of the rat, shows little repair,
and may therefore be linear in incidence down to levels of 20 rad
or less. The actual human experience, even at 50 rads, is not
however adequate to demonstrate such a linear relation. The
Nagasaki experience suggests some diminution in the risk per rad
at low doses, partly as a result of the unexpectedly low incidence
in the zero dose control population, and partly because of the low
incidence in the group with about 55 rads average dose. The
Western studies are also weak in the dose range below 100 rads
where the incidence is not significantly elevated above the control
level. These questions may be clarified in the future as evidence
of breast cancer in a large Canadian study of fluoroscoped tuberculosis patients is analyzed and as the follow-up of the Nagasaki
population is extended. In the interim it is prudent to believe
that, for breast cancer induced by x-irradiation, the risk estimate
derived from considerably higher dose levels is applicable to the
doses employed in mammography.

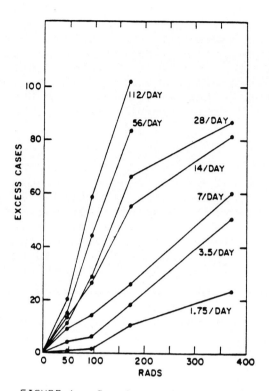

FIGURE 1. Ovarian tumors in mice as
a function of dose for different
gamma-ray dose-rates.
(courtesy of J.M.Yuhas and Radiation
 Research)

FIGURE 2.
Incidence of
myeloid leukemia
in RF male mice
receiving
x-irradiation:
effect of dose
rate.
(A.C.Upton et al)

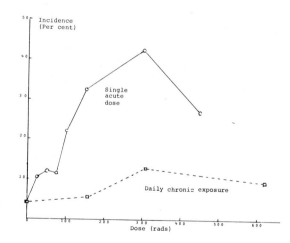

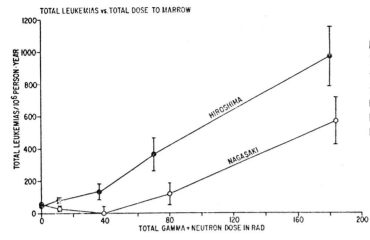

TOTAL LEUKEMIAS vs. TOTAL DOSE TO MARROW

FIGURE 3.
Total leukemias
versus total dose
to bone marrow
Courtesy:
H.H.Rossi and
Health Physics)

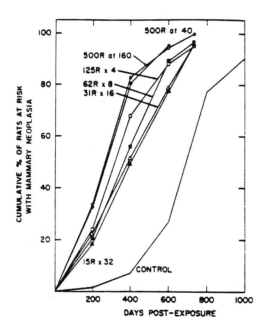

Figure 4. Mammary tumors in rats
after single or multiple doses of
gamma rays from 40th to 160th day
of age plotted against time.
(courtesy of C.J.Shellabarger and
Cancer).

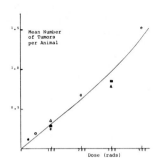

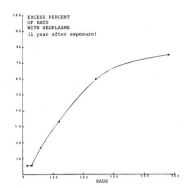

FIGURE 5. Mammary tumor incidence
in Sprague-Dawley rats following
x-irradiation (200-250 kVp)
corrected for spontaneous incidence.
(redrawn from Rossi and Kellerer, 1972)

FIGURE 6. Acceleration of
mammary neoplasms in Sprague-
Dawley rats after total-body
Co-60 irradiation (control
incidence subtracted). (After
Shellabarger et al, 1969)

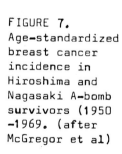

FIGURE 7.
Age-standardized
breast cancer
incidence in
Hiroshima and
Nagasaki A-bomb
survivors (1950
-1969. (after
McGregor et al)

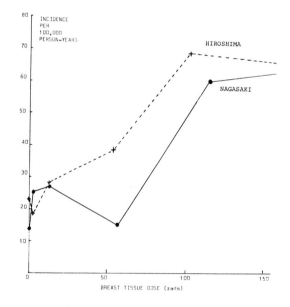

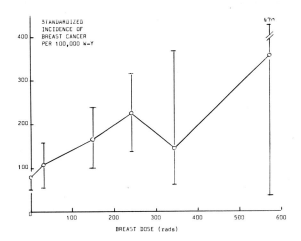

FIGURE 8. Massachusetts fluoroscopy study.
Standardized incidence of breast cancer
as a function of estimated average breast
dose. Error bars are 80% confidence limits.
(courtesy of J.D.Boice, Jr. and Journal of
  the National Cancer Institute)

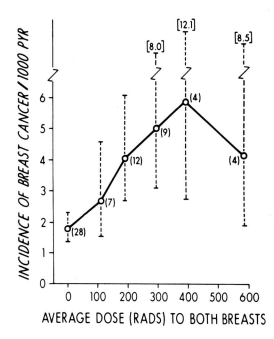

FIGURE 9. New York mastitis study.
Breast cancer incidence by average dose
to both breasts for period 10-34 years
after irradiation. Error bars represent
80% confidence intervals and number of
breast cases/dose group in parentheses.
(courtesy R.E.Shore and Jour. Nat.Cancer Institute)

45

REFERENCES

1. Mays,C.W., Lloyd,R.D. Bone sarcoma risk from ^{90}Sr. (In) Biomedical Implications of Radiostrontium Exposure, editors M.Goldman and L.K.Bustad. USAEC CONF-710201 pp. 352-375, 1972.
2. Rossi, H.H., Mays, C.W. Leukemia risk from neutrons. Health Phys. 34: 353, 1978
3. Yuhas, J.M. Recovery from radiation-carcinogenic injury to the mouse ovary. Radiat. Res. 60: 321, 1974
4. Upton, A.C., Randolph, M.L., Conklin, J.W. Late effects of fast neutrons and gamma rays in mice as influenced by the dose rate of irradiation: induction of neoplasia. Radiat. Res. 41: 467 1970
5. Shellabarger, C.J. Radiation carcinogenesis. Laboratory studies. Cancer 37: 1090, 1976
6. Shellabarger, C.J., Bond, V.P., Aponte, G.E., Cronkite, E.P. Results of fractionation and protraction of total body radiation on rat mammary neoplasia. Cancer Res. 26: 509, 1966
7. Rossi,H.H., Kellerer, A.M. Radiation carcinogenesis at low doses. Science 175: 200, 1972.
8. Shellabarger, C.J., Bond,V.P., Cronkite,E.P., Aponte,G.E. Relationship of dose of total-body Co-60 radiation to incidence of mammary neoplasia in female rats. (In) Radiation-Induced Cancer. International Atomic Energy Administration, Vienna,1969
9. Advisory Committee on the Biological Effects of Ionizing Radiations, National Academy of Sciences-National Research Council. The effects on populations of exposure to low levels of ionizing radiation. Washington, D.C: U.S.Government Printing Office,1972
10. McGregor,D.H.,Land,C.E., Choi,K. et al. Breast cancer incidence among atomic bomb survivors, Hiroshima and Nagasaki, 1950-69. J.Natl. Cancer Inst. 59: 799, 1977
11. Boice,J.D.Jr., Monson,R.R. Breast cancer in women after repeated fluoroscopic examinations of the chest. J.Natl. Cancer Inst. 59: 823, 1977.
12. MacKenzie, I. Breast cancer following multiple fluoroscopies. Brit. J. Cancer 19: 1, 1965
13. Shore, R.E., Hempelmann,L.H., Kowaluk,E., et al. Breast neoplasms in women treated with x-rays for acute post-partum mastitis. J.Natl.Cancer Inst. 59: 813, 1977
14. Baral, E., Larsson,L-E., Mattson,B. Breast cancer following irradiation of the breast. Cancer 40: 2906, 1977
15. Shellabarger,C.J. Modifying factors in rat mammary gland carcinogenesis. p.31 in Biology of Radiation Carcinogenesis, editors J.M.Yuhas, R.W.Tennant and J.D.Regan. Raven Press, New York, 1976
16. Final Reports of National Cancer Institute Ad Hoc Working Groups on Mammography Screening for Breast Cancer. Report on Mammography Risks, p.24. U.S.Dept. of Health, Education and Welfare, National Institutes of Health. DHEW Publication No.(NIH) 77-1400,March 1977

DEPTH DOSE DATA FOR MAMMOGRAPHY

G. Richard Hammerstein
Northeast Center for Radiological Physics
Memorial Sloan-Kettering Cancer Center
New York, New York

INTRODUCTION

Until rather recently, comparisons of relative risk for different mammographic imaging systems were based on entrance exposure measurements, and assessments of carcinogenic risk generally were based on estimated doses which were taken to be some fixed fraction of the entrance exposure.[1,2,8] Employing entrance exposure in either of these ways is inappropriate. While exposure measurements provide essential physical information, the use of exposure as a risk indicator can be seriously misleading. For example, consider Figure 1, which shows energy fluence per Roentgen for monochromatic beams: a 1R exposure with 35 kV x-rays carries ten times more energy into the breast than a 1R exposure with 17 kV x-rays.

Estimation of carcinogenic risk requires determination of the total energy absorbed in radiosensitive tissue. This in turn requires knowledge of breast tissue densities and atomic compositions, the spatial distribution of different tissue types, and the relation of absorbed dose in tissue at depth to entrance (or receptor) exposure and to x-ray beam quality. Various physical quantities which can be derived directly from available depth dose data—midplane dose or mean dose to a standard phantom or total energy absorbed in tissue like material—are useful parameters for comparing relative risks associated with different imaging systems and techniques. They can also be used, at least on an interim basis, in estimates of carcinogenic risk to an "average" patient. Nonetheless, the goal of mammographic dosimetry should be the ability to make accurate statements of risk to individual patients, since this is the information which is directly relevant in balancing the demands of patient safety and high image quality. Despite significant progress, this goal has yet to be achieved fully, primarily for lack of detailed, quantitative evidence on the spatial distribution of high risk tissue.

DEPTH DOSE RESULTS

Calculations of the energy absorption parameters applicable to risk estimates are based on measurements of absorbed dose. Dose as a function of depth can be determined for a given beam quality by measuring exposure as a function of depth in tissue simulating phantoms and applying calculated exposure-to-dose conversion factors, "f factors", which for a given x-ray energy are[3]

$$f = \frac{\Sigma P_i \frac{\mu_{en}}{\rho})_i}{\frac{\mu_{en}}{\rho})_{air}} \qquad (1)$$

where $\frac{\mu_{en}}{\rho})_i$ is the mass energy absorption coefficient[3,4] for atomic element i and P_i is the proportion by weight of that element in the tissue type for which f is calculated.

Information on tissue elemental compositions is necessary both for calculating f-factors and for relating the radiation interaction properties of dosimetry phantoms to the interaction properties of actual tissues. Densities and elemental compositions have been measured[5] recently for skin, adipose tissue, and mammary gland taken from fresh mastectomy specimens. f-factors for water, gland, and adipose tissue are shown in Table I as a function of energy for monochromatic beams. The f-factors' relatively weak energy dependence has useful consequences in simplifying subsequent analyses.

TABLE I

EXPOSURE-TO-DOSE CONVERSION FACTORS FOR
WATER, MAMMARY GLAND, AND ADIPOSE TISSUE

E(kV)	water	f(rad/R) gland	adipose
10	0.90	0.81	0.52
15	0.89	0.80	0.52
20	0.88	0.79	0.52
30	0.87	0.79	0.53
40	0.89	0.81	0.57
50	0.91	0.83	0.64

The phantoms used in the Northeast CRP measurements[5] were formulated[6] to match the radiation interaction properties of adipose tissue, water, and 50% water-50% fat.[7] The phantom materials have the same densities, linear attenuation coefficients, and mass energy absorption coefficients as the corresponding tissue materials to an accuracy of better than 3% at all energies of interest in mammography. The 50% water-50% fat material gives a better than 5% match to a 50% adipose-50% gland composition, which we will take to be representative of an "average" breast. The importance of the water and adipose tissue phantoms lies in the fact that those materials should closely match the extremes of radiographic density encountered clinically. Thus data for those phantoms bracket the range of dose variations arising from patient to patient variation in breast composition. Also, at a given beam quality accurate interpolations can be made between the measured depth exposure curves to obtain results appropriate for other tissue compositions, e.g. 75% adipose-25% gland.

Measured curves of exposure versus depth in phantom are shown in Figure 2. Details of the experimental procedures have been given elsewhere.[5] In each of the graphs 2a-2d the results for adipose tissue are given by the dotted curves, for 50% adipose-50% gland by long dash, and for water by a solid line. The irradiation techniques are given in Table II.

TABLE II

IRRADIATION TECHNIQUES FOR THE DEPTH-EXPOSURE
CURVES OF FIGURES 2a-2d

technique	target/filter	kVp	HVL (mmAl)
a	W/Al	50	1.21
b	W/Al	40	0.79
c	W/Al	30	0.36
d	Mo/Mo	28	0.31

Figure 3 shows dose per unit entrance exposure (including backscatter) as a function of depth in a) adipose tissue, b) water, and c) 50% adipose-50% gland.

for each of the four irradiation techniques. The f-factors employed were those appropriate for mammary gland; i.e., in each case these results represent dose to a small mass of pure gland embedded in the otherwise homogeneous medium. This seems the most appropriate choice, since gland presumably is the tissue at risk, but other choices are, of course, possible. In Figure 3c, if f-factors for the homogeneous 50-50 medium had been adopted, the calculated doses would have been about 18% lower.

QUANTITATIVE RISK INDICATORS

MIDBREAST DOSE

For the sake of specificity, we assume the "average" breast to be 6cm thick under compression, so that midbreast dose is the dose to a point 3cm below the middle of the entrance surface. The choice of midbreast to represent overall risk is rather arbitrary; it would be preferable to adopt a quantity which takes into account variations in dose levels throughout the breast. Nonetheless, midbreast dose is worth considering for two reasons: first the concept is relatively simple and familiar; second, the widely publicized risk analyses by an NCI working group[1] and Bailar[8] were based on an assumption of 1 rad midbreast dose per view, and a re-examination of that assumption in light of current information is in order.

Consider Figure 3c. Midbreast gland dose per unit surface exposure is 0.29 rad/R for the 1.21 mmAl HVL beam, falls to 0.20 rad/R for the 0.79 mmAl beam, and is only 0.06 rad/R for the 0.31 mmAl beam. This indicates a strong dependence of midbreast dose on x-ray beam quality. To investigate the effect further, measurements were made for five additional beam qualities. The combined results are shown in Figure 4 in the form of midbreast gland dose per unit entrance exposure in air (no backscatter) versus x-ray beam first half value layer. The relatively small differences between results for W/Al and Mo/Mo systems, despite the large differences in incident x-ray spectra, indicate that the conclusions to be drawn from these results are essentially independent of a particular choice of target, filter, or waveform.

Clearly, midbreast dose per unit entrance exposure increases in direct proportion to HVL. The simplicity of the result is due primarily to the weak energy dependence of the f-factors: since f is nearly constant with beam quality, Figure 4 can be viewed as a graph of x-ray attenuation through tissue versus x-ray attenuation through aluminum, and the proportionality is then not especially surprising. A highly useful consequence of this simplicity is that the measured data can be interpolated (extrapolated) simply and accurately to any beam quality which might be of interest clinically.

The strong beam quality dependence of dose at depth implies that caution should be exercised in the use of hard beams. While increased kVp and filtration can reduce entrance exposure, comparable reductions in dose at depth are not obtained and soft tissue contrast deteriorates.

The results of Figure 4 have been used to analyze clinical data taken by the Centers for Radiological Physics at the ACS/NCI Breast Screening Centers. Each pair of exposure and HVL data used in the analysis represented the technique most commonly employed for imaging a 5cm breast on a given Screening Center x-ray unit. Calculated midbreast doses are shown in Table III. Two major points can be made:

1) Primarily because of the hard beams employed in Xeromammography, current

midbreast doses associated with Xerox imaging at the Centers are substantially higher than the doses with film/screen work (eight times higher on average). 2) The assumption of 1 rad midbreast dose per view promulgated in references 1 and 8 represents a significant overestimate of the doses currently being delivered at the Screening Centers (on average, three times too high for Xerox, twenty five times too high for film/screen).

TABLE III

MIDBREAST DOSES AT THE ACS/NCI SCREENING CENTERS
(data as of June, 1978, from the CRP's)

Receptor	Case	Exposure* (R)	HVL (mmAl)	Midbreast Dose (rad, 1 view)
Xerox	lowest dose	0.59	1.05	0.15
	highest dose	1.23	1.79	0.50
	average (34 x-ray units)	--	--	0.32
film/ screen	lowest dose	0.28	0.42	0.024
	highest dose	0.96	0.32	0.064
	average (14 x-ray units)	--	--	0.040

*including backscatter

ENERGY ABSORBED PER UNIT AREA

Another quantity which has been proposed[9] as a risk indicator is total energy absorbed per unit cross sectional area irradiated. For a homogeneous medium of area A, thickness t, density ρ_{med}, and f-factor f_{med}

$$E_{abs}/A = \rho_{med} \int_{o}^{t} f_{med} \, X \, (z) \, dz \qquad (gm \cdot rad/cm^2) \qquad (2)$$

where $X(z)$ is the exposure as a function of depth. Values of E_{abs}/A calculated for the 50% adipose-50% gland data were found to be in good agreement with the results of reference 9. Figure 5 shows E_{abs}/A per unit entrance exposure in air (no backscatter) versus x-ray beam first HVL. As with midbreast dose, E_{abs}/A increases in direct proportion to HVL, indicating a relative risk advantage for soft beams.

E_{abs}/A is an improvement on midbreast dose as a risk indicator, in the sense that it takes into account variations of dose with depth. However, it fails to account for possible variations in the amount and distribution of high risk tissue, and by implicitly assuming all tissue to be at equal risk includes significant amounts of energy which in an actual patient would be absorbed in skin, fat, and other low risk tissues.

TOTAL ENERGY ABSORBED IN GLAND

The physical quantity which is most directly relevant to risk estimates for the individual patient is total energy absorbed in high risk tissue, which we have assumed to be mammary gland. No quantity stated in terms of a ratio such as energy absorbed per unit area or energy absorbed per unit mass (dose) can account in a consistent way for individual variations in the amount and distribution of high risk tissue. If $\rho_g (\overline{y})$ is the mass of gland per unit volume (not the density of pure gland) in the inhomogenous medium surrounding point $\bar{y}$, and if f_g is the f-factor for gland, then

$$E_g = \iiint \rho_g (\bar{y}) \, f_g (\bar{y}) \, X (\bar{y}) \, d^3y \qquad \text{(gm·rad)} \qquad (3)$$

where $x (\bar{y})$ is the exposure at point $\bar{y}$. Sufficient dosimetry data is available for calculations of E_g to be undertaken once $\rho_g (\bar{y})$ is known for a variety of cases, but to our knowledte little quantitative information on ρ_g is presently available. Quantitative studies of mammograms and actual breast specimens should be undertaken.

MEAN GLAND DOSE

In lieu of detailed information on $\rho_g (\bar{y})$ recourse can be made to models of an "average" breast as a basis for calculating risk to an "average" patient or the relative risk of different techniques in terms of mean dose to glandular tissue. A model which is closely related to the NECRP dosimetry data assumes that the "average" breast is 6cm thick under compression, including a 0.5cm layer of skin and adipose tissue, and has an interior volume containing a total mass M_g (av) = 175gm of gland distributed uniformly through a medium equivalent to 50% adipose-50% gland. The mean gland dose to this "average" breast is then

$$\bar{D}_g(av) = \frac{E_g (av)}{M_g (av)} = \frac{1}{M_g (av)} \iint dxdy \int \rho_g f_g X(z)dz$$

$$= \frac{\rho_g}{\rho_g} \frac{A}{V} \int f_g X(z)dz$$

$$= \frac{1}{5} \int_{0.5}^{5.5} f_g X(z)dz \qquad (4)$$

Figure 6 shows mean gland dose per unit entrance exposure in air (no backscatter) versus HVL. As with midbreast dose and E_{abs}/A, mean gland dose displays a strong linear dependence on beam quality. The corresponding graph for midbreast dose is shown for comparison. Quantitative differences between mean gland dose and midbreast dose are model dependent; as the thickness of the region assumed to contain gland decreases, $\bar{D}_g$ (av) reduces to midbreast dose.

CONCLUSIONS

Currently available dosimetry data allow the calculation of various quantitative indicators for estimating carcinogenic risk to an "average" patient and relative risks associated with different mammographic imaging systems. Midbreast dose, energy absorbed per unit area, and mean gland dose all display a strong, linear dependence on x-ray beam quality, indicating a substantial relative risk advantage for soft beams. Analysis of clinical data from the ACS/NCI Screening Centers shows midbreast doses at the Centers to be substantially lower than the 1 rad per view estimated in several earlier analyses.

The physical quantity which is directly relevant to calculations of individual risk is total energy absorbed in glandular tissue, E_g. Calculations of E_g require detailed, quantitative data on the amount and distribution of glandular tissue, $\rho_g (\bar{y})$, for individual cases, and effort should be directed toward obtaining such data. Ideally, once data on $\rho_g (\bar{y})$ and calculations of

E_g become available, the radiologist could

1. on the basis of a physical examination and possibly a low dose baseline mammogram, place a given patient in one of a range of narrowly defined categories related to breast size and radiographic density and amount and distribution of high risk tissue,
2. consult precalculated tables of dosimetry and risk, and
3. arrive at a reliable estimate of the risk to that patient associated with any particular choice of mammographic technique.

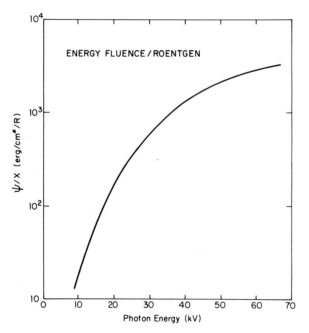

Figure 1.   Energy fluence per Roentgen versus x-ray energy for mono-chromatic beams.

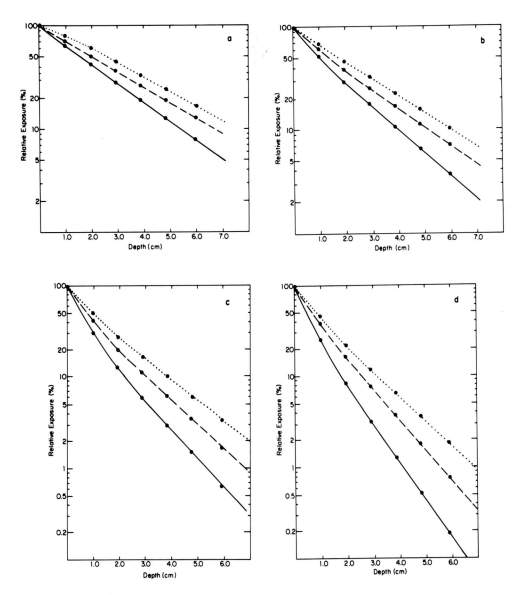

Figure 2.   Relative exposure versus depth in phantom for adipose tissue
            (dots), 50% adipose-50% gland (dashes), and water.   Irradiation
            techniques for cases a-d are given in Table II.

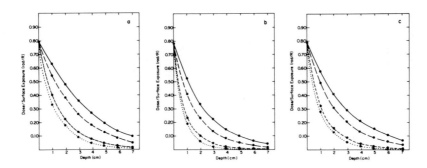

Figure 3. Dose to a small mass of gland per unit surface exposure
(including backscatter) versus depth in a) adipose tissue,
b) wqter, c) 50% adipose-50% gland.   The solid curves give
results for the highest HVL beam, the dotted curves give
results for the lowest HVL beam.   Irradiation techniques
are given in Table II.

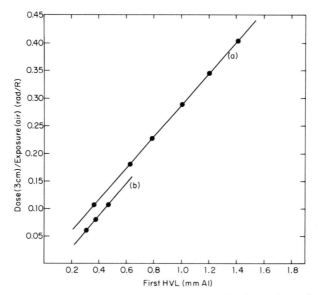

Figure 4. Dose to a small mass of gland embedded at 3cm depth in
50% adipose-50% gland per unit entrance exposure in air
(no backscatter) versus x-ray beam first half-value layer.
Target/filter combinations are a) W/Al and b) Mo/Mo.

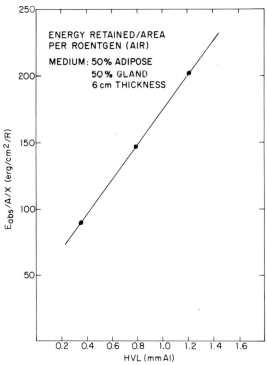

Figure 5. Energy absorbed per unit area in 50% adipose-50% gland
per unit entrance exposure in air (no backscatter) versus
x-ray beam first half-value layer. W target/ Al filter.

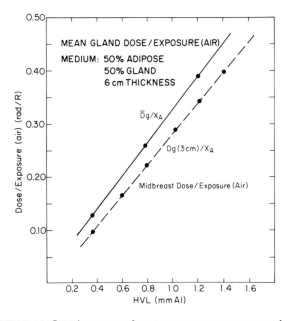

Figure 6. Mean dose to gland per unit entrance exposure in air
(no backscatter) versus x-ray beam first half-value layer.
Model assumptions are discussed in the text. The
corresponding graph for midbreast gland is shown for
comparison.

REFERENCES

1. Report of the NCI ad hoc working group on the risk associated with mammography in mass screening for the detection of breast cancer. July, 1976.
2. Lester, R.G.: Risk versus benefit in mammography. Radiology 124: 1-6, July, 1977.
3. Johns, H.E., Cunningham, J.R.: The Physics of Radiology. Springfield, Ill. Thomas, 3rd ed, 1969, p. 275 and pp. 742-744.
4. Hubbell, J.H.: Photon mass attenuation and mass-energy absorption coefficients for H,C,N,), Ar, and seven mixtures from 0.1 keV to 20 MeV. Radiation Res. 70, 58-81, April, 1977.
5. Hammerstein, G.R., Miller, D.W., White, D.R., Masterson, M.E., Woodard, H.Q., Laughlin, J.S.: Radiation absorbed dose in mammography. Submitted for publication in Radiology.
6. White, D.R.: The formulation of tissue substitute materials using basic interaction data. Phys. Med. Biol. 22: 889-899, Sept.,1977.
7. White, D.R., Martin, R.J., Darlison, R.: Epoxy resin based tissue substitutes Br. J. Radiol. 50: 814-821, November, 1977.
8. Bailar, J.C.: Mammography: a contrary view. Ann Intern Med. 84: 77-84, January, 1976
9. Boag, J.W., Stacey, A.J., Davis, R.: Radiation exposure to the patient in xeromammography. Br. J. Radiol. 49: 253-261, March, 1975.

AVERAGE, MID-PLANE, ENTRANCE AND OTHER HYBRID DOSES IN MAMMOGRAPHY

E.P. Muntz, Ph.D.
University of Southern California

INTRODUCTION

In this volume as well as in a number of other publications, breast mid-line or mid-plane dose is used by many authors as a convenient indicator of carcinogenic risk due to irradiation in mammography. Mid-plane dose has even been adopted in certain guidelines for mammography. The purpose of this very brief note is to point out that the use of mid-plane dose as an indicator of carcinogenic effect in mammography can be very misleading, particularly for the softer beams used with screen-film systems.

METHOD AND MATERIALS

The depth dose and depth exposure data of Hammerstein (this volume and Ref. 1), Boag (Ref. 2) and BJR Suppl. II (Ref. 3) can all be correlated as shown in Fig. 1. Here the λ'_i in the abscissa is the distance required for an individual depth dose or exposure profile to drop to e^{-1} (0.368) of its initial value. The λ'_i's are a function of the beam half-value layer and the type of material being penetrated. Values of λ'_i for different materials and half-value layers are given in Fig. 2. More details of this work are presented in Ref. 4, to which the reader is referred. Based on the data correlation in Fig. 1, the average and mid-plane doses for a variety of phantom thicknesses and λ'_i's have been calculated and are shown in Fig. 3. The second abscissa in Fig. 3 was obtained by finding the half value layers corresponding to λ'_i's for a 0.5 adipose, 0.5 water mixture as given in Fig. 2. The solid lines in Fig. 3 represent mid-plane doses, the broken lines average doses, normalized by entrance dose in both cases, for phantom thickness ranging from 3 to 6 cm. Note that for a 0.5 adipose, 0.5 water, 6 cm thick phantom (refer to Ref. 1 for phantom details) and a 0.3 mm Al HVL, the average dose is about three times the mid-plane dose. On the other hand, for a hard beam, the differences are much smaller.

DISCUSSION

The results shown in Fig. 3 indicate that the appropriate measure for the significant dose in mammography should be considered very carefully. The tendency to quote mid-plane dose as a representative measure of dose may be seriously in error for the softer beams. A more extensive analysis of this question along with a consideration of non-linear dose-effects curves appears in Ref. 4. A further complication arises because some authors refer to an average dose as defined by Hammerstein, et al (Ref. 1) which includes a 0.5 cm layer of insensitive adipose tissue surrounding the radio-sensitive glandular tissue. The effect of this "adipose shielding" (see Ref. 4) is to cause the average dose and the mid-plane dose to come closer together than indicated by Fig. 3 for the case of glandular tissue distributed uniformly about the breast mid-plane. Glandular tissue distribution is not quantitatively known although it is not thought to be uniformly distributed about the mid-plane

(Ref. 5). Until this distribution is better determined some caution should be exercised in assuming specific distributions. These matters are also discussed in more detail by Muntz in Ref. 4.

In any event, the doses quoted at various places throughout this volume should be treated carefully, keeping in mind the several ways in which the authors have chosen to generate their numbers. One should be particularly wary of mid-plane doses calculated from measured entrance exposures by assuming an average 6 cm thick phantom. Most modern film-screen mammography for instance uses significant compression giving average compressed breast thickness nearer 4.5 or 5 cm. For a given entrance exposure with a 0.3 mm HVL beam, assuming an average breast had a thickness of 6 cm for a mid-plane dose calculation when it actually had a 5 cm thickness would lead to a factor of 1.7 underestimate of the mid-plane dose (see Fig. 3). Average glandular doses are probably more appropriate but then one has to be specific about the breast configuration.

SUMMARY

It is important to realize that "dose" in mammography may be calculated in various ways, using basic entrance exposure data, that can differ by large numerical factors. When composing results in mammography it is important to establish how quoted doses were obtained. In the future it is to be hoped that all investigators will quote the following parameters which are essential for determining accurately the relevant doses:

1. entrance beam half-value layer
2. compressed breast thickness
3. entrance exposure
4. explictly state any assumptions about adipose shielding and glandular tissue distribution

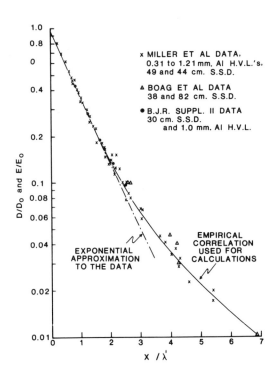

Figure 1: Correlation of Depth Dose and Exposure Data from Hammerstein et al and Boag et al, and Cohen et al.

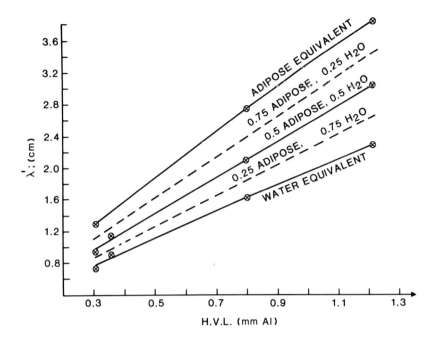

Figure 2: Characteristic Dimension λ'_i as a Function of Beam Quality.

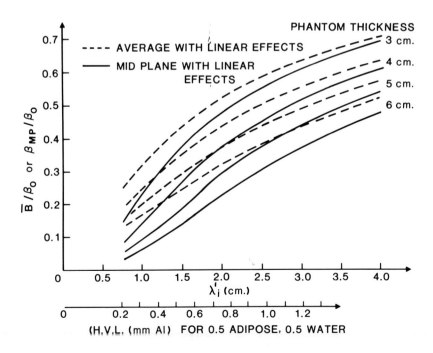

Figure 3: Comparison of Average ($\bar{B}$) and Mid-Plane (β_{MP}) Doses Relative to Entrance Dose ($\beta(o)$) as a Function of λ'_i and H.V.L. for a 50% Water, 50% Adipose Phantom.

REFERENCES

1. G.R. Hammerstein, D.W. Miller, D.R. White, M.E. Masterson and J.W. Laughlin: "Radiation Absorbed Dose in Mammography." To be published, Radiology, 1979.

2. J.W. Boag, A.J. Stacey, and R. Davis: "Radiation Exposure to the Patient in Xeroradiography." Brit. J. Radiol., 49:253, 1976.

3. M. Cohen, D.E.A. Jones, D. Greene (editor): "Central Axis Depth Dose Data for Use in Radiotherapy." Brit. J. Radiol., Suppl. II, 1972.

4. E.P. Muntz: "On the Relative Carcinogenic Effects of Different Mammography Techniques." To be published, Medical Physics, May/June 1979.

5. S.A. Feig: "Anatomic and Pathologic Basis of Radiation Related Human Breast Cancers" in "Reduced Dose Mammography." eds. W.W. Logan and E.P. Muntz, Masson, N.Y., 1979.

RISK-BENEFIT ANALYSIS FOR REDUCED DOSE MAMMOGRAPHY

by

Richard P. Chiacchierini, Ph.D.
and
Frank E. Lundin, Jr., M.D., Dr.P.H.

Epidemiologic   Studies Branch
Division of Biological Effects
Bureau of Radiological Health, FDA

INTRODUCTION

Since 1975, tighter control of technique factors and the introduction of new methods have led to a substantial reduction in breast radiation exposures associated with mammography (1,2). These exposure reductions are accompanied by reductions in the average radiation dose absorbed in breast tissue, though the size of the dose reduction is technique dependent. In previous analyses (3,4) the risk-benefit balance was estimated for the exposures associated with the earlier procedures and for benefits derived from the clinical trial of the Health Insurance Plan of Greater New York (5).

The present analysis estimates the breast cancer risks associated with the reduced dose mammographic procedures. It does so, however, by contrasting those risks with hypothetical 5-year breast cancer mortality reductions for women between the ages of 35 and 50 years of age. The resulting risk-benefit balance is estimated for 5-year screening programs beginning at the ages of 35, 40, and 45 and for three levels of average absorbed doses.

It should be noted that these analyses refer only to screening mammography. The distinction here is between screening mammography, which pertains to large numbers of asymptomatic women, and diagnostic (or referral) mammography, which applies to a much smaller group of symptomatic women. Because of the small number of women in this group of patients referred for diagnostic examination and the benefits of determining the type and degree of disease present, the small radiation risk associated with the examination is thought to be justified (6).

MATERIALS AND METHODS

The risk-benefit analysis of screening for breast cancer using mammography is accomplished by use of a computerized abridged life table model which allows the estimation of the lifetime risks and benefits experienced by hypothetical populations. In Figure 1, the flow chart of the steps or calculations necessary for each age interval in the lifetable is presented. The mathematical details of the model are described in other papers (3,4) and are reproduced in the Appendix for reference. Only a brief description of the methodology is given here. The steps are straight-forward beginning with a population alive at some exact age, say 35, and ending with the number who survive five years to age 40.

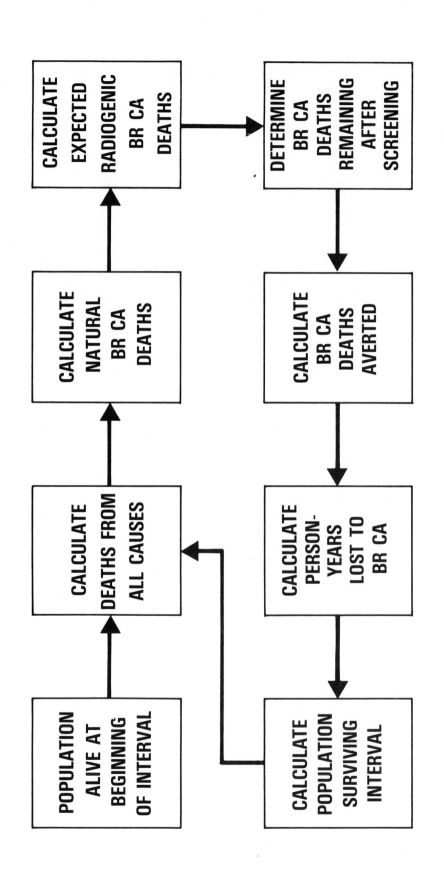

LIFE TABLE MODEL FLOW CHART

FIGURE 1.

Intermediate calculations include the number of deaths from all causes, from naturally occurring breast cancer, and from radiogenic breast cancer; and the number of lives saved by the breast cancer treatment initiated by the screening program. This process is repeated until all members of the population have died which for our purposes occurs at age 100. The model begins with 100,000 women at age 35, whose total and breast cancer mortality experience is assumed to follow the United States female population, and traces their breast cancer mortality experience under different risk and benefit assumptions. In this manner, the effects of various factors, including radiation dose, on breast cancer mortality in hypothetical populations can be estimated.

The benefits used in this analysis are hypothetical 5-year mortality reductions between 10 percent and 50 percent after adjustment for leadtime. This range of percentages reflects an upper limit similar to the benefit observed in the HIP Study (5) for women age 50-59. It is felt that the mortality reductions to be experienced among women between 35 and 50 years of age will lie in the range used in this analysis.* The use of hypothetical benefits is necessitated by the paucity of reliable data to estimate the mortality reductions associated with modern mammographic techniques.

In Figure 2, the time line of the cancer is schematically presented. Leadtime is the difference between the time the cancer would be detected by mammography and the time it would be discovered by other clinical means such as palpation. The adjustment for leadtime is necessary because survival rates to a given point in time are measured from the time of detection and the true measure of survival is taken from the time the cancer would have been found had mammography not been used. Thus, unless survival time for women whose cancers were detected by mammography exceeds the survival time plus leadtime for women whose cancers were detected by other clinical means, no advantage is gained by the earlier diagnosis.

In the present and previous analyses, the use of 5-year mortality reductions has overestimated the benefit to some degree. In the operation of the model, women surviving five years after detection are considered cured and are at risk of death only from the natural age-specific mortality from that point on. It is well-known, however, that 10-year survival in women with breast cancer is about 20% lower than at 5-years after diangosis, indicating that these women are still at increased risk of dying from their cancer. A similar effect has been noted after 9 years of follow up in the HIP study (8). Therefore, caution should be exercised in the use of the estimates given here for purposes other than the internal comparisons made in this report.

In addition, the hypothetical benefits presented have represented the mortality reduction which must be associated with mammography over and above that attributable to physical examination alone. Since mammography is thought to be associated with an increased risk of breast cancer whereas physical examination is not, that risk needs to be offset by mammography above the level of benefit demonstrated for physical examination alone.

The risk estimates used in this analysis were derived from the BEIR report absolute risk estimates (9) as modified by Upton et al, (10). In that modification, a range of risk between 3.5 and 7.5 cases per 10^6 person-year-rem is given with a 10-year latent period and a lifetime period of risk. We have chosen to use an estimate of 6 cases per 10^6 person-year-rem with a 10-year latent period and a lifetime period of risk which lies about in the middle of this range.

*Suggested from data found in the Beahrs Committee Report (7) on the 27 Breast Cancer Demonstration Detection Centers pages 56 and 58.

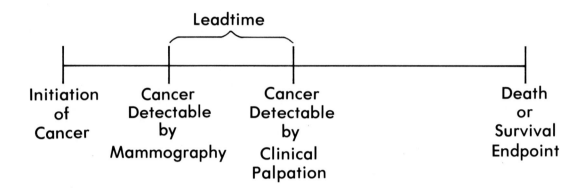

FIGURE 2. **Time-Line of Cancer Development**

RESULTS

The results are given in terms of two variables: breast cancer deaths averted and person-years gained. The latter variable includes a weighting factor related to the age at death while the former weights all deaths equally.

The next three figures exhibit the results in terms of breast cancer deaths averted for 5-year screening programs which include mammograpy begun at ages 35, 40, and 45 respectively. For each age, the results are shown for 0.1, 0.3 and 0.5 rads average absorbed dose to each breast per total examination. These doses are consistent with those reported by Hammerstein (11). Note that the appropriate dose parameter is the average breast tissue dose, not the mid-plane or mid-point dose. For the sake of brevity, the graphs showing the same information for the person-years gained variable were not included. Summary tables are presented, however, to show the lowest mortality reduction needed to just offset the assumed radiation risk based on deaths averted and person-years gained respectively. An important additional assumption used here is that the given dose reductions do not seriously impair image quality.

In Figure 3, the breast cancer deaths averted at given reductions in mortality for screened women between the ages of 35 and 39 are presented. Note that the net benefit exceeds the assumed risk if the mortality reduction attributable to mammography is between 0 percent and 10 percent for 0.1 rads, between 10 percent and 20 percent for 0.3 rads, and between 20 percent and 30 percent for 0.5 rads.

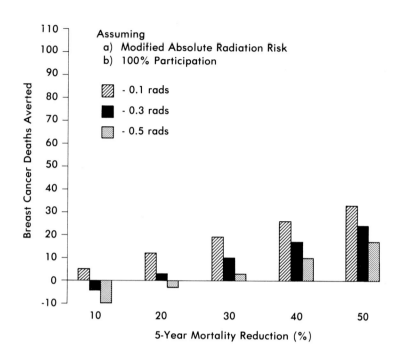

FIGURE 3.   Estimated Breast Cancer Deaths Averted by
Screening Women 35 - 39 Inclusive

In Figure 4, similar data are presented for screened women between the ages of 40 and 44. Both the 0.1 and 0.3 rad doses are offset by mortality reductions below 10 percent. For the 0.5 rad dose, a reduction of between 10 percent and 20 percent is needed. It should also be noted that the numbers of breast cancer deaths averted are larger due to the greater incidence of cancers available for early detection and cure.

In Figure 5, the breast cancer deaths averted are presented for women screened from age 45 through age 49. Note here that all three doses are offset by reductions in mortality of less than 10 percent.

Table 1 gives a summary of the three previous graphs by showing the estimated percentage of 5-year mortality reduction necessary to just offset the assumed radiation risk. Note that two higher dose levels have been included in this analysis because there are still some facilities operating at levels which would exceed the given doses.

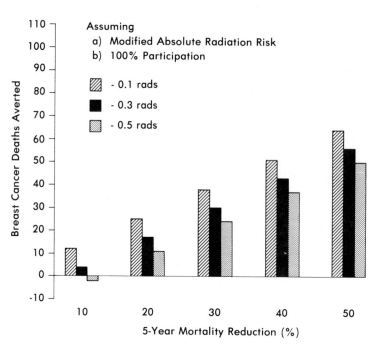

FIGURE 4. Estimated Breast Cancer Deaths Averted by
Screening Women 40 - 44 Inclusive

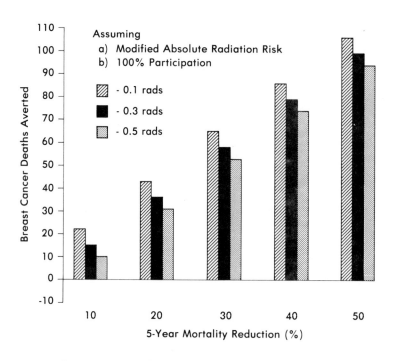

FIGURE 5. Estimated Breast Cancer Deaths Averted by
Screening Women 45 - 49 Inclusive

Table 1. Estimated minimum percentage of breast cancer mortality reduction needed to offset the assumed radiation risk (deaths averted variable)

Screening Ages	Dose (rads)				
	0.1	0.3	0.5	1.0	1.5
35 - 39	3	16	25	52	76
40 - 44	1	7	12	25	35
45 - 49	0.5	3	5	12	17

This table indicates the trends in the relationships between dose, age of screening and mortality reduction. For a dose of 0.1 rads, only small reductions in mortality need to be realized to offset the assumed radiation risk. For 0.3 rads small to moderate reductions are needed depending on age at screening. For 0.5 rads and above, moderate to large mortality reductions are required. For screening between 35 and 39 years of age, these estimates indicate that facilities giving 1 or more rads for an average absorbed dose to each breast per examination need to demonstrate mortality reductions in excess of maximum found in the HIP study. Such mortality reductions could be demonstrated only with drastic improvements in therapy as well as in detection.

In Table 2, similar data are presented for the person-years gained variable. These estimates are approximately one half as large as those given for the deaths averted variable due to the greater weights given to the breast cancers cured in younger women.

Table 2. Estimated minimum percentage of breast cancer mortality reduction needed to offset the assumed radiation risk (person-years gained variable)

Screening Ages	Dose (rads)				
	0.1	0.3	0.5	1.0	1.5
35 - 39	2	7	11	22	34
40 - 44	0.5	3	5	11	15
45 - 49	0.2	1	2	5	7

Thus whether one uses the unweighted results of deaths averted or the weighted results of person-years gained, the effect of dose reduction on the risk-benefit balance is dramatic so long as image quality is preserved. Furthermore, by considering the decreasing trend of the necessary mortality reductions with advancing age of screening, one can see the effect of breast cancer yield. For the age groups considered here, the older the population is when screening is begun, the more cancers there are to be found and, hence, the more productive and beneficial is the screening procedure.

DISCUSSION

This analysis attempts to circumvent the problems of using the results of the HIP study for benefit estimation by using mortality reductions which are hypothetical but reasonable. Besides the intended purpose of studying the relationships among risks, benefits, and screening age, a byproduct of this analysis is the suggestion of areas of study in which clincial investigators may expect to find the greatest chance for a successful implementation of screening mammography in women under 50 years of age. For all doses, the benefits necessary to offset the risk are smallest for screening women aged 45 through 49 as might be expected. However, if the dose is sufficiently low, say below 0.1 rads, it may be reasonable to screen women aged 35 through 39 provided that a mortality reduction on the order of 5 percent or greater can be realized. Thus, the data target ranges of benefit for a given screening age and dose which should be achieved as a minimum to discount the radiation risk.

That the lower radiation doses are possible without severe degradation of image quality, has been demonstrated at this conference. It is now up to the clinical research community to determine the extent to which the necessary mortality reductions can be achieved by use of mammography at the lower doses to permit a net overall benefit for women aged 35 to 50 years of age.

APPENDIX I

The equations and variables which constitute the life table model presented here are deterministic in nature and are based on the following notation. Let

x_i = exact age of the population at the beginning of the ith interval.

l_i = number of women alive at the beginning of the ith interval.

q_i = proportion of women alive at the beginning of the ith interval who die in that interval from all causes.

d_i = the number of women alive at the beginning of the ith interval who die from all causes in the interval.

M_i = the age specific mortality rate from all causes corresponding to the ith interval.

$M_{i\delta}$ = the age specific mortality rate from cause R_δ (in this instance breast cancer) corresponding to interval i.

L_i = the number of person-years lived in interval i by women who were alive at the beginning of the interval.

a_i = the fraction of interval i lived by women who died in that interval.

n_i = the number of years spanning the ith interval.

$Q_{i\delta}$ = proportion of women alive at the beginning of the ith interval who die from breast cancer in that interval.

$d_{i\delta}$ = number of women alive at the beginning of the ith interval who would naturally die of breast cancer in the interval in the absence of a screening benefit.

R_{ik} = increased risk per rad in the ith interval under risk model k.

$M'_{i\delta}$ = age specific mortality rate due to radiogenic breast cancer corresponding to interval i.

$I_{i\delta}$ = age specific incidence rate of breast cancer corresponding to interval i.

D_i^{Eff} = the dose in rads which is effective in interval i for induction of breast cancer.

$Q'_{i\delta}$ = proportion of women alive at the beginning of the ith interval who die of radiogenic breast cancer in the interval.

$d'_{i\delta}$ = number of women alive at the beginning of the ith interval who die of radiogenic breast cancer.

$d^*_{i\delta}$ = total number of deaths from breast cancer occurring in spite of screening in interval i.

$F^*_{i\delta}$ = fraction dying despite screening in the ith interval

$s_{i\delta}$ = number of deaths from breast cancer prevented by the screening procedure in the interval.

$P_{i\delta}$ = person-years of life lost by women who died from breast cancer in the interval.

q_i^* = derived proportion of those entering the ith interval adjusted for deaths caused by radiation and lives saved by screening.

z_i = expectation of years of life lost by women who die in the interval.

The life table equations utilized here are essentially those given by Chiang (12) with some modifications. Beginning with l_i, the computation of the number dying in the interval is given by

$$d_i = l_i \, q_i \tag{1}$$

To obtain an estimate of the subset of d_i who died from breast cancer, we utilize a formulation given by Chiang (12) for the probability of death from specific causes

$$Q_{i\delta} = \frac{n_i \, M_{i\delta}}{1 + (1-a_i) \, n_i \, M_i} \tag{2}$$

where

$$n_i = x_{i+1} - x_i \tag{3}$$

and

$$a_i = \frac{L_i - n_i \, l_{i+1}}{n_i d_i} \tag{4}$$

The L_i, l_{i+1} and d_i values are taken from the U.S. Life Tables for 1973. The number of deaths from the specific cause is given by

$$d_{i\delta} = l_i Q_{i\delta} \tag{5}$$

The risk data are then utilized to form the mortality rate in the ith interval from radiogenic breast cancer. For the absolute risk model we obtain

$$M'_{i\delta} = \frac{D_i^{Eff} \, R_{i1} \, M_{i\delta}}{I_{i\delta}} \tag{6}$$

where for purposes of this paper

$$R_{i1} = 6 \text{ cases/million women/rad/year.}$$

For the relative risk model we obtain

$$M'_{i\delta} = D_i^{Eff} \, R_{i2} \, M_{i\delta} \qquad (7)$$

where

$$R_{i2} = 0.008/\text{rad.}$$

Equation (7) assumes that a proportionate increase in the incidence will be accompanied by an equally proportionate increase in the mortality within each age interval. The probability of death from radiogenic breast cancer and the number of deaths are computed from M_i by

$$Q'_{i\delta} = \frac{n_i \, M'_{i\delta}}{1 + (1 - a_i) \, n_i \, M_i} \qquad (8)$$

and

$$d'_{i\delta} = l_i \, Q'_{i\delta} \qquad (9)$$

The number of breast cancer deaths which remain in spite of the screening procedure is computed by

$$d^*_{i\delta} = (d_{i\delta} + d'_{i\delta}) \, F^*_{i\delta} \qquad (10)$$

The gross number of lives saved then is given by

$$s_{i\delta} = (d_{i\delta} + d'_{i\delta}) - d^*_{i\delta} \qquad (11)$$

and the adjusted probability of death accounting for deaths caused and lives saved is calculated as

$$q^*_i = \frac{d_i + d'_{i\delta} - s_{i\delta}}{l_i} \qquad (12)$$

The number of women surviving to the next interval is obtained by

$$l_{i+1} = l_i (1 - q^*_i) \qquad (13)$$

Finally, the person-years of life lost in interval i by women who died from breast cancer in that interval is given by

$$P_{i\delta} = d^*_{i\delta} \, z_i \qquad (14)$$

The l_{i+1} then becomes the new l_i and is fed back into the process beginning with equation (1). The process is repeated until the final age interval computations have been completed. It is assumed that the last age interval for women 85 years of age and over is 15 years long implying that all women have died by age 100.

REFERENCES

1. Jans, R. This volume.

2. Bates, L. This volume.

3. Chiacchierini, R., F. Lundin, and P. Scheidt. 1976. A risk benefit analysis by life table modeling of an annual breast cancer screening program which includes x-ray mammography. Proceedings of the Third International Symposium on the Detection and Prevention of Cancer, New York, New York April 26 - May 1.

4. Chiacchierini, R. and F. Lundin. 1977. Benefit/risk ratio of mammography. In Breast Carcinoma: The Radiologists' Expanded Role. W. Logan (ed.). John Wiley and Sons, Inc. New York: 15-28.

5. Shapiro, S., P. Strax, L. Venet and W. Venet. 1973. Changes in 5-year breast cancer mortality in a breast cancer screening program. In Seventh National Cancer Conference Proceedings. American Cancer Society. New York:663

6. Lester R. 1977. A radiologist's view of the benefit/risk ratio of mammography. In Breast Carcinoma: The Radiologist's Expanded Role. W. Logan (ed.). John Wiley and Sons, Inc. New York: 29-33.

7. Beahrs, O. et al. 1977. Report of the working group to review the NCI/ACS Breast Cancer Demonstration Detection Projects. Presented at NCI Consensus Panel Meeting. Bethesda, MD September 14-16.

8. Shapiro, S. 1977. Evidence on screening for breast cancer from a randomized trial. Cancer 39: 2772-2782.

9. National Academy of Sciences - National Research Council 1972. The Effects on populations of exposure to low levels of ionizing radiations. Report of the Advisory Committee on the Biological Effects of Ionizing Radiations. Washington and Ottawa: 136-145.

10. Upton, A. et al. 1977. Final reports of National Cancer Institute ad hoc working groups on mammography screening for breast cancer and a summary report of their joint findings and recommendations. USDHEW (NIH) 77-1400. Washington.

11. Hammerstein, R. This volume.

12. Chiang, C. 1968. Introduction to Stochastic Processes in Biostatistics. John Wiley & Sons, Inc., New York: 313.

MAMMOGRAPHIC AND CLINICAL ACCURACY IN BREAST CANCER DETECTION: RELATIONSHIP TO PARENCHYMAL PATTERNS, LESION LOCATION, AND BREAST SIZE

Stephen A. Feig, M.D., Gary S. Shaber, M.D., Arthur S. Patchefsky, M.D., Gordon F. Schwartz, M.D. and Rudolph Nerlinger, B.S.

Department of Radiology, Thomas Jefferson University, Phila., Pa.

The relative effectiveness of mammographic and clinical examinations depends on many factors including breast parenchymal density and duct pattern, breast cancer location, and breast size. The ability of each of these two modalities in breast cancer detection will vary independently according to these parameters.

Material for this analysis consists of data for 167 breast cancers detected in a National Cancer Insititute funded screening program at our institution. All women were screened by physical examination of the breast performed according to the Haagensen technique (3) by a clinical physician specializing in breast diseases. All patients had been screened by xeromammography interpreted by one or two radiologists. Both mammography and clinical examination were interpreted with no knowledge of findings from the other modality.

If a mammographic reader recommended biopsy or if two readers differed in their recommendation for 6 month or 2 year follow-up, the case was reviewed by a highly experienced mammographer who did have access to clinical data. However, if both readers recommended 6 month follow-up or if both recommended 2 year follow-up, the case would not be reviewed by the experienced mammographer.

Although all patients received a single initial clinical examination, re-commendation of either biopsy or 6 month follow-up would result in re-examination by a more experienced clinical examiner who did have access to the mammographic findings.

Mammographic and clinical examiners were drawn from a pool of many individuals. For a case to be counted as positive on either initial clinical or mammographic examination, the most experienced clinician or radiologist must have advised biopsy. The study protocol has been more detailed in previous papers (1, 2). For all cancers, 53% (89/167) were detected on clinical examination and 78% (131/167) on xeromammography.

According to protocol, many biopsy proven carcinomas were not reviewed by the most experienced reader. Because of this, all lesions were reviewed by him following biopsy. These results are listed as the "retrospective" mammographic evaluation in figures 1-4. Overall, 87% (146/167) of all cancers could be seen on xeromammography.

BREAST DENSITY AND DUCT PATTERN

To evaluate the effect of breast structure on accuracy of mammographic and clinical detection, mammograms of the opposite (normal) breast were graded without knowledge of clinical and/or radiographic findings in the cancerous breast (Figs. 1, 2). Overall breast density was rated from 1(completely fatty) to 5(severely dense, fibrous, and glandular breast of nearly homogenous opacity

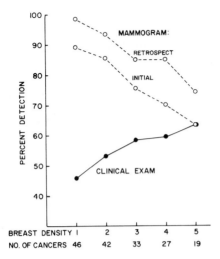

Figure 1. Effect of breast
  density on cancer detection.

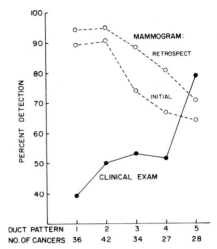

Figure 2. Effect of duct
  pattern on cancer detection.

throughout the entire breast). In addition, one component of overall breast
density, ductal pattern, was singled out and graded independently from 1(no
visible ducts) to 5(marked ductal prominence throughout the entire breast).
Grading was based not only on extent of glandular and ductal tissue but also on
its density. Thus, ducts extending throughout the entire breast would be graded as 4 or 5, depending on the degree of periductal collagenosis.

Mammographic accuracy was highest in fatty breasts with little or no ductal, fibrous, or glandular tissue (density and duct patterns 1 and 2), but decreased in a fairly linear manner with increasing parenchymal density. Although more cancers were seen on retrospective evaluation by the most experienced reader, the inversely proportional relationship between mammographic detection and breast density was maintained. Initial and retrospective mammographic curves closely paralleled one another.

Although these curves have been obtained for a screening type situation,
their applicability to a referral type mammographic practice is evident. An
experienced mammographic reader should be capable of detecting 93-98% of cancers occurring in fatty breasts (density and duct pattern 1 and 2,representing
approximately 50% of all cancer patients in our series) but only 74-79% of
cancers occurring in extremely dense fibrous and glandular breasts (density or
duct pattern 5, representing 12-17% of all cancer patients in our series).

CANCER LOCATION

Similarly, when cancers were analyzed according to location within the
breast (Fig. 3), mammographic accuracy was highest in the upper inner quadrant
which usually contains the least amount of glandular and ductal tissue. All 25
cancers (100%) occurring in this region were detected by mammography on both
initial and retrospective evaluation.

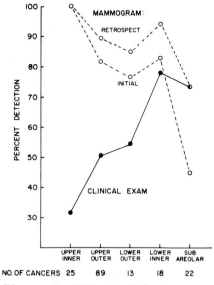

NO. OF CANCERS   25   89   13   18   22

Figure 3. Effect of lesion
location on cancer detection.

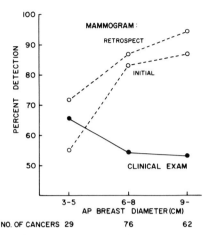

NO. OF CANCERS 29   76   62

Figure 4. Effect of breast
size on cancer detection.

Among upper and lower outer quadrant and lower inner quadrant lesions, mammographic accuracy differed little, detecting 85-94% on retrospective evaluation.

Mammography was least successful in detecting cancers located in the sub-areolar region (usually opaque from a convergence of ducts and periductal collagen tissue). Even on retrospective analysis, only 73% of all cancers occurring here were associated with mammographic findings indicating the need for biopsy.

BREAST SIZE

In a related analysis, the anteroposterior breast diameter on the craniocaudal mammogram was measured to determine the relationship of breast size to mammographic and clinical accuracy (Fig. 4). Mammography was most reliable for medium and large size breasts. A minority of cancers (17% or 29/167) occurred in small breasts with an AP diameter of 5 cm or less. Here there was a decrease in mammographic detection from that observed in medium and large breasts. This decrease was more pronounced on initial than on retrospective analysis.

This may be due to: 1. the tendency of small breasts to show dense areas of severe dysplasia on mammography; 2. imaging difficulties related to compression and the greater proportion of breast tissue located close to the chest wall in small breasts; 3. improved clinical accuracy in small breasts because of decreased lesion depth.

CONCLUSION

In nearly all instances where mammography shows no evidence of malignancy in a fatty area of the breast, suspicious or questionable clinical findings should be subject to appropriate follow-up or re-examination rather than biopsy. On the other hand, clinical evidence of cancer should not be dismissed because of a mammographic report of "no malignancy seen" if the area in question contains high parenchymal density or is in the retroareolar region.

Mammographic reports should convey an indication of mammographic accuracy appropriate to the particular situation. In all cases, discussion and consultation between clinician and radiologist is essential. Once a cancer is found or suspected on clinical or mammographic examination, medical decision making must be based on proper realization of the advantages and limitations of both modalities.

1. Feig, S A, Shaber, G S, Patchefsky, A S, et al: Analysis of clinically occult and mammographically occult breast tumors. Am J Roentgenol 128: 403-408, 1977

2. Feig, S A, Shaber, G S, Schwartz, G F, et al: Thermography, mammography, and clinical examination in breast cancer screening, review of 16,000 studies. Radiology 122: 123-127, 1977

3. Haagensen, C D: Diseases of the Breast. Philadelphia: W B Saunders, 1974

4. Wolfe, J N: Mammography, errors in diagnosis. Radiology 87: 214-219, 1966

5. Wolfe, J N: Analysis of 462 breast carcinomas. Am J Roentgenol 121: 846-853, 1974

EFFECT OF EARLY BREAST CANCER DETECTION: THEORY AND EXPERIENCE

Stephen A. Feig, M.D.

Department of Radiology, Thomas Jefferson University Hospital, Phila., Pa.

It is well established that breast cancer survival depends on lesion size and lymph node status at time of treatment. Smaller lesions with no histological evidence of axillary metastases have the best prognosis. Among patients studied by Fisher (21), 5 year survival was highest (85%) in tumors measuring less than 2cm with negative nodes (Figure 1). More recently, it has been demonstrated that current mammographic techniques provide the most effective means of detecting early lesions (15, 17-19, 47). Thus it would appear that mammographic screening could greatly diminish the effects of a disease which now afflicts 1 of every 14 women in her lifetime. Its impact on breast cancer could be similar to that which the Pap smear had in reducing mortality from cervical carcinoma (34).

That the role of mammographic screening in women over 35 years of age has not been universally recognized, relates to two specific issues. First, concern has been expressed about the hypothetical risk incurred from low doses of radiation (2, 3). This hypothetical risk now appears extremely low when compared to expected benefits (15, 36) as has been shown in several rigorous mathematical analyses derived from actual screening results (23, 32, 41, 48).

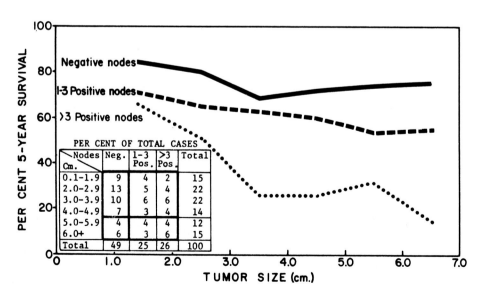

Nodes \ Cm.	Neg.	1-3 Pos.	>3 Pos.	Total
0.1-1.9	9	4	2	15
2.0-2.9	13	5	4	22
3.0-3.9	10	6	6	22
4.0-4.9	7	3	4	14
5.0-5.9	4	4	4	12
6.0+	6	3	6	15
Total	49	25	26	100

Figure 1. Breast cancer 5 year survival percentages in relation to primary tumor size and axillary node status among 1,105 operable cases (from ref. 40 with permission).

Secondly, a distinction can be made between favorable survival in cancers detected on screening and decreased mortality in the entire population screened. It has been said that observation of favorable survival does not necessarily predict occurrence of decreased mortality.

Several arguments have been proposed which can be understood by means of figure 2. This illustrates some possible relationships of breast cancer mortality to stage of disease at detection time. A tumor rises at point 0 and enlarges over time. It can be detected after points A, B, and C for mammographic screening, clinical screening, and non-screening respectively. The locations of these points depend on the size threshold of each modality.

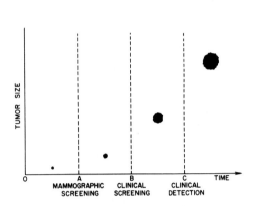

Figure 2. Relationship of breast cancer size to detection modality. Some theoretical relationships of breast cancer mortality to detection modality (see text).

Those who question the validity of mammographic screening raise several questions related to benefit (2, 3, 20, 56-58):
1. Do highly aggressive lesions metastasize prior to mammographic detection (at point A), thus predetermining the course of disease? Mammography would then advance the time of detection but not affect the time of demise (lead time bias).
2. May some histological malignancies be of such low biological aggressiveness that they will not metastasize during the patient's lifetime?
3. If a lesion of intermediate biological aggressiveness does not metastasize until after point B or C, then detection by some other means could be as effective as detection by mammography (length biased sampling).

For these reasons, it has been argued that prognostic pathologic factors do not confer the same degree of proof and quantitative measurement of decreased mortality as would be obtained from a randomized clinical trial involving study and control populations. The purpose of this chapter is to evaluate these problems in terms of current knowledge and concepts.

DEFINITION OF LEAD TIME AND MEAN PRECLINICAL DURATION

At present, approximately 90% of all breast cancers are first detected by the patient herself when the tumor mass reaches sufficient size to come to her attention (38). Nearly always, this occurs not as a result of periodic breast self examination but rather by chance recognition. Lesions discovered in this manner are referred to as clinical disease. Before the mass attains this size, there is a period when it can be recognizable through mammographic or clinical screening. This early stage of the disease is referred to as "preclinical disease". As defined by Hutchinson and Shapiro (35), lead time refers to the interval by which diagnosis is advanced by screening (Figure 3).

The incidence of preclinical disease is defined as the rate at which new cases develop (cases / 1,000 women / year). If all cases eventually advance into the clinical stage, then the incidence of preclinical disease must be identical to the incidence of clinical disease. Prevalence refers to the number of women in a population with disease at a given time (cases/1000 women).

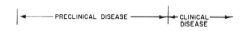

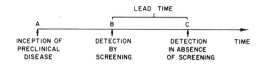

Figure 3. Diagrammatic representation of lead time.

Preclinical disease can persist for a given length of time (duration) before clinical recognition. Prevalence (P), incidence (I), and average duration (d) of preclinical disease are related as follows: d=P/I. For example, if each year one new case of preclinical breast cancer develops in 1,000 women and persists as preclinical disease for 2 years thereafter, then at any point in time, 2 cases of preclinical disease can be expected in every 1,000 women.

The relationship of lead time to mean preclinical duration can be seen in figure 4. Let us assume a mean preclinical duration of 2 years represented by the length of arrows A, B, or C. Initial screening of this population will result in lead time measured from time of screening to the arrow point. For cases A, B, and C lead times will be equal to 2, 6, and 18 months respectively. The average lead time for all cases will be 12 months or half the mean preclinical duration.

ESTIMATE OF LEAD TIME GAINED BY DIAGNOSTIC SCREENING(HIP PROJECT)

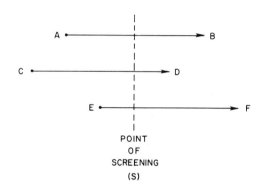

Figure 4. Relationship of lead time to point of screening and duration of preclinical disease.

A randomized clinical trial of breast cancer screening was begun by the Health Insurance Plan of Greater New York in 1963 under the direction of Strax, Shapiro, and Venet (50, 51, 54, 55). The study involved 62,000 women between 40 and 64 years of age. These women were allocated to study and control groups of 31,000 women each. Only the study group was offered four annual clinical and mammographic examinations. When breast cancer mortality rates were tabulated, a one third reduction in breast cancer mortality in the study group compared to the control group was evident. This result is all the more impressive considering that only 65% of the study group (21,000/31,000) participated in the initial screening examinations and only 41% (12,600/31,000) completed all four annual examinations.

Based on a breast cancer prevalence at the first screening of 2.7 cases/ 1000 women screened and an incidence of 1.6 cases/ 1000 women/ year in the control population, Hutchinson and Shapiro have estimated the average duration of preclinical disease to be 20 months. Lead time would be 10-20 months depending on the distribution of the total duration of preclinical disease (35). When applied to the HIP data, other statistical models would also result in a lead time estimate within these bounds (56, 58).

Assuming that breast cancer is a composite of cases of varying preclinical durations, cases detected on screening (prevalence series) will contain a higher proportion of long duration cases and a lower proportion of short duration cases than will an incidence series of clinical disease. Therefore, for screening an average lead time of 1/2 the mean duration of disease should be considered a minimal estimate.

LEAD TIME BIAS

Lead time refers to the fact that the point from which survival is measured is shifted backward in time as a result of screening. Lead time bias refers to the theory that screening results only in an advancement in the time of diagnosis but not delay in the time of death. The disease is presumed to be fatal despite early detection. If the disease is detected two years earlier, patients live two years longer from diagnosis to death but the actual length of life from inception of disease to death remains unaltered. This type of biological predeterminism is based on the contention that systemic spread has occurred prior to diagnosis.

Table I Comparison of Lesion Size and Lymph Node Status for Breast Cancers Encountered in Clinical Practice and Those Detected by Screening

Per cent of Cancers[5]	Screening[2]		Clinical Practice[1]
	Subclinical[4] Cancers	Clinical[3] Cancers	
Lesion Size Less than 2.0cm	94%	54%	30%
Negative Axillary Nodes	92%	49%	49%

1. 2578 cancers from National Surgical Adjuvant Breast Project (ref.21)

2. 183 cancers from Jefferson Breast Diagnostic Center detected on clinical and mammographic screening by both clinical examination and mammography or clinical examination alone (98 cancers) (3) and 85 subclinical cancers detected by mammography alone (4) (ref. 18)

5. Lesion size and nodal status determined by pathological examination

Evidence that lead time bias does not apply to most subclinical cancers is provided in table I. Axillary lymph nodes are free of disease in about half of all cases encountered in clinical practice. Among non-palpable cancers detected on mammographic screening, 92% were found to have negative axillary nodes. Since pathological examination of axillary lymph nodes provides the best indication of metastasis beyond the breast, it follows that progression of disease has been intercepted at a curable stage.

A lead time of 2-3 years could account for improved short term survival but as follow up periods of 10 years or more are considered, lead time of this duration no longer provides a tenable explanation. Among 176 patients with minimal breast cancer as defined by Gallager and Martin (28) a 20 year actuarial survival of 93% has been reported (24). All but 21 of these lesions were in situ and 95% were associated with negative axillary nodes.

Similarly, when women with cancers of identical histologic grade were followed for 15 years, improved survival persisted among those whose cancers were detected at an early clinical stage. This was true for grade I, II, and III ductal carcinomas as well as medullary carcinomas (18).

Long term follow up of 20 years should compensate for even the longest lead time estimate for invasive ductal carcinomas. Among Berg's patients, survival at 20 years still depended on the stage at time of treatment (Figure 5).

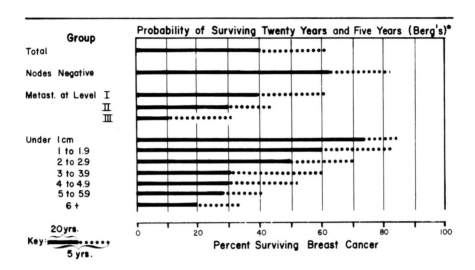

Figure 5. Breast cancer survival at 5 years and at 20 years after treatment of 1,458 women by radical mastectomy. Patients are grouped according to lymph node status and lesion size (from refs. 4, 48 with permission).

Recently, Shapiro has calculated the cumulative breast cancer death rates in study and control groups of the HIP project through Dec. 31, 1975 (50). These have been for the period of 2 to 9 years from date of entry. Only women diagnosed as having breast cancer within 5 years after entry have been included. For these reasons, results should not be influenced by lead time bias. At the end of 9 years, deaths due to breast cancer in the total study group were still about 30% less than those in the control group.

POSSIBLE BENEFIT OF SCREENING IN WOMEN BELOW 50 YEARS OF AGE

H.I.P. Study

When the entire screened group of HIP women is compared to the control, a one third reduction in breast cancer mortality can be found. When further classified according to age at time of detection, a 40% mortality reduction is seen in women over 50 years of age but no reduction is demonstrated for women between 40 and 50 years of age. Thus the entire observed benefit was confined to women over 50 at time of detection. Shapiro has stated that because of the relatively small number of breast cancers detected in women below 50 years of age, "a 20-30% reduction in mortality in women below 50 could be missed in a study of this size" (50). Nevertheless, because a substantial proportion of breast cancers occur in this age group, alternative explanations should be considered.

The most plausible reason for the failure to demonstrate benefit in screening women below 50 years of age can be found in the distribution of tumor sizes and cases with positive nodes among the various age groups in the HIP study. A statistically significant percentage of larger cancers was found in the control group compared to the study group for women aged 50-59 and 60+ but not for the 40-49 year age group. The number of cancers with positive nodes was significantly greater in the control versus study group for women age 60+ but not for those in the 40-49 and 50-59 year age groups (46).

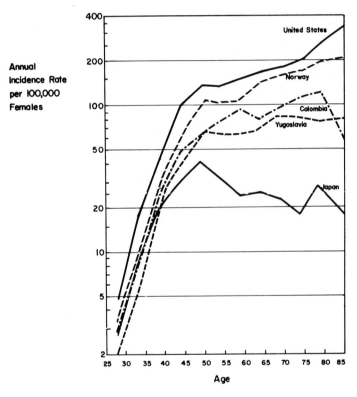

Figure 6. Female breast cancer incidence rates by age in selected areas, periods around 1965 (From ref. 48 with permission).

Pre and Post Menopausal Breast Cancers

Western women exhibit a progressive increase in breast cancer risk with advancing age which continues into the eighth and ninth decades of life. Among Asiatic populations, breast cancer incidence is not only considerably lower, but risk increases only until around age 45 after which it plateaus or falls (Figure 6). These findings have led to the proposal that there may be two types of breast cancer: premenopausal (found in both Western and Asiatic women) and postmenpausal (confined to Western women). Occurrence of a trough in the incidence curve of some European populations between 50-55 years of age could represent a gap between incidence curves of the two types of tumors (14). Alternatively, it might be due to slowing of tumor growth around the time of menopause (12). One could postulate that premenopausal breast cancer because of its inherent biological potential or its immunological and endocrinological environment, represents a disease whose prognosis might be unaffected by early detection and treatment.

However, for women whose breast cancers are detected and treated in clinical practice, survival among those below 50 years of age is no worse than in older women (6, 10, 16, 38, 44) (Figure 7).

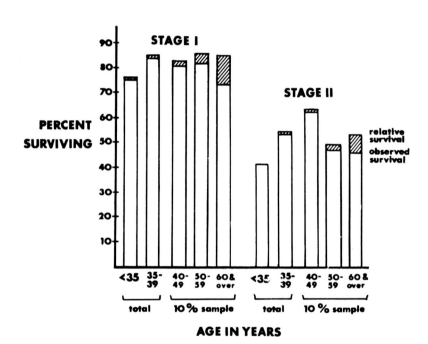

Figure 7. Breast cancer survival according to age at time of radical mastectomy. Stage I was disease without lymph node involvement. Stage II was disease with histologic evidence of axillary metastases but no evidence of distant metastases. (From ref. 38 with permission)

Stoll observed scar recurrences within 3 years in 20% of 74 breast cancer patients under 50 years of age and in 23% of 107 patients between 50 and 69 years of age. This would suggest that breast cancer growth rate as measured by growth of cancer cells in the scar from microscopic to clinically detectable size is similar in these groups (53).

Comparison of HIP and BCDDP Studies

One may ask whether mammographic detection at the HIP study was less effective in women under 50 years of age. Could the use of current mammographic equipment lead to benefit in this younger age group? Data from the HIP study indicate that breast cancer fatality rates were lowest among cancers detected on mammography alone. They were approximately half those of cancers detected only on clinical examination (Table II). Of course, the implications of this observation may be subject to the theory of length biased sampling. Nevertheless, nearly all of these were invasive cancers to which the length bias argument would seem most tenuous. The fact remains that cancers detected by mammography alone have exceptionally low case fatality rates. Shapiro has estimated that approximately 30% of the reduction in breast cancer mortality found in the HIP study was due to mammographic detection (50).

Table II   Cumulative Breast Cancer Fatality Rates 8 Years Following Diagnosis on H.I.P. Screening Study

Detection Modality	Fatality Rate
M+ C+	41.4
M- C+	31.8
M+ C-	14.4

Source: ref 50

Supportive evidence that the quality of breast cancer detection has improved coincident with advances in mammographic imaging can be found by comparing breast cancer detection rate on initial screening in the HIP and BCDDP studies. Although there are large differences between the populations screened, detection rates at the BCDDP centers have been approximately twice as high as those from the HIP (Table III).

Table III   Breast Cancer Detection Rates at First Screenings for H.I.P. and BCDDP Studies

	H.I.P.	BCDDP
Cancers/ 1000 Women Screened	2.73	5.54

Source: ref 47

The Breast Cancer Detection Demonstration Projects (BCDDP) are 27 National Cancer Institute (NCI) and American Cancer Society (ACS) supported centers begun in 1973 to complete 5 annual screenings of 270,000 women between 35 and 74 years of age by physical examination and mammography (47). The relative contribution of mammography to breast cancer detection at different age groups in both studies is shown in Table IV. Several observations can be made. First, for each age group, a greater proportion of cancers detected were clinically occult in the BCDDP than in the HIP study. Secondly, in the HIP series the per cent of breast cancers detected only on mammography fell considerably below 50 years of age, whereas the per cent remained virtually unchanged among all age groups at the BCDDP.

Detection in the 40-49 year age group has been further analyzed in Table V. Mammography alone or in association with positive physical examination detected over 90% of breast cancers in the BCDDP study but less than 40% of those in the HIP study.

Mammography was particularly effective in detecting minimal cancers (defined as all infiltrating cancers less than 1cm and all in situ cancers) at the BCDDP (Table VI). At least 95% of such lesions were detected on mammography but only 33% on clinical examination. It is apparent that mammography was responsible for the high proportion of minimal cancers among all cancers detected at the BCDDP.

Table IV Per cent of Breast Cancers Detected Only on Mammography Compared to Patient Age at Time of Diagnosis for HIP Study and First 2 BCDDP Screenings

	Age		
	40-49	50-59	60-64
HIP	19.4%	41.5%	30.6%
BCDDP	45.3%	46.7%	44.1%

Source: refs 47, 50

Table V Relative Contributions of Mammography and Clinical Examination to Breast Cancer Detection in 40-49 Year Age Group. Comparison of HIP Study and First 2 BCDDP Screenings

	Per cent	Detection
	HIP	BCDDP
M- C+	61.2%	9.1%
M+ C+	19.4%	45.3%
M+ C-	19.4%	45.6%
Total M+	38.8%	90.9%

Source: refs 47,50

Considering the overall detection rates (minimal and non-minimal cancers) from both studies, there were approximately 7 times as many minimal cancers detected per 1000 patients screened at the BCDDP than at the HIP study. Possibly, some in situ lesions included among the minimal cancers may not possess the same malignant potential as do invasive lesions. Still, detection of minimal cancers is an excellent indicator of ability to detect small cancers of all types, many of which undoubtedly do have significant metastatic potential.

Pursuing this line of reasoning, it would seem that significantly decreased breast cancer mortality through mammographic screening could be expected in women both above and below 50 years of age based on cancer detection rates and proportion of clinically occult early lesions found in the BCDDP projects. However, this does not constitute the same degree of proof as would be found in a randomized clinical trial (Table VII).

EFFECT OF LATER CLINICAL DETECTION

It might be proposed that clinical detection at a later, palpable stage would be as effective as earlier mammographic diagnosis if metastases had not occurred in the interval (between points A and B of figure 2). As seen in Table VIII, however, metastatic spread frequently occurs before most lesions

Table VI Detection of Minimal Breast Cancers for BCDDP (First 2 Screenings) and HIP Studies

	HIP	BCDDP
Minimal Cancers/ Total Cancers	8%(5/61)	28%(374/1336)
Per cent Detection by Modality		
M+ C-	40%(2/5)	65%(244/374)
M+ C+	0%(0/5)	30%(110/374)
M- C+	60%(3/5)	3%(12/374)
Total M+	40%(2/5)	95%(354/374)

Source: refs 46,47

Table VII Mammographic Screening in HIP and BCDDP Studies: Observed and Expected Results

	HIP		BCDDP	
Age at Detection	40-49	50-64	40-49	50-64
Significant Mammographic Detection	No	Yes	Yes	Yes
Decreased Mortality	No	Yes	Expected but not demonstrated through a randomized clinical trial	

Table VIII Relationship of Clinical Detection to Lesion Size and Lymph Status

Cancer Size (Cm)	Number of Cancers	Per cent of Cases with Axillary Metastases	Per cent Clinical Detection
-1	68	7%	30%
1-2	54	20%	53%
2-3	24	63%	88%

Source: ref 17

are identified on physical examination.

Although it is often stated that an experienced clinical examiner can identify lesions as small as 1cm, this opinion originated in an earlier era before
mammography provided a standard by which clinical misses could be appreciated.
Moreover, clinical recognition depends as much on breast size and lesion location within the breast as on the examiner's skill.

A precise estimate of the independent contributions of mammography and clinical examination towards decreased breast cancer mortality could be obtained through a randomized clinical trial involving 4 groups of women;
1. Control group
2. Study group screened by mammography and clinical examination
3. Study group screened by mammography only
4. Study group screened by clinical examination only

This would involve periodic screening over several years. Short and long term breast cancer mortality could then be monitored in each group.

BREAST CANCER SPECTRUM

Breast cancer represents a spectrum of tumors of various biological potentials as demonstrated by breast cancer growth rates as seen on serial mammography. Gershon-Cohen described a range of doubling times between different tumors from 23-209 days (mean = 115) (29). Lundgren reported a variation of 42-397 days (mean = 211)(37).

Another indication that breast cancer is not a disease of uniform clinical behavior can be seen in the application of histologic grading to prognosis. Based on regularity of nuclear size and shape, staining, and degree of tubule formation, Bloom classified breast cancers as grade I (low), II (moderate), and III (high) malignancy. Even when tumors of similar size, axillary lymph node status, and treatment are considered or when untreated breast cancers are compared, survival will hold a close correlation to histologic grade (5-9).

Estimation of breast cancer growth rates can also be based on the interval between mastectomy and mastectomy scar recurrence assuming the implant of a single cell or clone occurred at the time of mastectomy. These studies suggested that approximately 50% of tumors were rapidly growing, having growth rates of up to 25 days; 35% were of intermediate growth rate with doubling time of 26-75 days; and 15% grew slowly with doubling time of 76 days or longer (43, 45). It should be noted that none of these studies suggests that tumor doubling time remains constant within the life time of the tumor.

LENGTH BIASED SAMPLING

The term length biased sampling refers to the theory that breast cancers detected on screening may contain a greater proportion of slow to fast growing lesions than do breast cancers which are brought to medical attention in the usual non-screening situation of clinical practice. Let us assume that 3 cancers of slow, medium, and rapid growth rates arise at time 0 in figure 8. By time X, each will have attained a larger size proportional to its individual growth rate. Only the most rapidly growing would have reached sufficient size to be noted by the patient herself. Clinical screening would detect this lesion plus the one possessing a medium growth rate. Mammographic screening could detect these two as well as the slowest growing lesion.

Of course, in the more complex "real world", cancers would arise at multiple points in time. Some slow growing lesions arising before time 0 would be found by the patient herself or detected on clinical screening. Nevertheless, the highest proportion of slow to fast growing lesions would always be present in the situation employing the most sensitive detection modality.

Another way of understanding length biased sampling is through duration of preclinical disease represented as horizontal lines in figure 9. These

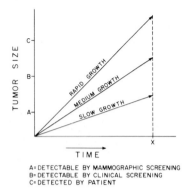

A=DETECTABLE BY MAMMOGRAPHIC SCREENING
B=DETECTABLE BY CLINICAL SCREENING
C=DETECTED BY PATIENT

Figure 8. Effect of breast cancer growth rate on lesion size and mode of detection.

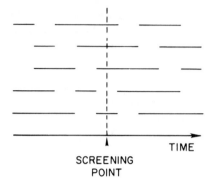

SCREENING
POINT

Figure 9. Effect of duration of pre-clinical disease on mode of detection (length biased sampling).

lengths correspond to the shorter and longer preclinical durations in faster and slower growing lesions respectively. Since slow growing lesions remain at a smaller, subclinical size longer than do faster growing lesions, smaller size ranges will contain a greater proportion of slowly progressing lesions.

Thus, cancers detected on screening might contain relatively large numbers of slowly progressing lesions which might have above average survival rates even in the absence of screening. It is conceivable that some lesions may be so slow growing as not to exert any effect on the patient's life span. Critics therefore contend that the favorable cure rates obtained through screening will not necessarily be translated into a reduction of breast cancer deaths.

Before one accepts these implications, it should be remembered that smaller lesions consist not only of less aggressive cancers but also more aggressive detected at an early stage. Some smaller lesions may never metastasize because of low inherent biological potential. Other aggressive lesions may not yet have reached the critical size at which most metastases occur. The net benefit from screening would depend on the number and proportion of different types detected from the breast cancer spectrum.

Data from Feig (17) suggest that less aggressive lesions as defined by low histologic grade or well defined tubule formation represent only a minority of clinically occult lesions below 1 cm. Based on observation of early invasive growth in smaller lesions, he found no evidence to suggest that substantial numbers of early lesions are biologically inert.

Further insight into this problem can be found in observation of untreated breast cancers. All of the lesions followed were ultimately lethal to the patients.

UNTREATED BREAST CANCERS

One method of evaluating the effect of early diagnosis and treatment is through analysis of survival rates in treated and untreated breast cancer patients. Most untreated mammary carcinomas are found in patients who refuse treatment or those who entered institutions when their disease was too advanced for treatment. Most such reports were collected from medical records dating from 1805 to 1933 prior to the widespread use of radiotherapy and hormonal therapy. These studies were undertaken by Bloom (17), Daland (13), Forber (22), Greenwood (31), and Nathanson (42). They reveal remarkably similar 5 years survival rates from first recognized symptoms ranging from 16-22%.

Because of bias in case selection, no totally valid comparison can be made between survival in treated and untreated patients. Nevertheless, comparison can best be made by dating survival from onset of symptoms rather than from the time of surgery. This has been done by Donegan (16) utilizing data on 460 patients from Ellis Fischel State Cancer Hospital treated with radical mastectomy between 1940 and 1952 (Figure 10). Treated patients have been staged according to the Columbia Clinical Classification (33). Stage A and B show no skin edema, ulceration, or solid fixation of tumor to the chest wall. In stage B patients, the axillary nodes are clinically involved but are less than 2.5cm. Stage C and D represent more advanced disease.

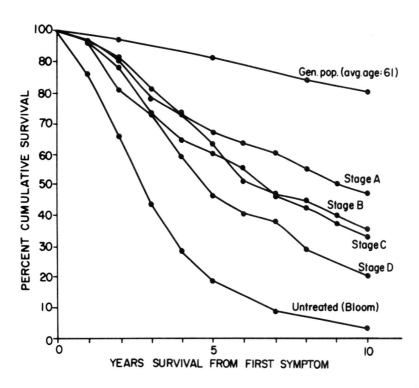

Figure 10. Survival of 460 patients reported by Donegan, treated with radical mastectomy and grouped by clinical stage, compared with survival of 250 untreated patients reported by Bloom. (From ref 16 with permission).

From these studies, one may arrive at the following conclusions:
1. Untreated breast cancer patients have a poorer 5 and 10 year survival than

those with any stage of treated disease including stage D. Survival for treated patients depends on stage of disease. These observations support the assumption that treatment can alter the natural course of breast cancer. The magnitude of this effect depends on stage of disease at time of treatment.

2. Among the untreated patients, the proportion of tumors which did not result in death within several years of onset was insignificant.

3. If a significant fraction of untreated tumors was of low biological potential, this would have been reflected in a 10 year survival higher than the 5% recorded.

4. Although there is variation in breast cancer behavior, it was not sufficiently broad to prevent nearly all untreated cancers from resulting in death within several years. All or nearly all untreated cases studied thus far are fatal.

5. Bloom reported that among his untreated breast cancers graded histologicaly graded as I, II, or III, practically none survived 10 years though length of survival depended on the grade of each lesion (5-9).

IN SITU CARCINOMAS

In situ carcinoma may represent 20-25% of all cancers detected at the BCDDP. Of these, approximately 4/5ths were in situ ductal and 1/5th in situ lobular lesions (47). This prevalence of in situ carcinoma can be contrasted to an incidence series as in the SEER Report where in situ lesions represented only 5% of all breast cancers (11). At present, the significance of detecting this high a prevalence of in situ lesions is not fully known.

It is obvious that all invasive breast cancers must exist as in situ lesions at some early stage. It is also fairly certain that detection and proper treatment at this early stage should result in complete cure. The few treatment failures are probably due to undetected invasive foci. Ten year survival rates for in situ ductal carcinomas have ranged from 90-100% (1,11, 30, 39).

However, it is not certain what proportion of in situ lesions will ultimately become invasive and it is possible that some in situ lesions may never do so. The prevalence of in situ disease within the breast tissue, the duration of ductal carcinoma in the in situ phase, and the rate of progression to invasive carcinoma are not known. Because of these questions, it may be that the concept of length biased sampling is more applicable to in situ than to invasive lesions.

Silverberg found no correlation between tumor size and degree of marginal infiltration. However, his study contained very few cancers in the smaller size categories (52).

Taking ductal carcinomas detected on screening, most of which measured from 0-2cm, Feig plotted the proportion of intraductal to infiltrative growth as a function of lesion size (17). Lesions were classified as in situ, minimally invasive (less than 10% invasive growth), moderately invasive (10-75% invasive growth), and maximally invasive. The relationship between these curves suggested that most lesions undergo a transition from in situ to invasive growth between 0-0.5cm size.

Another observation of his study was that most in situ ductal carcinomas were of histologic grade II or III which may be considered an indication of moderate or high metastatic potential. These findings suggest that in situ ductal carcinoma does not represent an indolent biological disease but rather an early stage in a continuous progression to invasive carcinoma.

Similarly, whole breast section studies by Gallager and Martin (26-28), strongly support the relationship of in situ to invasive disease. In patients with invasive ductal carcinoma, breasts were found to contain multiple widely distributed foci with a wide range of histologic abnormalities ranging from cellular atypia and in situ carcinoma to minimally invasive carcinoma. If in situ carcinoma does not occur as an isolated focus, then the chance of transition from in situ to infiltrative growth would represent the sum of probabilities from all foci.

It is apparent that detection of in situ disease would advance lead time considerably further than would detection of infiltrating ductal carcinoma. Because in situ lesions represented only 7% of HIP cancers (46), their contribution to lead time calculations for that study was insignificant. If a breast contains multiple foci of in situ disease with each focus having a different lead time, then the effective lead time would be equal to that of the most advanced focus.

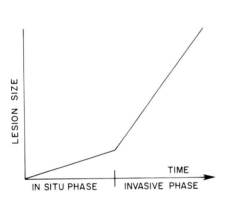

Figure 11. Hypothetical relationship of breast cancer growth rate to phase of disease. (Adapted from ref 25).

Gallager has suggested that the growth rate of ductal carcinoma may be slower in its in situ phase because immunologic and other host defense mechanisms are more effective at that time (25) (Figure 11). If this hypothesis is correct it would extend the period during which mammography could detect breast cancer prior to metastatic spread.

Detection of in situ carcinoma did not contribute to decreased mortality in the HIP study because very few in situ lesions were found. Nearly all mortality reduction resulted from detection of invasive disease at an earlier stage (46). Based on an analysis of incidence and prevalence data from screened and unscreened women at the Cincinatti BCDDP, Moskowitz indicates that removal of minimal cancer from the population can alter the natural history of the disease (40).

CONCLUSION

Arguments of lead time and length biased sampling notwithstanding, mammography had a significant role in decreasing breast cancer mortality in women over 50 years of age in the HIP study. Current data from the BCDDP suggest that the magnitude of this contribution could be increased among older women and extended to those between 35-50 years of age. This benefit could accrue from either detection of infiltrating carcinoma at an early stage and/or detection of in situ carcinoma.

All or nearly all invasive ductal carcinomas will eventually result in patient death (though at different time courses) if left untreated. Early detection can alter prognosis. The reality of this effect cannot be denied by lead time bias since favorable survival persists for over 20 years.

Analysis of infiltrative ductal carcinomas suggests that the chance of metastases having occurred becomes less and less as smaller sized lesions are considered. It is likely that most of these lesions could not have been detected by clinical examination while still confined to the breast.

Efforts at dose reduction consistent with acceptable image quality should be pursued since they could result in more frequent screening intervals permitting earlier detection of fast growing tumors.

Although the proportion of in situ carcinomas which progress to invasive disease is not known, it is reasonable to assume that all invasive lesions must originate from in situ disease. Several studies suggest that mammographic detection of in situ disease holds enormous promise for substantial reduction in breast cancer mortality. Because of the finite duration of in situ disease, decreased mortality from its detection might not appear until a later time during followup than would decreased mortality from early detection of invasive disease.

The concepts of lead time and length bias do not negate the existence of benefit of early detection. They do point out that though survival data can indicate potential benefit, only a randomized clinical trial can measure actual benefit. Since mammography has become a more effective modality since the HIP Study began, a new randomized trial would be indicated to validate reduction in mortality among women 35-50 years of age. Such a trial should be constructed to document the relative contributions of mammography and clinical examination.

The past several years in mammography have been an edifying experience. They have produced new knowledge stirring much hope and encouragement regarding its role in early detection. They have also raised new questions causing us to take a hard look at the assumptions underlying breast cancer screening. There have been reductions in radiation dose and improvements in image quality, though these have not always gone hand in hand. The issues raised are not simple ones but peering through the complexities, it appears that further reduction in mortality can and will be demonstrated.

REFERENCES

1. Ashikari R, Huvos A G, and Snyder R E: Prospective study of non-infiltrating carcinoma of the breast. Cancer 39: 435-439, Feb 1977

2. Bailar J C: Mammography, a contrary view. Annals of Internal Med 84: 77-84, Jan 1976

3. Bailar J C: Screening for early breast cancer, pros and cons. Cancer 39: 2783-2795, Jun 1977

4. Berg J W, and Robbins G F: Factors influencing short and long term survivals following operations for breast cancer. Surg Gynecol Obstet 122: 1311-1316, Jun 1966

5. Bloom H J G: Prognosis in carcinoma of the breast. Br J Cancer 4: 259-288, Sept 1950

6. Bloom H J G: Further studies on prognosis of breast carcinoma. Br J Cancer 4: 347-367, Dec 1950

7. Bloom H J G: The natural history of untreated breast cancer. Ann N Y Acad Sci 114: 747-754, Apr 1964

8. Bloom H J G, and Field J R: Impact of tumor grade and host resistance on survival of women with breast cancer. Cancer 28: 1580-1589, Dec 1971

9. Bloom H J G and Richardson W W: Histological grading and prognosis in breast cancer. Br J Cancer 11: 359-374, Jul 1957

10. Byrd D F, Stephenson S E, Burch J C, et al: Type of mastectomy in cancer of the breast. Ann Surg 163: 746-750, May 1966

11. Cancer Surveillance, Epidemiology and End Results (SEER) Program. Prepublication data. National Cancer Institute, Bethseda, Maryland

12. Clemmesen J: Carcinoma of the breast. Results from statistical research. Br J Radiol 21: 583-590, Dec 1948

13. Daland E M: Untreated cancer of the breast. Surg Gynecol Obstet 44: 264-268, Feb 1927

14. DeWaard F, Baanders-van Halewijn E A, and Huizinga J: The bimodal age distribution of patients with mammary carcinoma. Cancer 17: 141-151, Feb 1964

15. Dodd G D: Present status of thermography, ultrasound, and mammography in breast cancer detection. Cancer 39: 2796-2805, June 1977

16. Donegan W L: Staging and end results. [In] Cancer of the Breast, ed by Spratt J S and Donegan W L. Philadelphia: W B Saunders, 1967

17. Feig S A, Patchefsky A S, Shaber G S, et al: Prognostic factors in breast cancers detected by mammographic and clinical screening. Paper presented at the 64th Scientific Assembly and Annual Meeting of the Radiological Society of North America, Chicago Ill, Nov26-Dec 1, 1978

18. Feig S A, Shaber G S, Patchefsky A, et al: Analysis of clinically occult and mammographically occult breast tumors. Am J Roentgenol 128: 403-408, Mar 1977

19. Feig S A, Shaber G S, Schwartz G F, et al: Thermography, mammography, and clinical examination in breast cancer screening. Review of 16,000 studies. Radiology 122: 123-127, Jan 1977

20. Feinleib M, and Zelen M: Some pitfalls in the evaluation of screening programs. Arch Environ Health 19: 412-415, Sept 1969

21. Fisher B, Slack N H, and Bross I D J: Cancer of the breast: Size of neoplasm and prognosis. Cancer 24: 1071-1080, Nov 1969

22. Forber J E: Incurable Cancer. Ministry of Health Reports on Public Health and Medical Subjects, No. LXVI. London, England: His Majesty's Stationery Office, 1931

23. Fox S H, Moskowitz M, Saenger E L, et al: Benefit/risk analysis of aggressive mammographic screening. Radiology 128: 359-365, Aug 1978

24. Frazier T G, Copeland E M, Gallager H S, et al: Prognosis and treatment in minimal breast cancer. Am J Surg 133: 697-701, June 1977

25. Gallager H S: View from the giant's shoulder. The fifth annual Wendell G Scott lecture. Cancer 40: 185-194, Jul 1977

26. Gallager H S and Martin J E: The study of mammary carcinoma by mammography and whole organ sectioning. Cancer 23: 855-873, Apr 1969

27. Gallager H S and Martin J E: Early phases in the development of breast cancer. Cancer 24: 1170-1178, Dec 1969

28. Gallager H S and Martin J E: An orientation to the concept of minimal breast cancer. Cancer 23: 1505-1507, Dec 1971

29. Gershon-Cohen J, Berger S M, and Klickstein H S: Roentgenography of breast cancer moderating concept of "biologic predeterminism ". Cancer 16: 961-964, Aug 1963

30. Gillis D A, Dockerty M B, and Clagett O T: Preinvasive intraductal carcinoma of the breast. Surg Gynecol Obstet 110: 555-562, May 1960

31. Greenwood M: The natural history of cancer. Ministry of Health Reports on Public Health and Medical Subjects, No. XXVI. London, England: His Majesty's Stationery Office, 1926

32. Gregg E C: Radiation risks with diagnostic x-rays. Radiology 123: 447-452, May 1977

33. Haagensen C D: Diseases of the Breast. Philadelphia: W B Saunders, 1971

34. Hammond E C and Seidman H: Progress in control of cancer of the uterus. Arch Environ Health 13: 105-116, Jul 1966

35. Hutchinson G B and Shapiro S: Lead time gained by diagnostic screening for breast cancer. J Natl Cancer Inst 41: 665-681, Sept 1968

36. Lester R G: Risk versus benefit in mammography. Radiology 124: 1-6, July 1977

37. Lundgren B: Observations on growth rate of breast carcinomas and its possible implications for lead time. Cancer 40: 1722-1725, Oct 1977

38. Mausner S J, Shimkin M B, Moss N H, et al: Cancer of the breast in Philadelphia hospitals 1951-1964. Cancer 23: 260-274, Feb 1969

39. Millis R R, and Thynne G`S J: In situ intraduct carcinoma of the breast. A long term follow up study. Br J Surg 62: 957-962, Dec 1975

40. Moskowitz M: The importance of finding minimal breast cancer. See this volume.

41. Moskowitz M, Keriakes J, Saenger E L, et al: Breast cancer screening. Benefit and risk for the first annual screening. Radiology 120: 431-432 Aug 1976

42. Nathanson I T and Welch C E: Life expectancy and incidence of malignant disease. Carcinoma of the breast. Amer J Cancer 28: 40-53, Sept 1936

43. Pearlman A W: Breast cancer - influence of growth rate on prognosis and treatment evaluation. Cancer 38: 1826-1833, Oct 1976

44. Peters M V: The role of local excision and radiation in early breast cancer [In] Breast Cancer Early and Late. Year Book Medical Publishers, Chicago, 1970

45. Philippe E, and LeGal Y: Growth of 78 recurrent mammary cancers. Cancer 21: 461-467, Mar 1968

46. Report of the NCI Ad Hoc Pathology Working Group to Review the Gross and Microscopic Findings of Breast Cancer Cases in the HIP Study (Health Insurance Plan of Greater New York). J Natl Cancer Inst 59: 497-541, Aug 1977

47. Report of the Working Group to Review the NCI/ACS Breast Cancer Detection Demonstration Projects. National Cancer Institute, 1977

48. Seidman H: Cancer of the Breast. Statistical and Epidemiological Data New York: American Cancer Society, 1072

49. Seidman H: Screening for breast cancer in younger women. Life expectancy gains and losses. An analysis according to risk indicator groups. Ca-A Cancer Journal for Clinicians. 27: 66-87, Mar/Apr 1977

50. Shapiro S: Evidence on screening for breast cancer from a randomized trial. Cancer 39: 2772-2782, Jun 1977

51. Shapiro S, Strax P, and Venet L: Periodic breast cancer screening in reducing mortality from breast cancer. JAMA 215: 1777-1785, Mar 1971

52. Silverberg S G, and Chitale A R: Assessment of significance of proportions of intraductal and infiltrating tumor growth in ductal carcinoma of the breast. Cancer 32: 830-837, Oct 1973

53. Stoll B A: Effect of age on growth pattern. [In] Risk Factors in Breast Cancer. ed by Stoll B A, Year Book Medical Publishers, Chicago, 1976

54. Strax P: Results of mass screening for breast cancer in 50,000 examinations. Cancer 37: 30-35, Jam 1976

55. Strax P, Venet L, and Shapiro S: Value of mammography in reduction of mortality from breast cancer in mass screening. Am J Roentgenol 117: 686-689, Mar 1973

56. Zelen M: Problems in the early detection of disease and the finding of faults. Bull Intern Stat Inst 44: 649-661, 1972

57. Zelen M: Theory of early detection of breast cancer in the general population. [In] Breast Cancer. Trends in Research and Treatment, ed by Heuson J C, Mattheiem W H, and Rozencweig M. New York: Raven Press 1976 pp 287-300

58. Zelen M, And Feinleib M: On the theory of screening for chronic disease. Biometrika 56: 601-614, 1969

THE IMPORTANCE OF FINDING MINIMAL BREAST CANCER

Myron Moskowitz, M.D.

University of Cincinnati, College of Medicine

Benefit for screening asymptomatic women over the age of 50 was proven in the Health Insurance Plan study performed in the early 1960's (67). No such benefit was demonstrated by that study for women under 50. Since that time, the efficacy of mammography and clinical exam for detecting early breast cancer has improved remarkably (50,41,62). Since no controlled clinical trial has been or is being performed, and if one were to be started immediately an answer would not be known for 10-15 years, it is in order to ask if a reasonable estimate of the value of screening asymptomatic women can be made from available data generated by an aggressive screening program.

BENEFIT/RISK ESTIMATES OF SCREENING ASYMPTOMATIC WOMEN FOR BREAST CANCER

BENEFIT MODELS

There are extant several previous models that have gained wide circulation and are worthy of comment.

By use of a life table model, Chiacchierini (22) has calculated that maximum benefit to screening, both in terms of person years gained and lives saved, occurs when screening begins at age 50. As in any model, however, results depend on the basic assumptions. Since this model's benefits estimates are based on the age specific benefits of HIP, it is obvious that the model cannot generate any benefit for screening women younger than age 50. Additionally, this model uses as the risk estimate the level given in the BEIR report for younger women. If one uses the age specific risk factor, the net benefits demonstrated over age 50 will increase. The major importance of Chiacchierini's model is that it graphically demonstrates the magnitude of the effect of dose reduction on the net benefit of any mammographic screening program. For example, according to this model, if screening were begun at age 50 and an absorbed dose per year was 10 rads, 8,838 person years would be gained by annually screening 100,000 people 5 years. If the dose were 1 rad, 14,458 net person years would be gained. Today, an annual absorbed dose of 1 rad is easily achievable with no loss in detection yield. Lower doses are possible, but high detection yield of smaller cancers for the lower doses has not yet been shown.

The model for screening of Blumenson (9) is a sophisticated mathematical one which has many appealing features. The application of this model, however, depends upon certain assumptions made about the natural history of breast cancer. A major assumption is based upon initial size of tumor and growth rate estimates derived from observations of patients with advanced disease. From these observations, two families of tumor growth rates were deduced: fast (25 days) and slow (1½ months). It was presumed that the slope of growth rates was constant from the inception of the disease, and that the frequency distribution of these growth rates was representative of the disease in the population as a whole.

Little hard data is available concerning linearity of tumor growth rates when the tumors are very small. The shape of the curve of growth rate may indeed be linear, it may be exponential, it may have multiple shoulders and varying slopes. Thus, while any one of a number of assumptions can be inferred, none should be presented as being absolute. In point of fact, there is evidence that volumetric growth rates are not constant. Silvestrini's (69) observations of potential doubling times in cell culture, as measured by Thymidine incorporation does indicate that there are different growth rate tumors; that the frequency distribution of potential doubling times is exponential; and that there is a definite cell loss which occurs in vivo varying from 92 to 96%. Furthermore, her work demonstrates that correlation exists with the log volume of the primary tumor, while none exists between labeling index and duration of symptoms. This could be taken to explain the "clinical observation that the recurrence rate within the patients with or without metastases is inversely dependent on the primary tumor size".

Another point against the constancy of growth rates is the observation noted in Table I.

VOLUME DOUBLING TIME OF HUMAN MAMMARY TUMORS*

Material	Range	Mean	Median Value	
Recurrent tumors	3-211		40	Philippe et al
Primary tumors	6-540		105	Kusama
Primary tumors	23-209		85	Gershon-Cohen
Cincinnati data				
Age 50		100		
Age 50		150		

*Adapted from Silverstrini et al, Cancer 34:1252-1258, 1974

It can be seen that the median value of doubling times based upon observations of recurrent tumor growth is 40 days. In the reported series where doubling times were based upon observation of primary tumors, the median doubling times were 85 to 105 days. This could be taken to mean:

(a) growth rates change once host resistance has been overcome,

(b) tumors of rapid doubling times tend to recur more quickly,

(c) it is a statistical fluctuation due to sampling size.

While all of these are possible, the difference at least indicates the dangers of extrapolating back to point zero from observations based on a population of advanced disease.

These data, it seems to me, suggest strongly that growth rates observed in advanced disease are very likely not reflective of growth during the developmental phase of the tumor.

In Bross's attempt to use his natural history model to supply data for Blumenson's screening model, an assumption of tumor growth rates had to be made. Since the distribution initially postulated did not fit the interval cancer rate for HIP (which was 41%), an alteration in the assumption of the frequency distribution of tumor growth rates was necessary. Since interval cancer rate in at least two of the screening centers of the BCDDP is 10%, it can only be presumed that this estimate will have to be altered once again to fit the observed facts.

Another observation concerning the model of Bross and Blumenson is in order here.

Doubling time observations based upon direct measurement of skin recurrences, metastases or radiographic changes, can only be used to indicate that there are indeed tumors of different growth rates. To assume that detailed mathematical models can be based reliably on these observations renders the quantification of the model suspect. For example, it is generally accepted by those who favor the concept of doubling time based upon Collin's work, (23) that it requires 30 doublings from inception before a tumor reaches one centimeter in size. From one cm to death of the patient is generally accepted as being an additional 17 to 20 doublings. If one assumes the distribution of tumor growth rates as measured by Pearlman, (56) Phillipe and LeGal, (59) Rigby-Jones (63) and the observed survival rates that they have noted, (56) an obvious disparity exists. For example, if one considers their intermediate growth tumors with doubling times ranging from 26-75 days, and assumes all had the maximum doubling time of 75 days, and all were detected at 1 cm in size, then no patient should have been alive 3½ years after initial detection. If they were all 5 mm at time of detection, none should have been alive at 4 years. Yet the observed, 5-year survival rate was over 60% in these series for this intermediate growth rate cancer.

As Post et al (60) have pointed out, the "growth of the breast cancer mass is a resultant of the proliferative patterns of the tumor cells plus the contribution of an indeterminate amount of connective tissue in which they may be growing. Thus, it is not possible to ascribe the growth of the tumor mass to the tumor cell population alone. This can only be done in a neoplasm composed only of tumor cells. Hence, the validity of the estimation of the actual doubling time which may be ascribed to tumor cell increase is questionable."

These measurements are, therefore, at best, biological approximations. As far as screening is concerned, a better estimate of the frequency of distribution of rapidly growing tumors in an otherwise well, asymptomatic group of patients can be determined from the interval rate of advanced cancer and the frequency of higher stage cancers occurring in the incidence years of an aggressively performed screen.

An assumption which is of key importance to the model of Bross and Blumenson (10,14,15) holds that metastasis occurs very early in the inception of the tumor, and the ultimate course thereafter is biologically foreordained despite diagnostic and therapeutic intervention. This assumption is shared by others (12,20,55).

The maximum force of mortality exerted by rapidly growing tumors occurs within five years of initiation of treatment. Thereafter, the post treatment survival differences between tumors of rapid and intermediate growth rates disappear. Long-term survivorship then is representative of the effects of diagnostic and therapeutic intervention. To deny that any benefit exists for finding and treating breast cancers at Stage I and II is contrary to reasonably well established medical observations.

While eradication of disease is the ultimate goal, if such is not possible, one would hope to be able to (1) alter the course of the disease and (2) improve the quality of survival. It would appear that both of these goals are possible with breast cancer. Bond, (12) while believing the disease to be widespread at time of initial detection, and speaking primarily of invasive cancers, has presented regression analyses of available data which suggest that simple removal of the primary tumor affects the outcome of the disease in all Stage 1 cases, and he has indicated that even 30% of Stage 4 cases will benefit. This may be due to either (a) reduction in the rate of metastatic release when the primary tumor is removed, or (b) its removal enhances host defense in some way. Growing evidence would tend to support the latter concept (21). If there is the likelihood that Bond's analysis has a better than even chance of being correct, it would seem that unless the risks involved are unequivocal, absolute and of large magnitude, the medical imperative for diagnosis at the lowest possible stage is quite clear.

As indicated previously, much of the furor that has arisen concerning the breast cancer screening controversy stems from the fact that the Health Insurance Plan screen conducted in the early 60's failed to demonstrate a benefit to screening women under the age of 50, while a 1/3 decrease in case fatality rate was obtained after the age of 50. This has been attributed to a different biologic behavior of cancers in younger women. However, as Shapiro points out, (67) "the results from the HIP study must be interpreted in terms of the screening procedures used. As discussed previously, mammography added relatively little to the physical examination in detecting breast cancer in younger women. The significance of this lies in the very low case fatality rates (italics mine) among cases in which the initial basis of biopsy recommendation was mammography alone. If mammography has indeed become a more effective modality in recent years, a new set of circumstances may exist."

The data from the Cincinnati and Milwaukee Centers demonstrate that from 8-73 through 6-77 in the age group under 50, 48/81 (59%) of cancers detected were found by mammography alone. In the HIP study in this age group, fewer than 20% of the cancers were found by mammography alone. Taken at face value, this suggests that mammography has become a more effective modality. It might be postulated that this is less a reflection of mammography efficiency, than rather a reflection of inept physical examination.

At this juncture, suffice it to say that the fact that 60% of the cancers detected by mammography alone were minimal breast cancer suggests that the basic change is in mammography.

Thus, it seems there is a need to model the possible benefit of screening, or lack thereof, on current detection capabilities, dose delivered and observed distribution of tumor growth potentials in a recently screened population.

Based on the results of aggressive screening of 20,000 women at the Cincinnati and Milwaukee Centers of the ACS/NCI Breast Cancer Demonstration Project (BCDP) and a delivered annual average midbreast absorbed dose of 1 rad per year, a model has been developed by Fox et al (26) for estimating the benefit/risk ratio for mammography in screening populations of asymptomatic, randomly selected women. The model includes corrections for self-selection bias and the presence of symptomatic women in the BCDP population. Benefit, expressed in terms of breast cancer deaths averted over not screening, is estimated based on distribution of cancers by pathological stage of detection.

The "worst case" estimate of Fox et al (26) of the benefit/risk ratio for five annual mammographic examinations on randomly selected, asymptomatic women age 35 to 49 at the start of screening is 3.4 $\pm$ 1.1 to 1. The corresponding "most probable" estimate is 8.0 ± 3.1 to 1. The most likely estimate is not the most favorable estimate. This benefit/risk ratio is derived from 10-year survival data from the Third National Cancer Survey. In either case, worst or most likely, benefit exceeds the risk significantly, clinically, and statistically.

If one calculates the person years gained as a result of screening, based upon this model, a different appreciation of the effect of screening can be obtained. It is estimated that, above the mean age of 40, for every age group screened for 5 years, 60,000 net person years will be gained per 10^6 people screened.

From mean age 40-60, two-thirds of this person year salvage is due to mammography alone. It is not until mean age 70 that person year salvage by physical examination and mammography are equal.

It should be remembered when estimating presumed risk versus presumed benefit, that the additional risk of each subsequent rad of irradiation diminishes with increasing attained age. On the other hand, benefit for each year of screening increases with each year of attained age. Since these curves are changing in opposite directions, once their point of decussation has been passed, the cumulative benefit to cumulative risk ratio can only increase.

Our model estimates that by aggressive screening of asymptomatic, randomly selected women under the age of 50, annual physical examination for five years could increase the relative survival of patients with breast cancer to approximately 59% plus or minus 4% from a national average of 50% unscreened. Mammography, added to this regimen, could increase the relative survival to 78% plus or minus 5%.

THE NATURAL HISTORY OF MINIMAL BREAST CANCER

It has been presumed that minimal and intraductal (in situ ductal) and in situ lobular cancers do not have the same life-threatening potential as larger, well established, invasive breast cancers that are detected in the usual course of clinical case finding.

Although it is true that wide gaps exist in our knowledge of the natural history and precursors of carcinoma of the breast, there is a general consensus (1,16,20,27,28,29,30,34,35,38,44,47,65,70,75) that intraductal carcinoma and in situ lobular carcinoma do represent early malignancy. Full agreement as to what constitutes the premalignant disease spectrum has not yet been reached. There is growing sentiment that atypical hyperplasia is, quite likely, premalignant, perhaps "nonobligate" preneoplasia. There is less agreement concerning the role of hyperplasia without atypia, and there are those who believe that patients with gross fibrocystic disease are at greater risk than the general population, although this does not seem to be the prevailing opinion.

We have previously analyzed biopsies obtained from our prevalence year (52). Those data suggested to us that there is a natural progression of the disease from ductal epithelial hyperplasia, and/or adenosis without atypia, into atypical epithelial hyperplasia, thence into carcinoma. It was felt that very likely hyperplasia represented the last form of nonobligate preneoplasia.

We now have available longitudinal data which allows us to begin to test some of the assumptions made thus far concerning the natural history of the disease.

The risk for development of a frank cancer within two years of a previous proliferative biopsy is 9 times the risk of a woman with a bland biopsy in our patient population.

Implicit in this criticism of the lack of knowledge of the natural history of the disease, is that the minimal cancers being detected are truly "very early", in the genesis of neoplasia. Actually, since our detection and diagnostic methods are crude, it is far more likely that these lesions are much further developed than is generally accepted. The evidence for this statement is as follows:

(1) In our screen, the average lead time gained by screening varied with the age at the time screening was begun. Under age 50, the mean detection lead time was 2.2 years, $\pm$ 0.4, and over age 50 it was 3.2 years, $\pm$ 0.4. This calculation is based upon observed prevalence data from two BCDDP's.

(2) Thirty-two percent of our minimal cancers are already demonstrably invasive, while 54% are intraductal, 7% are frank tumors with good prognostic characteristics and only 7% are in situ lobular cancer (Table II).

TABLE II

DISTRIBUTION OF MINIMAL BREAST CANCER BY PATHOLOGY

	#	%
IN SITU LOBULAR	4	7
INTRADUCTAL	31	54
INTRADUCTAL 10% INVASIVE	9	16
INVASIVE<5 MM.	9	16
CYSTOSARCOMA PHYLLOIDES	1	
INTRACYSTIC	1	7
TUBULAR	2	
	57	100%

The distribution of these minimal breast cancers in our own data follow closely the distribution of invasive carcinoma by histologic type described in the SEER data in 1975 (72). This again would suggest to us that there is little intrinsic difference in the biologic behavior, or pathologic characteristics of these early carcinomas vis-a-vis their more advanced counterparts.

If, in fact, these cancers are so far along, is there any evidence to suggest that detecting them, and offering treatment, is likely to alter their course? We have previously reported the 25-year survival of 75 patients with intraductal neoplasm treated with mastectomy in Cincinnati from 1950 to 1969 (49). Twenty percent of these patients are dead of their disease in 15 years (absolute survival). No increase in mortality due to breast cancer occurs in this population over the following 10 years. The numbers are small, and the potential for statistical fluctuation are wide. The 10-year crude survival figures reported by Urban and Wanebo (72,74) for 162 such patients is 95%, again no deaths from breast cancer having occurred in this group. Twenty-year data from M.D. Anderson Hospital (25) indicate 97% relative survival.

The implications of these data (i.e., that some cancers can be cured) are extremely important, particularly in contrast to the conflicting data reported by Campos (20) and Mueller and Jeffries (55) for invasive cancers. Campos' analysis of women treated for breast cancer at the University of Michigan from 1940-1965 suggests that (1) the chance of dying of cancer does not diminish with time for those patients that are to die of it; (2) whatever the mechanism that brings a patient to her death, that mechanism is acting more slowly in the cases without axillary metastases than in those with them; and (3) younger women (under 40) with axillary metastases, have a worse prognosis than older women with axillary metastases, and such women at the time of mastectomy have virtually complete dissemination.

Mueller and Jeffries (55) analyzed the mortality data from the Syracuse-Upstate Medical Cancer Registry, randomly selected patients from the Ontario Cancer Foundation and a group from the Syracuse Cancer Registry dying after 10 years. These were essentially all cancers, all stages. Although not specifically stated, based upon national figures available at that time, and our analysis of comparable data from the Cincinnati Tumor Registry, it is unlikely that more than 3% of the cancers were intraductal. The data of these two authors is interpreted by them to indicate that any woman who develops carcinoma of the breast has an 85% chance of dying of it; the force of this mortality is operative over a period of at least 15 years and the effect increases with age.

If these authors are correct in concluding that the course of invasive breast cancer is essentially predestined, then the survival analysis of intraductal carcinoma can be viewed in one of two ways:

(a) intraductal carcinoma of the breast is the last stage of the disease where complete cure can be achieved, or
(b) intraductal cancer is not really cancer at all.

Let us examine question b in some detail.

Most physicians would agree that microinvasive cancer is indeed real or potentially lethal disease. Some, perhaps, will retain reservations about the significance of in situ cancer.

In situ lobular cancer has been termed by some pathologists as "lobular pre-neoplasia". Indeed, while patients who harbor it have a definite propensity to develop invasive cancer, that time interval may be very long. Further, it is very likely, because of this duration to invasion, many such patients will not develop invasive cancer in their lifetime. Pennisi has reported that 15% of 419 patients who had subcutaneous mastectomy for non-malignant conditions had this pathological diagnosis (58).

Does this situation hold true for intraductal (in situ ductal) carcinoma (i.e., is the prevalence of intraductal cancer high in the general population?) There is no data presented to date which demonstrate that a high prevalence of such tumors exists in the general population.

In the data reported above by Pennisi et al (58) there were no cases of intraductal cancer in 419 subcutaneous mastectomies performed. One could argue that failure to detect these intraductal lesions represented a sampling problem due to their small size. Neither in situ lobular cancer nor intraductal cancer have distinguishing gross characteristics which would attract the attention of the attending pathologist. It should be borne in mind that invasive cancer of ductal origin occurs four times as often as cancer of lobular origin. Yet, in this particular population of women, not even one intraductal cancer was found, while 60 in situ lobular neoplasms were detected. This distribution, it seems, would attest to (a) the slow growth and low neoplasia potential of lobular neoplasia, (b) there are not an inordinate number of intraductal cancers "lying around", waiting to be discovered, and (c) the time in residence for intraductal cancer must be relatively short, else in this high risk population surely more such lesions would have been uncovered. These findings would be consistent with observations we have previously reported concerning lead time estimates and natural history of breast cancer and its precursors.

If 10-15% of our screened population were harboring intraductal cancer during the prevalence year, then our screening would have an efficiency rate of 2% in detection of these small cancers. This would suggest that guided biopsy has little more effect in detection than random chance. There is no support for this assumption by any hard data available today. Furthermore, the presumption that such a high percentage of intraductal cancers exist in a prevalence pool requires that: (a) all the intraductal cancers which will present in the lifetime of this screened population are present in intraductal form when first seen and, (b) there are no precursor lesions; or (c) intraductal cancer is not cancer, or (d) the lead time to invasion is such that intraductal cancer is effectively not cancer. There is no evidence to suggest that (a) is correct; there is ample evidence (1,5,17,30,34,35,37,44,47,52,75) to suggest that (b) in incorrect, and (c) is speculative. As to (d), analysis of lead time based upon our own data suggest that lead time gained by detection of intraductal cancer is probably on the order of months to at most 2-3 years.

To our knowledge, no large scale prospective autopsy study of coroners' cases with guiding radiography has been done to establish the frequency of intraductal cancer. In 1962, however, Sandison (64) reported the results of a study he conducted on 800 consecutive autopsies, performed over a 5-year period. The cases were not randomly selected, and histologic examination was limited in general to only one or two selected blocks from each case. Further, selection of areas for histologic sampling was not aided by radiography of the breast removed. Therefore, one could presume that unless the lesion were grossly demonstrable, this study would represent essentially a random sampling of the breasts examined with respect to microcancer. In this particular study, one patient with intraductal cancer was uncovered out of 776 women without clinical cancer. Since autopsy studies are, by their very nature, prevalence studies, a higher yield would have been expected, but, as indicated, failure to demonstrate more such lesions could have been a sampling problem.

What is immediately striking about Sandison's work is not the number of clinically occult invasive cancers detected (6/776), but rather their distribution. The fact that 5 cancers occurred in 17 women over the age of 80, and only 1 was found in 677 women between the age of 36-75 raises serious question about the validity of the study. Certainly, it is possible for there to be a backlog of slow growing cancers accumulating in older women in a prevalence study. However, one would expect some stepwise gradation. In other words, certainly some slow growing tumors would be expected to be present between the ages of 50-65 and none were found. It is more likely that this skewed distribution is a function of the nature of the study itself, the patient population selected or the premortem screening than it is a true representation of the underlying natural history of the disease.

Sandison's work, however, is extremely important in that it points up a great void in our knowledge of the natural history of the disease. A similar study of national scope of the breasts of women coming to autopsy as a result of foul play or trauma might be of great importance. This study, which must be carefully planned, should include, at a minimum, whole organ radiography as well as the most modern, meticulous pathology techniques for detecting minimal and microinvasive disease.

Our data (52) suggest that, in breast cancer, the nonobligate premalignant pool is hyperplastic disease, and that intraductal breast cancer is obligate cancer which will very likely present during the lifetime of younger women, if left to pursue its natural course.

It has been suggested that because a far larger number of in situ cancers have been found in routine studies of thyroid and prostate glands than will present clinically, such a situation exists with respect to breast cancer. At this time, this is pure speculation.

Furthermore, prostate cancer and thyroid cancer are not good models for breast cancer. Carcinoma of the prostate does not begin to present as a clinically significant lesion until the sixth decade of life, while breast cancer begins to significantly affect mortality a full 20 years earlier. Thyroid cancer, on the other hand, exerts only a very limited influence on mortality at any age. Thus, the natural history of these two diseases is not comparable to the natural history of breast cancer. While it is dangerous to extrapolate from one cancer model to another, there are many more similarities of clinical expression, i.e., natural history, between breast cancer and cervical cancer than there are between breast cancer and thyroid cancer, or breast cancer and prostate cancer. Therefore, if one were to select a biolgoical model, cervical cancer would seem to be a more viable candidate.

Recent work from Japan (39) presents us with a model of the natural history of carcinoma of the cervix. Of 151 patients with histologically proven mild to moderate dysplasia followed culdoscopically for 1-8 years, 64% regressed, while 10% progressed to invasive cancer. For 74 patients with severe dysplasia, regression was 58%, and progression 16%; for 32 with severe dysplasia-borderline cancer in situ, 25% regressed and 31% progressed. Of 37 patients with frank carcinoma in situ, only 3% regressed in 1-7 years of follow-up, and 54% developed invasive disease. Thus, we have a clinical model which demonstrates the natural progression of this form of cancer from nonobligate preneoplasia through obligatory, early cancer. It is very likely that all cancers pass through similar stages, but rates of change to clinical disease vary with the biology of the cancer and the immune status of the host.

CONCLUSIONS

The data we present here suggest that many patients with microcancers are in essence cured of breast cancer. For patients with invasive disease, it seems that if death due to breast cancer cannot be completely averted, it can be deferred if detected while limited to the breast. This seems to be so for tumors of all growth rates. While this is not ideal, such a situation is not unique in medicine. Many chronic diseases cannot be cured, but can be reasonably controlled. Until we have either new diagnostic/prognostic tools that can tell us which tumors will behave poorly and/or therapeutic tools which can treat all grades, and stages, of tumor equally well, "early" diagnosis seems to be our only hope of reducing the death rate from this disease.

In the meantime, mass hysteria concerning the dangers of screening mammography is simply not justified on the basis of available data, such as presented here.

As Cramer (24) has stated concerning cervical cytology screening, "Though the evidence is impressive, it remains largely circumstantial...

For those who would demand (a controlled clinical trial) before accepting a causal relationship between invasive and in situ cervical cancer, it must be conceded this is not available. For those who deal on a practical level with these lesions, the proof available may be sufficient."

To admit our ignorance is not equivalent to saying we know nothing.

To say we are partially ignorant and, therefore, impotent to act, foredooms failure.

To carelessly discard the potential gains unearthed thus far by the BCDDP's would, in our considered opinion, be very unwise.

REFERENCES

1. Ashikari, R., Huvos, A.G., Snyder, R.E., Lucas, J., Hutter, R.V.P., McDivitt, R.W., and Schottenfeld, D.: A clinicopathologic study of atypical lesions of the breast, Cancer, 1974, 33, 310-317.

2. Bailar, J.C. III, Personal Communication, Sept. 1, 1977.

3. Baral, E., Larsson, L.E., and Mattson, B.: Breast cancer following irradiation of the breast, Cancer, 1977, 40, 2905-2910.

4. Baum, M.: The curability of breast cancer, in Breast Cancer Management - Early and Late, ed. Basil Stoll, Heinemann Medical and Year Book, 1977.

5. Bhagavan, B.S., Patchefsky, A., and Koss, L.G.: Florid subareolar duct pappillomatosis (nipple adenoma) and mammary carcinoma: report of three cases, Human Pathology, 1973, 4, 289-295.

6. Black, M.M., Barclay, T.H.C., Cutler, S.J., Hankey, B.F., and Asire, A.J.: Association of atypical characteristics of benign breast lesions with subsequent risk of breast cancer, Cancer, 1972, 29, 338-343.

7. Bloom, H.J.G.,: The influence of delay on the natural history and prognosis of breast cancer. A study of cases followed for 5 to 20 years, British Journal of Cancer, 1965, 19, 228-262.

8. Blood, H.J.G., and Field, J.R.: Impact of tumor grade and host resistance in survival of women with breast cancer, Cancer, 1971, 28, 1580-1589.

9. Blumenson, L.E.: When is screening effective in reducing the death rate? Mathematical Biosciences, 1976, 30, 273-303.

10. Blumenson, L.E., and Bross, I.D.J.: A mathematical analysis of the growth rate and spread of breast cancer, Biometrics, March, 1969, 95-109.

11. Boice, J.D., and Monson, R.R.: Breast cancer in women after repeated fluoroscopic examinations of the chest, Journal of National Cancer Institute, Sept. 1977, 59, 823-832.

12. Bond, W.H.: Natural history of breast cancer in Host Defence in Breast Cancer, ed. Basil Stoll, William Heinemann Books Limited, Great Britain, 1975.

13. Brinkley, D., and Haybittle, J.L.: The curability of breast cancer, Lancet, 1975, 2, 95-97.

14. Bross, I.D.J. and Blumenson, L.E.: Screening random asymptomatic women under 50 by annual mammographies: Does it make sense?, Journal of Surgical Oncology, 1976, 8, 437-445.

15. Bross, I.D.J. and Blumenson, L.E.: Statistical testing of a deep mathematical model of human breast cancer, Journal of Chronic Disease, 1968, 21, 493-506.

16. Brown, R.W., Silverman, J., Owens, E., Tabor, D.C., and Lawrence, W.: Intraductal "non infiltrating" carcinoma of the breast, Archives of Surgery, 1976, III, 1063-1067.

17. Cardiff, R.D., Welling, S.R., and Faulkin, L.J.: Biology of breast preneoplasia, Cancer, 1977, 39 (Supplement, pp. 3734-3746).

18. Campos, J.L.: Observations on the mortality from carcinoma of the breast, British Journal of Radiology, 1972, 45, 31-38.

19. Cancer Patient Survival, Report #5. Edited by L.M. Axtell, A.J. Asire, and M.H. Myers: A report from the cancer surveillance, epidemiology and end results program (SEER), U.S. Department of Health, Education and Welfare, DHEW Publication No. (NIH)-77-992, NIH National Cancer Institute, Bethesda, Maryland, 20014, 1976.

20. Carter, D., and Smith, R.R.L.: Carcinoma in situ of the breast, Cancer, 1977, 40, 1189-1193.

21. Carter, R.L.: Immunological control of metastatic growth in host defence in breast cancer, ed. Basil A. Stoll, William Heinemann Medical Books Limited, Great Britain, 1975.

22. Chiacherrini, R., and Lundin, F.: The issues: benefit risk in mammography, 8th Annual National Conference on Radiation Control, HEW Publication (FDA)-77-8021, May 2-7, 1976, 209-229.

23. Collins, V.P., Loeffler, R.K., Tracy, H.: Observations on the growth rate of human tumors, American Journal of Roentgenology, 1956, 79, 988-1000.

24. Cramer, D.W.: The role of cervical cytology in the declining morbidity and mortality of cervical cancer, Cancer, 1974, 34, 2018-2027.

25. Dodd, G.P.: Position paper on mammography, American College of Radiology Committee on Mammography and Diseases of the Breast, November, 1976, as reported in Miscellaneous Information Relating to Breast Cancer Screening, Section B, NIH-NCI Consensus Development Meeting, DHEW Publication, available from Division of Cancer Control.

26. Fox, S., Moskowitz, M., Saenger, E.L., Kereiakes, J.G., Gardella, L., Milbrath, J., and Goodman, M.W.: Benefit/risk analysis of aggressive mammographic screening projected onto an asymptomatic randomly selected population, Radiology, Aug. 1978, 128, 359-366.

27. Gallager, H.S., and Martin, J.E.: The study of mammary carcinoma by mammography and whole organ sectioning, Cancer, 1969, 23, 855-873.

28. Gallager, H.S., and Martin, J.E.: Early phases in the development of breast cancer, Cancer, 1969, 24, 1174-1178.

29. Gallager, H.S., and Martin, J.E.: An orientation to the concept of minimal breast cancer, Cancer, 1971, 28, 1505-1507.

30. Gallager, H.S.: A view from the giant's shoulder, Fifth Annual Wendell Scott Lecture, Cancer, 1977, 40, 185-194.

31. Gershon-Cohen, J., Berger, S.M., and Klickstein, H.S.: Roentgenography of breast cancer moderating concept of "biologic predeterminism", Cancer, 1973, 16, 961-964.

32. Gordan, J., Reagan, J.W., Finkle, W.D., and Ziel, H.K.: Estrogen and endometrial carcinoma: pathological support of original risk estimates, N.E.J.M., 1977, 297 (Supplement, pp. 570-571).

33. Guenther, D.: Unpublished Data, 1977.

34. Gullino, P.M.: Natural history of breast cancer: Progression from hyperplasia to neoplasia as predicted by angiogenesis, Cancer, 39, (Supplement, pp. 2697-2703).

35. Hutter, R.V.P., and Foote, F.W.J.: Lobular carcinoma in situ: Long-term followup, Cancer, 1969, 24, 1081-1085.

36. Jensen, H.M., Rice, J.R., and Welling, S.R.: Preneoplastic lesions in the human breast, Science, 1976, 191, 295-297.

37. Kodlin, D., Winger, E.E., Morgenstern, N.L., and Chen, U.: Chronic mastopathy and breast cancer: a followup study, Cancer, 1977, 39, 2603-2607.

38. Kramer, W.M., and Rush, B.P.: Mammary duct proliferation in the elderly, a histopathologic study, Cancer, 1973, 31, 130-137.

39. Kurikawa, S.: Premalignant lesions of the uterine cavity, colon; especially on the benign and malignant nature of the borderline pathological alterations. Translated by T. Masukawa, from material presented to the Japanese academy of OB-GYN, 1972.

40. Kusama, P., Spratt, J.D., Jr., Donegan, W.L., Watson, F.R., and Cunningham, C.: The gross rates of growth of human mammary carcinoma, Cancer, 1972, 30, 594-599.

41. Lester, R.G.: Risk versus benefit in mammography, Radiology, 1977, 124, 1.

42. Letton, A.H., Wilson, J.P., and Mason, E.M.: The value of breast screening in women less than 50 years of age, Cancer, 1977, 40, 1-3.

43. Lynch, H.T., Guirgis, H., Albert, S., and Brennan, M.: Familial breast cancer in a normal population, Cancer, 1974, 34, 2080-2086.

44. McDivitt, R.W., Hutter, R.V.P., Foote, F.W., and Stewart, F.: In situ lobular carcinoma; a prospective followup study indicating cummulative patient risk, J.A.M.A., 1967, 201, 82-86.

45. McGregor, D.H., Land, C.E., Choi, K., Tokuoka, S., Wakabayashi, T., and Beebe, G.W.: Breast cancer incidence among atom bomb survivors, Hiroshima and Nagasaki, 1950-1969, J.N.C.I., Sept. 1977, 59, 799-811.

46. McGregor, D.H., Land, C.E., Choi, K., Tokuoka, S., Liu, P.I., Wakabayashi, T., and Beebe, G.W.: Risk of breast cancers in Japanese A bomb survivors, Radiation Effects Research Foundation, 5-2, Hijujima Park, Hiroshima 730, Japan.

47. McLaughlin, C.W., Jr., Schenken, J.R., and Tamisiea, J.X.: A study of precancerous epithelial hyperplasia and noninvasive papillary carcinoma of the breast, Annals of Surgery, 1961, 153, 735-744.

48. Moskowitz, M.: Clinical examination of the breast by non physicians: a viable screening option?, Accepted for publication, Cancer.

49. Moskowitz, M.: The issues: the need for mammographic screening appearing in radiation benefits and risks: facts, issues, and options, Proceeding of 8th Annual National Conference on Radiation Control, U.S. DHEW, Bureau of Radiological Health, Rockville, Maryland, 1976.

50. Moskowitz, M., Gartside, P., Gardella, L., deGroot, I., and Guenther, D.: Special lecture: the breast cancer screening controversy: a perspective, American Journal of Roentgenology, 1977, 129, 537-543.

51. Moskowitz, M., Gartside, P., Gardella, L., deGroot, I., and Guenther, D.: The breast cancer screening controversy: a perspective, In Breast Carcinoma, The Radiologists Expanded Role, ed. by W.W. Logan, John Wiley & Sons, New York, New York, 1977.

52. Moskowitz, M., Pemmaraju, S., Russell, P., Gardella, L., Gartside, P., and deGroot, I.: Observations on the natural history of carcinoma of the breast; its precursors and mammographic counterparts (Part I: Natural History), Breast: Diseases of the Breast, 1977, 3, 14-24.

53. Moskowitz, M., Pemmeraju, S., Fidler, J., Law, E.J., Sutorius, D.J., and Scheinok, P.: Minimal breast cancer in a screenee population, Cancer, 1976, 37, 2543-2547.

54. Moskowitz, M., Russell, P., Fidler, J., Sutorius, D., Law, E.J., and Holle, J.: Breast cancer screening: preliminary report of 207 biopsies performed in 4128 volunteer screenees, Cancer, 1975, 36, 2245-2250.

55. Mueller, C.B., and Jeffries, W.: Cancer of the breast: its outcome as measured by the rate of dying and causes of death, Annals Surgery, 1975, 182, 334-341.

56. Pearlman, A.W.: Influence of growth rate on prognosis and treatment evaluation: a study based upon mastectomy scar recurrences, Cancer, 1976, 38, 1826-1833.

57. Pellettierre, E.V.: The clinical and pathologic aspects of pappillomatous disease of the breast: a followup study of 97 patients treated by local excision, American Jouranl of Clinical Pathology, 1971, 55, 740-748.

58. Penisi, V., Capozzi, A., and Perez, F.A.: Subcutaneous mastectomy data. A preliminary report, Plastic and Reconstructive Surgery, 1977, 59, 53-56.

59. Phillipe, E., and LeGal, Y.: Growth of seventy-eight recurrent mammary cancers, Cancer, 1968, 21, 461-467.

60. Post, J., Sklarew, R.J., and Hoffman, J.: The proliferative patterns of human cancer cells in vivo, Cancer, 1977, 39, 1500-1507.

61. Report of the advisory committee on the biological effects of ionizing radiation: the effects on populations of exposures to low levels of ionizing radiation (BEIR Report) Division of Medical Sciences, National Academy of Sciences, National Research Council, 1972.

62. Report of the working group to review the NCI/ACS breast cancer demonstration detection projects, National Cancer Institute, Bethesda, Maryland, Sept. 6, 1977.

63. Rigby-Jones, P.: Prognosis of malgnant tumors of the breast in relation to rate of growth and axillary lymph nodes observed clinically, ACTA UICC, 1962, 18, 815.

64. Sandison, A.T.: An autopsy study of the adult human breast, National Cancer Institute Monography, No. 8, June, 1962, U.S. Department of HEW.

65. Schwerberg, S.G., and Chitale, A.R.: Assessment of significance of proportions of intraductal and infiltrating tumor growth in ductal carcinoma of the breast, Cancer, 1973, 32, 830-837.

66. Seidman, H.: Screening for breast cancer in younger women: life expectancy, gains, and losses, an analysis according to risk indication groups, Ca - A Cancer Journal for Clinicians, 1977, 27, 66-87.

67. Shapiro, S.: Evidence on screening for breast cancer from a randomized trial, Cancer, 1977, 39, 2772-2782.

68. Shore, R.E., Hempelmann, L.H., Kowalick, A., Mansur, P.S., Pasternak, B.S., Albert, R.E., and Haughie, G.E.: Breast neoplasms in women treated with x-ray for acute post partum mastitis, J.N.C.I., Sept., 1977, 59, 813-822.

69. Silvestrini, R., San Fillipo, O., and Tedesco, G.: Kinetics of human mammary carcinoma, and their correlation with the cancer and host characteristics, Cancer, 1974, 34, 1252-1257.

70. Toker, C.: Small cell dysplasia and in situ carcinoma of the mammary ducts and lobules, IV invasive carcinoma, The Mount Sinai Journal of Medicine, 1973, 40, 799-805.

71. Upton, A.C., Chairman: Report of National Cancer Institute ad hoc working group on the risks associated with mammography in mass screening for the detection of breast cancer, DHEW Publication, 1977.

72. Urban, J.A.: Changing patterns of breast cancer, Cancer, 1976, 37, 111-117.

73. Wallgreen, A., Silfversward, C., and Hultborn, A.: Carcinoma of the breast in women under 30 years of age, Cancer, 1977, 40, 916-923.

74. Wanebo, H.J., Huvos, A.G., and Urban, J.A.: Proceedings: Treatment of minimal breast cancer. Cancer, 1974, 33, 349-357.

75. Wheeler, J.E., Enterline, H.T., Roseman, J.M., Tomasulo, J.P., McIlvaine, C.H., Fitts, W.T., Jr., and Kirschenbaum, J.: Lobular carcinoma in situ of the breast. Long-term followup; Cancer, 1974, 34, 554-563.

76. Zelen, M.: Theory of early detection of breast cancer in the general population, appearing in breast cancer: trends in research and treatment, ed. by Heuson, J.C., Mattheien, W.H., and Rozencewei, N., Raven Press, NY, 1976.

THE BREAST CANCER DETECTION DEMONSTRATION PROJECT: AN ANALYSIS OF THE DATA

Richard G. Lester, M.D.
Professor and Chairman
Department of Radiology
The University of Texas
Medical School at Houston
Houston, Texas

An analysis of a proposed new procedure or method of diagnosis or therapy depends upon the evaluation of a variety of factors. Included among these are a) an evaluation of its effectiveness, b) a comparison with other available methodologies, c) an analysis of risk, and d) an estimation of cost. In my estimation, the experience of the Breast Cancer Detection Demonstration Project provides valuable evidence concerning the usefulness of mammography as a diagnostic tool and its effectiveness relative to physical examination. The factor of risk can be tested by relating the BCDDP experience to the estimates of risk derived from the NRC report on the Biological Effects of Ionizing Radiation (the BEIR Report)(1). The fourth aspect, that of cost, will not be considered in this presentation.

There are of course considerable elements of uncertainty. The absence of a control group in the BCDDP is a problem that can no longer be resolved. The fact that the approximately 270,000 women (261,059 screened by June 30, 1976) were volunteers adds a factor of indeterminacy as to the status of these women in regard to symptoms. (However, a substantial proportion of the women, 79%, were classified as asymptomatic by the Centers.)

The issue of the relevance of the available data in humans concerning mammary carcinogenesis derived largely from relatively high doses of radiation and applied to the very small quantities utilized in diagnostic mammography has also been questioned. For the purpose of this presentation, however, the straight line, no threshold hypothesis concerning mammary carcinogenesis has been adopted.

Despite these problems, however, the BCDDP program represents by far the largest collection of data available and valuable conclusions can, I believe, be drawn from it, though with due caution.

The gross and net benefits of mammography can be derived from an evaluation of the data presented in Table 1 (2). As can be seen, 1,597 cancers were found in the 270,000 screened once (including early recall). Of these, 711 (45%) were detected by mammography alone, this group representing the net diagnostic benefit of the procedure.

Approximately 50% of the patients screened were under 50 years of age. (Table 2). Approximately 31% of the cancers were found in this group. It had been suggested that mammography was relatively less useful in the detection of breast cancer in younger women. In fact, mammography was even more effective in finding cancers in younger women than in older ones. (Table 3).

In addition, the cancers found on mammography alone were significantly earlier (smaller) than those found by both mammography and physical examination. Particularly instructive in this regard is an evaluation of minimal breast cancer, defined as non-infiltrating cancers and infiltrating cancers under one cm diameter. Of 734 breast cancers, 278, or 37.9%, were defined as minimal. Of these, 153 were found by mammography alone. In 55% of the minimal breast cancers, physical examination was negative. (Table 4). (An interesting aside is the fact that in 9% of the minimal breast cancers, the physical examination was positive and mammography negative.)

Earlier breast cancer is positively associated with survival. (Table 5). The ten year survival rate for carcinoma localized to the breast was 74% in the period 1960-64, while with regional metastasis, ten year survival rate dropped to 39%. More recently, a study by Frazier and colleagues from M. D. Anderson Hospital showed a ten year survival rate for breast cancers one-half cm in diameter or smaller, including in situ carcinoma, of 96% (3).

The effectiveness of mammography in identifying breast cancers that cannot be found by physical examination seems proven. In addition, there is solid evidence that a substantial number of these breast cancers are relatively early or minimal in size and that diagnosis at this stage leads to significantly increased survival rates.

On the other hand, there is indubitable evidence implicating ionizing radiation as a weak but genuine breast carcinogen. It is not necessary to review this evidence here (1). For the purposes of this discussion, the estimate of the BEIR Report that radiation to the breast may induce cancer irrespective of dose (without threshold) and in linear fashion, even at very small doses, at the rate of approximately six cases per million per rad per year is accepted (although other hypotheses such as a decreasing rate of induction with decreasing doses at low levels can also be maintained from the data available).

In order to evaluate the significance of this, the quantity of radiation utilized for mammography in modern systems must be known. The significant dose is not the incident radiation to the skin but rather radiation to the mammary tissue. Table 6 shows the distribution of mid-line doses in the Breast Cancer Detection Demonstration Project. In the third year the average mid-line dose was approximately .22 rads, including all image receptor systems. There was substantial reduction in dose rates between the first and the third years. (5).

In my own department, a state of the art apparatus (Table 7) yields an average estimated mid-line dose of approximately 0.4 rad for a complete two exposure examination. (Table 8). Even greater reductions in radiation dose are obtainable utilizing other image receptor systems. (Table 9). For subsequent calculation purposes, however, an estimated mid-line dose of .4 rads is assumed.

From Table 10, it can be seen that approximately 19.4 cancers might be expected to be induced in 270,000 women examined by mammography at this dosage level. (Factors utilized for this calculation include the estimate of 6 cancers induced per rad per million patients per year and a thirty year average life expectancy for the women examined.) On the other hand, 711 cancers were identified by mammography alone in the BCDDP Program. This represents an excess of 691.6 cancers diagnosed to cancers induced.

The real test however is not diagnosis but effect on therapeutic effectiveness. Approximately 50% of patients with breast cancer initially diagnosed by physical examination will survive 10 years. Because the Breast Cancer Detec-

112

tion Demonstration Project began in the year 1973-74, 10 year statistics are not available. For purposes of evaluation, I have estimated the 10 year survival rate for those breast cancers diagnosed by mammography alone as 80%. (Table 11) This is a conservative figure because of the small size of the breast cancers, and the low incidence of regional and distant metastases identified in these patients.

Utilizing these survival estimates then, an estimate of increased survival for the whole group can be derived. (Table 12). Of 711 patients in the BCDDPs diagnosed by mammography alone, 568.8 will survive 10 years. Had mammography not been performed, these cancers would eventually have been diagnosed by physical examination. Utilizing the 50% 10 year survival rate, 355.5 would be alive at the end of that period had mammography not been performed. The net contribution of mammography is 213.3 patients.

In turn, a benefit/risk ratio for this group (Table 13) can be defined. Dividing the 213 patients representing the net contribution of mammography to survival by the 19 cancers induced, an 11 fold positive benefit/risk ratio is found. If the induced cancers are assumed to have a 10 year survival rate of 50%, the benefit/risk ratio for the whole group becomes approximately 22 times.

This marked balance in favor of benefit over risk is not surprising since two-thirds of the cancers were found in the 50% of patients 50 years of age and older.

More interesting is an analysis of the benefit/risk ratio in the women examined under age 50. Table 14 shows that 9.72 breast cancers can be expected to be induced in these women, while 199 cancers were diagnosed by mammography alone. In Table 15, the net contribution of mammography is seen to be 59.7 10 year survivors. In this group then, the benefit/risk ratio for mammography in the women under 50 years of age (Table 16) is 6.14, not taking into account the survivors with induced cancer or 12 times utilizing a 50% 10 year survival for this last group.

The case for regular mammography in women over the age of 50 is clinically proven and accepted. The usefulness of the baseline mammogram for women under the age of 50 is also established by this analysis.

A smaller data base is available for the determination of a favorable time to intitate mammographic examination in these younger women. However, data derived by the working group to review the BCDDPs (4) (Table 17) suggests a true incidence rate in women aged 35-39 of 1.58 per thousand, or 1,580 per million. Since 48% of these cancers are identified by mammography alone (Table 3) 758.4 such cancers will be diagnosed in this fashion in such a population. The 10 year survival rate will be 606.7 patients and the net contribution of mammography (606.7 minus the 379.2 patients who would survive 10 years after finally being diagnosed by physical examination alone) will be 227.5. In the same million patients, an estimated 72 induced breast cancers would be expected. In this group, then, the benefit/risk ratio is 227.5 divided by 72 or 3.16 times in favor of the base line mammogram in these women between 35 and 40 years of age.

There are unanswered questions. Why is the estimated incidence of breast cancer as derived from the BCDDP experience, based on the results of second screening plus known interval cases after the first screening so much higher than those of the third national cancer survey? (Since the BCDDP estimates are consistently higher, the possibility that programs based on women volunteering

113

to have the examination might be superior to mandated programs for all women must be seriously considered.) Can additional significant decreases in radiation dosage be expected in the foreseeable future? In women under the age of 50 what is an appropriate program of follow-up?

The analysis performed here was based on an estimated mid-line radiation dose of .4 rads per examination. Other systems, expecially those utilizing film/rare earth screen receptors today deliver even less radiation. Still further reductions in radiation might be achieved by single film follow-up examinations in asymptomatic women.

A prudent policy for the present is suggested in Table 18. The major indication for mammography is the clinical suspicion of cancer. In such women, mammography is recommended as a part of the initial workup. For women age 50 years and older, annual or other regular mammographic examination is recommended as a part of the regular health assessment. For women in the fourth and fifth decades of life, a base line mammogram is recommended at some point chosen between age 35 and 40. The need for additional mammography examination in the fifth decade should be determined by the physician in consultation with his patient and taking into account the findings of physical examination, the presence of historical risk factors such as maternal family history and the risk level assigned by the evaluation of the base line mammogram itself.

TABLE 1

PRELIMINARY ANALYSIS OF PROGRESS DATA
TOTAL DETECTED CANCERS BY AGE
GROUP, HISTORY, AND SYMPTOMS

	35-49			50-74			Other		
	Cancers*	Mammography Alone	P.E. Alone	Cancers	Mammography Alone	P.E. Alone	Cancers	Mammography Alone	P.E. Alone
History of Breast Cancer	15	4	1	58	32	2	2	1	0
Overt Symptoms	164	59	23	248	76	23	18	2	1
Asymptomatic	322	136	57	751	396	35	19	5	2
TOTALS	501	199	51	1,057	504	60	39	8	3

*All Modalities

114

TABLE 2

ANALYSIS OF DATA BY
5 YEAR AGE GROUPS

Age	Cancers Detected	Screenings
35-39	59	41,111
40-44	151	45,365
45-49	291	48,597
50-54	307	46,179
55-59	289	33,959
60-64	228	22,797
65-69	153	14,513
70-74	80	6,189
Other	39	4,138
TOTALS	1,597	262,848

TABLE 3

MODALITY FINDINGS BY AGE

(From Report of Working Group to Review BCDDPs)

MODALITY	35-39	40-49	50-59	60-64	65-74	TOTAL
Mammography Only	48%	43.5%	48%	39.5%	38.5%	43.9%
Physical Exam Only	4.0%	9.1%	8.1%	5.8%	5.4%	7.4%
Mammography and Physical Exam	48%	46.4%	42.1%	54.7%	55.4%	47.7%
Unknown						1.1%
SECOND SCREENING						
Mammography Only	57.1%	50.7%	42.9%	56.3%	54.5%	49.1%
Physical Exam Only	-	4.5%	2.2%	3.1%	3.0%	3.0%
Mammography and Physical Exam	42.9%	43.4%	54.9%	40.6%	39.4%	46.6%
Unknown						1.3%

115

TABLE 4

MINIMAL BREAST CANCER BY MODALITY
(From Report of Working Group to Review BCDDPs)

POSITIVE ON:	% of TOTAL	% MINIMAL
Mammography Alone	43.9%	55%
Mammography and Physical	47.7%	34.9%
Physical Alone	7.4%	9.0%
Unknown	1.1%	1.1%

TABLE 5

STAGE AND RELATIVE SURVIVAL RATES, CARCINOMA OF BREAST
(From Report of Working Group to Review BCDDPs)

STAGE OF DISEASE

Stage	1960-64	1970-73
Localized	47%	48%
Regional	41%	41%
Distant	9%	9%
Unknown	3%	2%

RELATIVE SURVIVAL RATES - 1960-64

Stage	10 Year Survival
Localized	74%
Regional	39%
Distant	2%
All Stages	52%
(Ca. in situ	90% -- 1955-64)

116

TABLE 6

DISTRIBUTION OF BREAST <u>MIDLINE DOSES</u> AT BCDD PROJECTS
Dose in rads at 3cm depth in a 6cm thick breast <u>per c-c image</u>

<u>All Units - All Detectors</u>

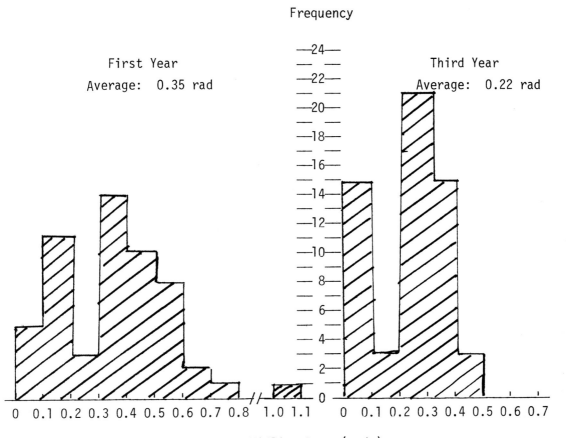

Midline Dose (rads)

TABLE 7

MAMMOGRAPHY SKIN DOSE MEASUREMENTS

X-RAY UNIT: Siemen's Mammomat
Tungsten tube, Be window
Three phase voltage, 0.6 mm focal spot
2.0 mm Al added filtration

IMAGE RECEPTOR: Xeroradiography
22 - inch target-image receptor distance
20 - inch target-chamber distance
For 2 - inch thick compressed breast

117

TABLE 8

TECHNIQUE	HVL (A1)	SURFACE DOSE (mrads)	ESTIMATED MIDLINE (3cm) DOSE (mrads)
42kVp, 80mAs	1.20	761	190
44kVp, 80mAs	1.22	834	208
46kVp, 80mAs	1.25	900	225

TABLE 9

DISTRIBUTION OF BREAST <u>MIDLINE DOSES</u> AT BCDD PROJECTS

Dose in rads at 3cm depth in a 6cm thick breast <u>per c-c image</u>

<u>FILM-SCREEN DETECTORS</u>

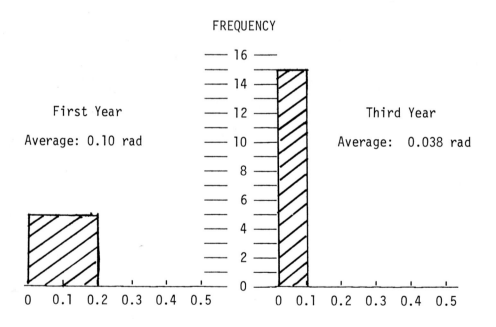

FREQUENCY

First Year

Average: 0.10 rad

Third Year

Average: 0.038 rad

TABLE 10

BCDDP RESULTS

				TOTAL
CANCERS INDUCED	$\dfrac{6 \times 270{,}000 \times .4 \times 30}{1{,}000{,}000}$		=	19.4

CANCERS DIAGNOSED BY MAMMOGRAPHY ONLY	Age 35 - 50	Age 50 - 74	Other	711
	199	504	8	

TABLE 11

ESTIMATE OF SURVIVAL

10 year survival rate for   50%
cancer dx by P.E.

10 year survival rate for   80%
cancer dx by Mammography

TABLE 12

ESTIMATE OF INCREASED SURVIVIAL
FOR WHOLE GROUP

By Mammography (711 x .80)	568.8
By P.E. (711 x .50)	355.5
Net Contribution of Mammography	213.3

TABLE 13

BENEFIT/RISK RATIO
FOR WHOLE GROUP

213.3/19.4   10.99

213.3/19.4
  (19.4 x .50 - 10 year
   survivors with induced
   cancer)   21.99

TABLE 14

BCDP RESULTS UNDER AGE 50

Cancers
Induced
$$\frac{6 \times 135{,}000 \times .4 \times 30}{1{,}000{,}000} = 9.72$$

Cancers Diagnosed by   199
  Mammography Alone

TABLE 15

ESTIMATE OF IMPROVED SURVIVAL
UNDER AGE 50

By Mammography   (199 x .80)   159.2

By P.E.   (199 x .50)   99.5

Net Contribution of Mammography   59.7

TABLE 16

BENEFIT/RISK RATIO
UNDER AGE 50

59.7/9.72   6.14

59.7/4.86
  (9.72 x .50 - 10 year
   survivors with induced
   cancer)   12.28

TABLE 17

BREAST CANCER DETECTION RATE PER THOUSAND
AND ESTIMATED INCIDENCE RATE
(From Report of Working Group to Review BCDDPs)

AGE	FIRST SCREENING	BCDDP ESTIMATE*	THIRD NATIONAL CANCER SURVEY
Total	4.80	2.97	1.59
35-39	1.14	1.58	0.53
40-44	2.47	1.66	1.03
45-49	5.05	3.21	1.56
50-54	5.05	3.74	1.68
55-59	6.81	3.23	1.88
60-64	6.51	4.05	2.22
65-74	10.29	3.65	2.40

*Determined from results of second screening and known interval cases.

TABLE 18

RECOMMENDATIONS FOR MAMMOGRAPHY

ALL PATIENTS

1) Signs, symptoms or other clinical suspicion of breast cancer.

AGE 50 AND OLDER

1) Annual or other regular mammographic examination with physical examination.

WOMEN FOURTH AND FIFTH DECADES

1) Baseline mammogram during age period 35-40 years.
2) Consideration of periodic mammography, frequency to be determined on the basis of risk factors, physical examination findings, and baseline mammographic findings.

121

REFERENCES

1. The Effects on Populations of Exposure to Low Levels of Ionizing Radiation. Report of the Advisory Committee on the Biological Effects of Ionizing Radiations. Division of Medical Sciences. National Academy of Sciences, November 1972.

2. Pomerance, William, late Chief of Diagnostic Branch, Division of Cancer Biology and Diagnosis. Personal communication.

3. Frazier, T. G., Copeland, E. M., Gallager, H. S., et al. Prognosis and Treatment in Minimal Breast Cancer. American Journal of Surgery 133:697-701, June 1977.

4. Final Report of National Cancer Institute Ad Hoc Working Group on Mammography Screening for Breast Cancer and A Summary Report of Their Joint Findings and Recommendations. National Institutes of Health, March 1977.

5. Gold, Richard H. Personal communication.

RESULTS OF THE CENTERS FOR RADIOLOGICAL PHYSICS' MEASUREMENTS AT THE BREAST CANCER DETECTION DEMONSTRATION PROJECTS

Lloyd M. Bates and Andrzej J. Demidecki

AAPM-CRP Coordination Office
Suite 307, 6900 Wisconsin Avenue
Chevy Chase, Maryland   20015

INTRODUCTION

In June, 1974, the Division of Cancer Control and Rehabilitation (DCCR) of the National Cancer Institute funded 6 Regional Centers for Radiological Physics (CRP). One of the tasks assigned to the CRP's was that of monitoring radiation exposures to persons being screened for breast cancer at Breast Cancer Detection Demonstration Projects (BCDDP) supported jointly by DCCR and the American Cancer Society.

Also in June, 1974, the American Association of Physicists in Medicine entered into contract with DCCR to coordinate the activities of the CRP's. One of the tasks of the Coordination Program established by this contract was to provide NCI with integrated reports on CRP activities. This point is made to emphasize the fact that while data assembly and a certain amount of calculation is carried out in the Coordination Office, the basic data on which the calculations are made were generated by CRP physicists.

Table I lists the CRP's, the instmitutions at which they are located, and the CRP Directors. Figure 1 shows the geographical area assigned to each CRP.

BCDDP MONITORING PROGRAM

In a program which has been in operation for about 4 years, the CRP's monitor the radiation output of approximately 60 mammographic x-ray units at the 27 BCDDP's. Monitoring is carried out through annual visits by CRP physicists to the BCDDP's in their region, at which time measurements of numerous x-ray machine parameters are made. Measurements are made in accordance with a detailed measurement protocol and with instrumentation whose calibration is traceable to the National Bureau of Standards. At the time of the visits, CRP physicists work with the BCDDP

Data assembly and calculations required for this report and the preparation of the report were carried out under contract NO1-CN-45162 with the Division of Cancer Control and Rehabilitation of the National Cancer Institute.

radiologists and technologists to reduce x-ray exposures in a manner which will not result in an unacceptable degree of image degradation.

Table I

The Centers for Radiological Physics

Mideast Center for Radiological Physics (MECRP)
Allegheny General Hospital, Pittsburgh, PA
Director: Dr. P. Shrivastava

Midwest Center for Radiological Physics (MWCRP)
University of Wisconsin, Madison, WI
Director: Dr. J. Cameron

Northeast Center for Radiological Physics (NECRP)
Memorial Hospital, New York, NY
Director: Dr. J. Laughlin

Northwest Center for Radiological Physics (NWCRP)
University of Washington, Seattle, WA
Director: Mr. P. Wootton

Southern Center for Radiological Physics (SCRP)
M.D. Anderson Hospital, Houston, TX
Director: Dr. R. Shalek

Southwest Center for Radiological Physics (SWCRP)
University of Colorado, Denver, CO
Director: Dr. W. Hendee

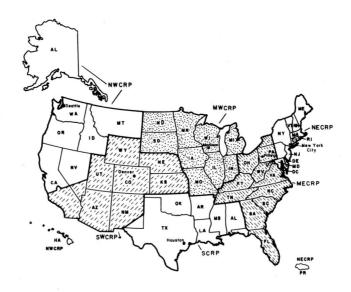

Figure 1: Regions assigned to the CRP's.

In the interval between visits to the BCDDP's, radiation exposure to screenees is monitored biweekly with thermoluminescent dosimeters (TLD). The TLD's are mailed to the BCDDP's, exposed there, and returned by mail to the CRP's for read-out and exposure calculation. The bi-weekly monitoring ensures that exposures are not varying or, alternatively, alerts the CRP and hence the BCDDP that a change in exposure has occurred. If a change is detected, the cause is investigated through a telephone call to the BCDDP or a visit to the Project by a CRP physicist. The BCDDP's are encouraged to consult with the CRP physicists on their imaging and dosimetry problems.

The data presented below are from the ionization chamber measurements made during actual visits to the BCDDP's. The results from the mailed TLD's agree remarkably well with these measurements.

BREAST SURFACE EXPOSURES

Exposure data are presented here as a series of histograms giving the distribution of exposures as measured during the first review visit (first year) and those as measured during the fourth review visit (fourth year). The exposure specified is that to the surface of a 6 cm thick compressed breast for a cranio-caudad image, when the image is made with the machine settings used at the BCDDP.

Figure 2 gives the distributions for all x-ray units at the BCDDP's. The exposure, averaged over all units, decreased from 3.3 R to 0.98 R, about 70%. A large reduction in the range of exposures is also evident.

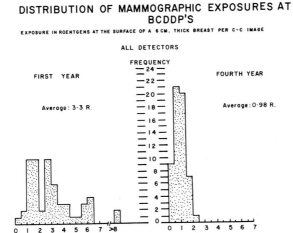

DISTRIBUTION OF MAMMOGRAPHIC EXPOSURES AT BCDDP'S

EXPOSURE IN ROENTGENS AT THE SURFACE OF A 6 CM. THICK BREAST PER C-C IMAGE

ALL DETECTORS

FIRST YEAR   FREQUENCY   FOURTH YEAR

Average: 3.3 R.   Average: 0.98 R.

EXPOSURE (R)

Figure 2: Distribution of surface exposures to breasts of women undergoing screening at BCDDP's. First and fourth years.

The data for the first year include exposures for x-ray units using film-screen combinations, xerox, and non-screen film as image receptors. At the time of the fourth visit, and, in fact, at the time of the third annual visit, the use of non-screen film at the one or two BCDDP's which had been using it had been discontinued. While the discontinued use of non-screen film did contribute to the reduction of average exposure and the range of exposures, it was not a major factor as can be seen from Figures 3 and 4.

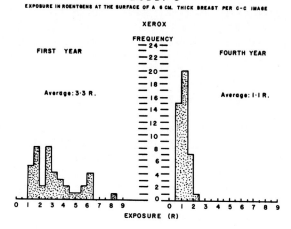

Figure 3: Distribution of surface exposures to breasts of women undergoing screening at BCDDP's using xerox image receptors.

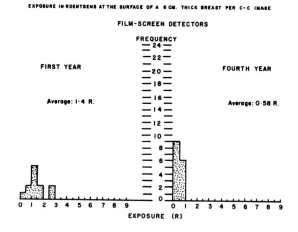

Figure 4: Distribution of surface exposure to breasts of women undergoing screening at BCDDP's using film-screen combinations as image receptors.

126

Figure 3 shows the distribution of exposures for mammographic units which use the xerox imaging system and Figure 4 those for units which use film-screen combinations. For the xerox system, a reduction in average exposure from 3.3 R to 1.1 R, about 65%, was achieved together with a reduction in exposure range comparable to that shown in Figure 2. For those units using film-screen combinations, a reduction of average exposure from 1.4 R to 0.58 R, again about 65% was achieved.

Reductions in exposure were achieved through the adjustment of x-ray machine exposure parameters to those more appropriate for the type of image receptor in use and through changes in focus-detector distances in some instances. Several of the BCDDP's began to use more sensitive film-screen combinations which had been developed for mammography, notably Dupont Lo-Dose II and Kodak MinR. This accounted for a considerable portion of the reduction demonstrated in Figure 4. As mentioned earlier, the discontinued use of non-screen film also contributed to the reductions. Reduction of exposure for units using xerox occurred in three steps: 1) The demonstration by the CRP's that, in many instances, exposures higher than necessary were being used. 2) The demonstration that an acceptable image could be achieved with beam filtrations greater than those used in many of the x-ray units. 3) A change at some of the BCDDP's from a negative to a positive imaging mode.

BREAST MIDLINE DOSES

From the initiation of the monitoring program, it was recognized that surface exposure was not an appropriate parameter to evaluate the risks of deleterious biological effects which might result from mammography. However, data were not available with which to make reliable calculations of doses at depth in the breast. Accurate back-scatter factors and depth dose data were required.

The Southwest CRP completed back-scatter measurements for beam qualities and beam geometries commonly used in mammography (1). These were confirmed by some additional measurements at the Northwest and Northeast CRP's. Following this, measurements made by the Northeast CRP yielded data on doses to tissues at depth in the breast for x-ray beam qualities and geometries used in mammography. From these data and the exposure data obtained at the BCDDP's, midline doses were calculated.

The distribution of midline doses are shown in Figures 5, 6 and 7 for all image receptors, xerox only and film-screen combinations only. The dose is quoted in rads to a sample of mammary gland lying on the midline of a 6 cm thick compressed breast. The chemical composition of the mammary gland and of the surrounding breast tissue is taken as that described by Hammerstein et al (2).

Figure 5 shows that the midline dose averaged over all units is 0.27 rads, having been reduced by about 35% from the 0.41 rads dose which existed at the time of the first review. Figures 6 and 7 show the comparable data for the xerox and film-screen combinations: a 20% decrease for xerox and a 60% decrease for film-screen combinations. The lesser reduction obtained with xerox is, of course, due to the fact that a reduction of surface exposure obtained by increasing x-ray beam filtration, does not result in a proportional reduction in dose at the midline because of "beam hardening."

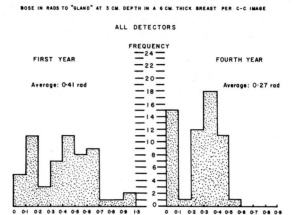

Figure 5: Distribution of breast mid-line doses to women undergoing screening at the BCDDP's. First and fourth years.

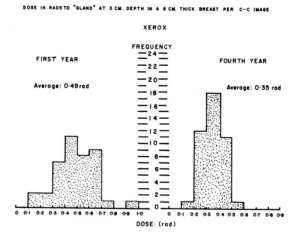

Figure 6: Distribution of breast mid-line doses to women undergoing screening at BCDDP's using xerox image receptors.

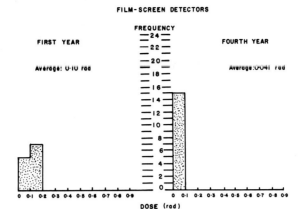

DISTRIBUTION OF BREAST MIDLINE DOSES AT BCDDP'S

DOSE IN RADS TO "GLAND" AT 3 CM. DEPTH IN A 6 CM. THICK BREAST PER C-C IMAGE

FILM-SCREEN DETECTORS

Figure 7: Distribution of breast mid-
line doses to women undergoing
screening at BCDDP's using film-
screen combinations as image
receptors.

BREAST AVERAGE DOSE

Hammerstein et al (2) described a model of tissue
distribution in the breast and provided depth dose data with which
the average dose to the more radiosensitive tissues could be
calculated. Using this model, the depth dose data, and the BCDDP
surface exposure data, breast average doses were calculated.
Table II provides a comparison of midline and breast average doses
and the reduction of these doses which was achieved between the
first and fourth years. In this table, the term "average" denotes
the breast average dose; the term "mean" denotes an average over a
number of x-ray units. Doses are given in rads to mammary gland
tissue as described by Hammerstein.

Table II

Comparison of breast midline and breast
average doses to women undergoing
screening at BCDDP's.

DETECTOR	QUANTITY	FIRST YEAR		FOURTH YEAR		RATIO: FOURTH/FIRST	
		MIDLINE	AVERAGE	MIDLINE	AVERAGE	MIDLINE	AVERAGE
FILM-SCREEN	MEAN	0·10	0·15	0·041	0·063	0·39	0·41
	RANGE	0·036 - 0·18	0·040 - 0·26	0·027 - 0·055	0·043 - 0·098		
XEROX	MEAN	0·49	0·61	0·35	0·39	0·72	0·65
	RANGE	0·19 - 0·94	0·18 - 1·3	0·18 - 0·56	0·18 - 0·61		
ALL DETECTORS	MEAN	0·41	0·53	0·27	0·31	0·66	0·58
	RANGE	0·036 - 1·2	0·040 - 1·9	0·027 - 0·56	0·043 - 0·61		

In Table II, it will be noted that with film-screen combinations the breast average dose is about 50% greater than the midline dose while for xerox it is from 12% to 20% greater. This reflects the change in the shape of depth dose curves from sharply concave upward for the lower energy beams used with film-screen combinations to the less pronounced curvature obtained with the higher energy beams used with xerox. The same effect can be seen in a comparison of average and midline doses for xerox in the first and fourth years. The trend during this time had been to increase the filtration on x-ray units using xerox.

Reductions in breast average doses are shown in the extreme right column of Table II: about 60% for units using film-screen combinations, about 35% for units using xerox, and an overall reduction of about 40%.

SUMMARY AND CONCLUSIONS

Data have been presented which summarize the radiation exposures and doses received by screenees at the BCDDP's, and the reductions achieved over the past four years through the cooperative efforts of CRP and BCDDP personnel.

Data on the results of the third year's measurements have not been presented because of time limitations. These would have shown that only minimal decreases in exposure and dose occurred between the third and fourth yearly reviews. This suggests that the doses at the BCDDP's are now at a practical lower limit and that any further reduction will be accompanied by image degradation unless achieved through some new imaging modality.

REFERENCES

1. Dubuque, G.L.; Cacak, R.K.; Hendee, W.R. Backscatter Factors in the Mammographic Energy Range. Med. Phys., Volume 4, #5, Sept./Oct., 1977

2. Hammerstein, R.G.; Miller, D.W.; White, D.R.; Masterson, M.E.; Woodard, H.Q.; Laughlin, J.S. Radiation Absorbed Dose in Mammography. In press: Radiology (March, 1979).

REDUCED DOSE MAMMOGRAPHY--RESULTS OF A NATIONWIDE STUDY

Ronald G. Jans* and Thomas R. Ohlhaber**

Bureau of Radiological Health
Food and Drug Administration
U.S. Department of Health, Education, and Welfare
5600 Fishers Lane
Rockville, Maryland   20857

INTRODUCTION

In order to minimize patient exposure from mammography and to improve image quality, the Bureau of Radiological Health, Food and Drug Administration, and the National Cancer Institute are supporting State radiation control agencies in implementing the Breast Exposure: Nationwide Trends (BENT) program. The BENT program, described in detail elsewhere (1,2,3), uses a survey card containing thermoluminescent dosimeters to determine the mammographic exposure levels and techniques within a State. The data are analyzed for suspected exposure and/or image quality problems. Followup surveys are then conducted in order to identify the problems and recommend corrections.

When we reported on the BENT program at the meeting held here in October of 1976, BENT was being pilot tested by five radiation control agencies. Currently, 42 States are implementing BENT. In addition to these States, the District of Columbia, New York City, Puerto Rico, Guam, Public Health Service Hospitals and Clinics, the U.S. Army, Navy, and Air Force, and two Canadian provinces have BENT programs. To date, 38 of these States and 4 of the other agencies have collected data on 2,379 x-ray units used for mammography (estimated to comprise 60 percent of the units used for mammography in the United States). These data were collected in either 1977 or 1978. This paper will present the results to date as they relate to the current status of reduced dose mammography.

DATA ON MAMMOGRAPHIC TECHNIQUES

For the purposes of the BENT program, the image receptors reported by mammography facilities have been categorized as direct exposure film (non-screen film), film/screen combinations, and Xeroradiography. The mammography facilities also reported workload data that have been used to estimate the percent of patients examined with each category of image receptor (Table 1).

*   Division of Training and Medical Applications
** Division of Electronic Products

TABLE ONE. Percent of X-ray Units and Percent of Patients
Examined by Type of Image Receptor in 38 States (1977-78)

IMAGE RECEPTOR	PERCENT OF X-RAY UNITS	PERCENT OF PATIENTS EXAMINED
Direct Exposure Film	11	4
Film/Screen Combinations	44	35
Xeroradiography	45	61

The direct exposure films were primarily those designed for automatic film processors, such as Kodak RP/M. Forty-five percent of the film/ screen combinations used were the newer (faster) DuPont LoDose II or Kodak Min-R systems. Both the direct exposure film and the film/screen categories include a few (2 percent of the units) film or film/screen combinations that are normally associated with general radiography rather than mammography; for example, a double emulsion film with par speed screens. The xeroradiography category includes units with both positive and negative mode xeroradiography. The positive mode was routine for 87 percent of the units used with the Xerox system.

Although Xerox and film/screen image receptors are used with approximately the same percentage of x-ray units, the Xerox system was used to examine 61 percent of the patients reported by the mammography facilities. Direct exposure film continues to be used with 11 percent of the x-ray units; however, because these facilities reported low workloads, only 4 percent of the patients are routinely examined with this image receptor.

Each mammography facility exposed a dosimetry card containing thermoluminescent dosimeters to the technique factors that would be used for a "medium-density, medium-size" breast. Table Two presents mean exposures for a single craniocaudal view, expressed as roentgens (R) free-in-air at the skin entrance site and the mean estimated half-value layer.

Currently, the mean craniocaudal exposure for all image receptors is 0.88R. The mean exposure for direct exposure film is twice that of Xerox systems, and four times that of film/ screen systems. Only the mean exposure for direct exposure film is greater than 1 R.

If the estimated half-value layers from the dosimetry cards are assumed to be reasonably accurate and if appropriate assumptions are made regarding backscatter and beam size, these exposure estimates can be converted into estimates of various measures of dose. Although average absorbed dose or integral dose would, most likely, be a better measure of biological risk, midline dose is also of interest because a report by National Cancer Institute working groups (4) recommended that the midline dose for a two-view examination be less than 1 rad. Table Three shows the results of applying the method developed by Miller et al (5) in order to develop estimates of the midplane dose to a 6 cm breast from a craniocaudal view.

TABLE TWO. Mean Exposure* per Craniocaudal View and Mean Estimate Half-Value Layer as Determined by Dosimetry Card (TLD) Measurements (manual mode techniques**)

IMAGE RECEPTOR	NUMBER OF X-RAY UNITS	EXPOSURE (R)		ESTIMATED HALF-VALUE LAYER (mmAl)	
		Mean	S.D.	Mean	S.D.
All	2,186	0.88	1.08	1.2	0.51
Direct Exposure Film	234	2.04	2.25	1.0	0.45
Film/Screen Combinations	900	0.49	0.74	0.8	0.38
Xeroradiography	1,052	0.95	0.64	1.5	0.40

* Exposure (R) free-in-air at the skin entrance site

** RAEC (radiation automatic exposure control, phototimed) units are not included because of differences in measurement techniques

TABLE THREE. Estimates of Midplane Dose (6 cm breast) per Craniocaudal View Calculated from Dosimetry Card (TLD) Measurements.

IMAGE RECEPTOR	ESTIMATED MEAN MIDPLANE DOSE (rads)
All	0.22
Direct Exposure Film	0.41
Film/Screen Combinations	0.08
Xeroradiography	0.30

FOLLOWUP SURVEYS

Data from the dosimetry cards were analyzed in order to identify mammography facilities where exposure appeared unnecessarily high or unusually low (Table Four). Forty-five percent of the x-ray units were suggested for followup by State personnel. Nine percent of the x-ray units were suggested for followup surveys because the exposure appeared too high for the image receptor being used. Surveys were suggested for 19 percent of the units because the exposure appeared too low and for 17 percent of the units because the technique factors, type of film processing or other reported data appeared unusual for the image receptor used. Both the low exposures and other indications for followup were of concern because they suggested that the image quality should be improved.

TABLE FOUR. Percent of X-Ray Units Suggested for
Followup Surveys

REASON FOR FOLLOWUP	PERCENT OF X-RAY UNITS
All	45
High Exposure	9
Low Exposure	19
Other Indication	17

Personnel from the State radiation control agencies have been conducting x-ray surveys at the suggested facilities. The most common reasons for high exposures have been:

1) the use of direct exposure film with high mAs and low kVp;

2) the overexposure of film/screen systems, producing higher than necessary densities; and

3) the conduct of xeroradiography with little or no added filtration.

Reevaluations of mammography exposures are underway in several States and have been completed in the radiation control agencies that pilot tested BENT. The pilot test results have shown a reduction in mean exposure from 1.48 R to 0.80 R. The percentage of x-ray units with exposures over 2 R was reduced from 21 percent to 7 percent. It is expected that the data from the States currently in the process of reevaluating exposures will also show that the efforts of radiologists, manufacturers, and other health professionals are succeeding in reducing high exposures.

The most common reasons for poor image quality in facilities with low exposures of unusual techniques have been:

1) the "wrong" x-ray spectrum for film or film/screen image receptors;

2) non-mammography film or film/screen systems; and

3) incorrect technique selection.

The "wrong" x-ray spectrum for film image receptors is illustrated in Table Five. Film mammography is normally conducted at 26 to 34 kVp with total filtration resulting in a first half-value layer of less than 1 mm of aluminum. Thirty-four percent of the x-ray units used with film are operated at 35 to 70 kVp or with total filtration that results in a first half-value layer greater than 1 mm of aluminum. Typically, the resulting films are very low in contrast and not able to illustrate all of the test objects in imaging phantoms. This problem occurs most frequently in low workload facilities that perform mammography with general purpose x-ray units that have not been or cannot be modified for lower kVp and removal of filtration.

TABLE FIVE. Percent of X-Ray Units by Nominal kVp and Estimated Half-Value Layer (HVL)--Direct Exposure Film or Film/Screen Image Receptors

	Estimated HVL (mm Al)		
Nominal kVp	$\leq$ 0.4	0.5-0.9	$\geq$ 1.0
$\leq$ 25	0	4	2
26-34	11	38	15
$\geq$ 35	2	4	11

kVp and/or HVL were unknown for 13 percent of the x-ray units

The solution of image quality problems is complicated by several factors:

1) the exposures associated with these problems are already low--very often less than 150 mR per film--and the reduction of high exposure is traditionally a major incentive for change;

2) unless dissatisfied with patient mammograms, the radiologist may tend to distrust the results of currently available breast imaging phantoms that tend to be more suitable to subjective rather than objective evaluation; and,

3) in most facilities, low patient workloads (Table Six)
    make the purchase of new equipment or the modification
    of existing equipment uneconomical.

TABLE SIX. Percent of X-Ray Units and Percent of Patients
            Examined by Patient Workload

FACILITY WORKLOAD (patients in one month)	PERCENT OF X-RAY UNITS	PERCENT OF PATIENTS EXAMINED
10 or less	38	6
11 to 20	20	10
21 to 40	20	19
41 to 100	18	33
101 or more	4	32

CONCLUSIONS

The BENT data show that the challenge to mammography facilities must be both image optimization and dose reduction, not just
dose reduction. Currently, there are a large number of facilities where exposures are too low, indicating poor image quality.
Correction is not simply a matter of increasing exposure; rather,
it is usually necessary to modify the x-ray equipment.

Because mammography is a difficult and exacting task, not
every x-ray facility can reasonably expect to perform good
mammography. Facilities that do conduct mammographic examinations must invest time in establishing quality assurance
programs, as well as invest resources in making necessary
improvements in their mammographic systems. If diagnostic
quality is to be maintained, then careful attention must be paid
to the utilization of proper equipment and techniques.

REFERENCES

1. Jans, RG: "Mammography Quality Assurance Program." Proceedings of the Eighth Annual Conference on Radiation Control. Springfield, Illinois. May 2-7, 1976. DHEW Publ. 77-8021.

2. Jans, RG: "A Federal/State Quality Assurance Program in Mammography," in Breast Carcinoma: The Radiologist's Expanded Role, Wende Westinghouse Logan, Ed. (John Wiley & Sons, Inc., New York, 1977) pp. 121-127.

3. Jensen, JE, Butler PF: Breast Exposure: Nationwide Trends; a Mammography Quality Assurance Program--Results to Date. Radiol. Techn.: To be published in December 1978.

4. Final Reports of National Cancer Institute Ad Hoc Working Groups on Mammography Screening for Breast Cancer and A Summary Report of Their Joint Findings and Recommendations, DHEW Publ. (NIH) 77-1400 (1977).

5. Miller DW et al.: "Radiation Absorbed Dose in Mammography," presented at AAPM 19th Annual Meeting. Cincinnati, Ohio. 1977.

BENEFIT-RISK PANEL
Wende Logan - Moderator

Gopalo Rao: Mr. Hammerstein in one of your slides you showed the energy absorbed in terms of ergs per square centimeter per roentgen, and that it increases progressively with increase in half value layer. Don't you think that the appropriate measure would be ergs per square centimeter absorbed within the breast (standard breast) for optimum image target as a function of half value layer rather than in terms of ergs per square centimeter per roentgen? Because there are other things that will change as the half value layer changes, that is penetration, image receptor sensitivity and other factors. It seems to me that a more appropriate quantity to plot would be ergs per square centimeter absorbed to obtain an optimal range against half value layer.

Dick Hammerstein: I would suggest that the information isn't in fact going to be any different. All that we are presenting there is simply energy absorbed per unit exposure and that presumably would be handled on the same basis as with mid breast dose or anything else, that is, the figures for half value layer and for exposure that would go into the analysis to determine the number of ergs per square centimeter being absorbed for a particular technique would presumably be derived from a clinical technique that the radiologist finds acceptable. That is, on the same basis as the BCDDP mid breast analysis one would use the value for half value layer for incident exposure corresponding to the technique that is actually used clinically. I would think that would be the most relevent way of dealing with that data.

Rao: It answers my question except that I do not want people to come to the conclusion that as the half value layer is increased there is indeed increased absorption of energy in the breast because if you do it the proper way I would suspect that you would come to a different conclusion.

Hammerstein: I would heartily agree that in any of these instances there is going to be a trade-off between exposure and half value layer at some point. And our intention certainly isn't to say that one ought to pay attention only to half value layer and let exposures go zooming back up or anything like that. We definitely don't intend that statement at all.

John Cameron: I would like to ask Dr. Moskowitz or Dr. Lester if they have any idea or any data available on the number of poor mammograms taken. The data you presented assumes that all the mammograms are of excellent quality, being looked at by a skilled mammographer and we certainly know that is not the true state of affairs. It would be nice if that were true but certainly the data on chest radiography indicates that a lot of technically poor chest radiographs are taken and one would expect that to be true of mammography also. Would you comment on that if you have any data or you have any suspicions from looking at mammograms that have been sent in.

Moskowitz: Well, I would try to answer that question perhaps by asking the same kind of question, when did you stop beating your wife? Certainly there are poor quality mammograms and there is difference in opinion even among experts about interpretation of mammography. Medicine is an inexact science. We're not dealing with a hard science, we're dealing with science where inter-observer agreement is considered excellent if we're talking 80-85%. We are not dealing with absolutes. Yes, there are poor quality mammograms; there are poor quality interpretations, but we can train technologists to be between 85-90% accurate in terms of agreement with me, based on our data at this point in time. So, we must always keep in mind that we don't want to throw away the baby with the bathwater. If we've got a problem but at the same time the modality is useful, we must use it to its maximum, train people to use it and get what we can from it until it can be replaced with something else which would do equally well. I think that's the approach that must be taken.

Dr. Lester: Let me add just a few words. I agree with what Mike said and what you're implying and I think that's a very important point. I think there are a number of factors that suggest that in this area we may have better quality and better levels in interpretation than in some other areas of radiology. I would like to adduce two of these: one has been the very consistent and extensive educational efforts sponsored by organizations like the American College of Radiology as well as governmental agencies in this area, which I think have been very impressive. Secondly, and I think very important has been the BENT program that the Bureau of Radiological Health has sponsored, which though it was directed specifically to radiation dosage, has had enormous spill-over in terms of quality examinations. Nonetheless I think this is an issue that radiologists must be alert to and that other clinicians must be alert to and one that needs to be constantly addressed because there is no 100% success in this area.

Ronald Ross from Cleveland: I agree with Dr. Lester that the pictures do look nicer but the dysplasias make it much more difficult to arrive at diagnoses. You can read a poor chest film perhaps and see a lesion in the chest. I would like to ask Dr. Moskowitz, of the 56 breast cancers how many were detected using the modality of suspicious calcification and how many were in fatty breast?

Moskowitz: In fact most of the cancers in the younger age group were not diagosed in fatty breasts. Most were detected in dense breasts and inter-estingly enough, 78% of those diagnosed came about as a result of breast biopsy of microcalcifications, alone. We biopsied lesions that other people might watch for a year. To get this kind of yield (whether this is cost effective and whether this is palatable or not) we have achieved, we accepted a biopsy yield rate of 1 cancer for every 9 to 10 biopsies performed (10-15%) and this is what we have maintained all along. We have compared our overall biopsy yield by surgeons, nurse palpators and by the general community of physicians in the city of Cincinnati who were biopsying, and there is only about a 5% yield on physical examination. So we're not terribly out of line. There is a big difference between screening, and diagnosis, where surgeons are used to seeing patients coming to them with "tell me what this lump is doctor".

Dr. Lester: But Mike, I think you do want to emphasize the point that this approach may be right, but it is a very aggressive biopsy policy and of course the yield of very very small cancers is directly related to this aggressive policy.

Moskowitz: It's not very palatable and not terribly acceptable to a lot of people but at the same time it's what we set out to do. As Wende says, neither is breast cancer particularly palatable to a lot of people. I think that our on-going yield and the longitudinal data are terribly impressive, and I can give you mortality data also by the way. With a 98% follow-up of all cancers up to now (and we have been in business since 1973) in the 35-49 year old age group, there are 2 patients dead of breast cancer, one of these being an interval cancer. That includes all the prevalent patients with breast cancer in that age group, some with quite far advanced disease.

Martin Braun: A question to Dr. Muntz. Have you compared the magnification systems with a low output, to the high output systems? Would that not change when you put a grid in? I think the low output system would gain by putting a grid in.

Muntz: Qualitatively you are correct. It all depends how much the grid absorbs and really it comes down to relative numbers. If you assume a perfect grid with no attenuation you get one answer, if you assume a practical grid you get a different answer. That analysis has not really been carried through for a practical grid.

Irwin Bross: This is a question for Dr. Lester. I believe he calculated the radiation induced cancers on the basis of a single examination, and the benefits from a series of examinations. Do you think this was a corect way to calculate the benefit-risk ratio?

Lester: I didn't do that. These are the statistics from one exam, and consequently one radiation dose.

Muntz: I think the answer was, if I'm not mistaken, that he used the number of cancers found from a single examination, not the number found for a whole series of examinations.

Dr. Rao: I just wanted to make a comment. I am quite impressed with the conclusions that Dr. Lester and Dr. Moscowitz have come to, as far as the importance of mammography in screening is concerned. However, at one time, I was very concerned with the therapeutic value of a diagnosis, and, in a crude way, to determine what was going on, I calculated the death rate and also the incidence rate. I took the ratio of the deaths to the incidence rate and plotted this as a function of time starting from the year 1900. I did this for various types of cancers, including breast cancer. Surprisingly, these graphs were almost straight lines in all cases of cancers except lung cancer where it was going up. On the other hand in the case of infectious diseases and others, where we have a better handle on how to deal with them the ratio fell progressively down to very small values in the year 1970. So does this not mean that we are far from attacking breast cancer in the therapeutic sense, in any satisfactory manner?

Moskowitz: I think that that is a terribly important point and it touches to the core of the argument of the paper that I wrote and why we analyzed the data and handled it as we have. Until now we have never had the ability to attack carcinoma of the breast at a stage when it is reasonably likely to truly be curable. Those data that you talk about and that I alluded to momentarily, a few moments ago, and alluded to by others is the ultimate fate of the patient with invasive breast cancer. That is, death from that disease, in no matter what stage it is detected. However, we have never in this country or any place in the world been able to find with regularity carcinoma of the breast when it is essentially in situ or minimal noninvasive cancer. Fewer than 3%, nationally (in our own data in Cincinnati over a 20 year period, less than 1½%) of cancers were minimal. We are talking about an entirely different ballgame where the 20 years survivability is 96% relative survival and, in our own series, with a 25 year follow-up, we have an 80%

141

absolute survival. This cannot be consumed by lead time if lead time is only 2½ years.

Chiacchierini: That type of a numerical gain is a very dangerous one, from the standpoint that regardless of whatever end point you use in survivability whether it be 5 years or 10 years, any change in the characteristic of the therapy of the disease will automatically alter that curve. You can take, for example, the survival rate for leukemia. Just recently in the past 4 or 5 years, the survival rate for leukemia due to the new chemotherapeutic techniques have increased dramatically. If you start taking your survival particularly on a 5 year level (the survival ratio to the incidence ratio), you are going to see a very different picture now than you saw 5 years ago. Similarly, if the disease course if being altered to the extent that Dr. Moskowitz says it is, you no longer have a true picture of incidence, by using old incidence data, so you really are talking about a rather fluid dynamic picture, than a static one.

Logan: Mike, I'm intrigued over the fact that many of the lesions that you recommended biopsies while not interpreted as carcinomas were in the "pre-malignant category" which is debatable. How do you feel this is going to affect the ultimate incidence of carcinoma in these women? We have a problem; we have a preselected group but you may have eliminated a lot of carcinomas these women will never get and we'll never prove they would have gotten it.

Moskowitz: Sixteen of them have already developed subsequent carcinoma and they are included in these data. They had prior biopsies technically inter-preted as benign, and subsequently in year 1, 2, 3 or 4 developed a carcinoma.

Logan: Are you implying then that the pathologist under-read these or that this was an incomplete removal of a premalignant lesion without borders included?

Moskowitz: These were suspicious, they had been biopsied, and the pathologists read proliferative disorder, severe atypia. One pathologist read one as an intraductal carcinoma and another said atypia, and four years later in the same breast, she developed an invasive carcinoma of the breast. We have 16 of those now. It's not a small number. I'm saying that this is a risk. That's why the whole breast has to be removed. I agree with Jerry Urban very much, there, based on the pathology work that has been done. If you've got a lesion one place in the breast, you've got to remove the whole breast because the whole breast is at risk[1].

Logan: This is why I feel very strongly that these women should be extremely closely followed, from all of these screening centers. All patients with premalignant lesions, as well as those that have been called malignant, should be followed extremely closely. I think we are going to gain a tremendous amount of information from this.

1. Rosen, PP, Lieberman, PH, Braun, DW, Kosloff, C, Adair, F, "Lobular carcinoma in situ, of the breast." Am. Jour. Surg. Path., 2(3):225-251, 1978.

PART II

TECHNICAL CONSIDERATIONS

MAMMOGRAPHY SYSTEMS CHARACTERISTICS:

HAVE WE IMPROVED IMAGE QUALITY WHILE REDUCING DOSE?

Arthur G. Haus, Gerald D. Dodd, and David D. Paulus

Departments of Diagnostic Radiology and Physics
Section of Experimental Diagnostic Radiology
The University of Texas System Cancer Center
M.D. Anderson Hospital and Tumor Institute
Houston, Texas 77030

INTRODUCTION

The field of mammography has changed dramatically during the past ten years. The introduction of new imaging techniques combined with renewed interest in breast imaging on the part of radiologists has given mammography a status comparable to other diagnostic radiology procedures. The technique has been utilized for mass screening and several controversial reports have implied that its use in asymptomatic women may produce more cancer than the technique is capable of detecting. While this result of radiation exposure to the breast is hypothetical (1,2), such reports have put mammography on the defensive, not only for the screening of asymptomatic women but also for the examination of those with symptoms. Therefore, during the past few years, considerable emphasis has been placed on dose reduction. This may be accomplished in several ways, but there is usually a concomitant decrease in image quality (3). In the following discussion some of the factors which affect image quality with the lower dose techniques will be reviewed in an attempt to provide greater insight into the present status of mammography.

MAMMOGRAPHY X-RAY UNITS

Table 1 lists some historical developments in mammographic x-ray units. Prior to the introduction of the molybdenum-target tube conventional tungsten-targets only were employed without added filtration. In 1969, the Senographe (4) became available in the United States. It was the first of a series of dedicated mammographic units. The Senographe contained a molybdenum-target tube with the beam filtered by either 0.03 mm of molybdenum or 0.5 mm of aluminum. This tube remains the most commonly used for mammography at the present time, although multiple variations on the basic mammographic unit have been marketed. Tungsten-target tubes are, for the most part, utilized only for Xeroradiography. A recent unit, which is used for magnification mammography, is also listed.

Table 1. Developments in mammographic x-ray units

DATE	UNIT	TARGET	FILTRATION (mm)
1950's-Present	Conventional Overhead Tubes	Tungsten (W)	Inherent
	DEDICATED UNITS		
1969	CGR Senographe	Molybdenum (Mo)	.03 Mo or .5 Al
1973	Siemens Mammomat	"	"
"	Philips Mammo Diag.	"	"
"	Picker Mammorex	"	"
1974	General Electric MMX	Mo/W	"
1977	Radiologic Sciences (Magnification)	W	.20 Al, 1.35 Al

Figures 1 and 2 illustrate the basic characteristics of molybdenum-target tubes. Figure 1 shows the x-ray emission spectra from a typical molybdenum

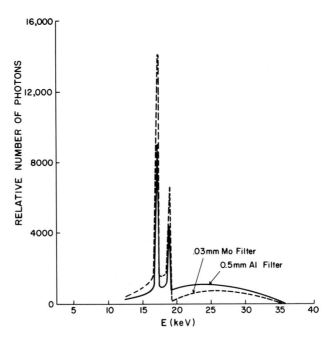

Fig. 1. X-ray emission spectra from a molybdenum anode tube with 0.03 mm molybdenum (Mo) and 0.5 mm aluminum (Al) filtration.

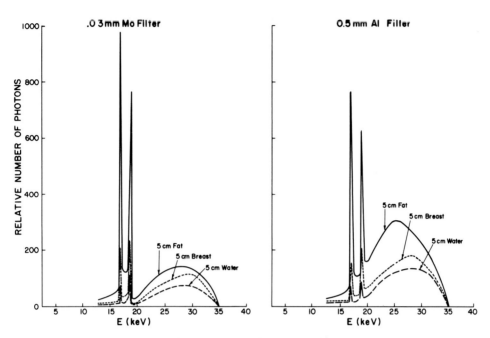

Fig. 2. X-ray spectra transmitted through 5 cm of fat, 5 cm of water, and 5 cm of breast tissue with 0.03 mm molybdenum (left) and 0.5 mm aluminum filters (right).

anode tube when the 0.03 mm molybdenum filter and 0.5 aluminum filter are used (5). The intense spectra lines at 17.9 and 19.5 keV are due to the characteristic Kα and Kβ radiations from the molybdenum target. When the 0.03 molybdenum filter is used, the spectrum is strongly suppressed at photon energies greater than 20 keV because of the K shell absorption edge of molybdenum at that energy. The use of such a concentration of low energy photons is especially important in film and screen-film mammography in order to provide high subject contrast.

The 0.5 mm aluminum filter is the minimal added filtration for Xeroradiographic systems. When used, the intensity of the characteristic lines is reduced relative to that of the higher energy portion. In essence, the aluminum filter causes hardening of the beam. Due to the inherent edge enhancement characteristics of the Xeroradiography system the subject contrast may not have to be as high as in film and screen-film mammography. Therefore, within limits, a harder x-ray beam may be used without appreciable sacrifice in image quality. In fact, the harder beam may be desirable in denser or larger breasts to obtain better penetration.

As more aluminum filtration is added, there will be a reduction in intensity of the characteristic lines relative to the number of photons in the higher energy portion of the spectrum. Therefore, as the beam becomes harder, the x-ray spectrum more closely simulates that of a tungsten target. The harder beam will not only reduce exposure to the breast surface but will also reduce contrast.

In order to better understand the useful beam quality and its relationship to dose, it is important to evaluate both the incident spectra and the spectra transmitted through the breast (5,6). Figure 2 shows spectra transmitted through 5 cm of fat and 5 cm of water representing the extremes of tissue composition in both breasts (5). Also shown are the spectra transmitted through a resected breast of a 35-year-old woman compressed to approximately 5 cm. On the left are the spectra using the 0.03 mm molybdenum filter and on the right are the spectra using 0.5 mm aluminum filter. The exposure conditions were the same for both measurements. Note the considerable difference between the spectra transmitted by fat and water with either filter. The spectrum transmitted by the resected breast more closely resembles the spectrum transmitted by water than that transmitted by fat. These spectra show that for fat a higher percentage of low energy photons is incident on the recording system; for breast tissue and water a higher percentage of low energy photons is absorbed and therefore does not contribute to formation of the image.

Clinically, for the predominantly fatty breast, a high percentage of low energy photons is transmitted and is utilized for the recording of the image when the molybdenum filter is used. The number of low energy photons is reduced considerably when the aluminum filter is used with a consequent reduction in contrast. For the denser, more glandular breast or for water the low energy characteristic lines are reduced considerably compared to fat if the 0.03 mm molybdenum filter is used. If the 0.5 mm aluminum filter is used, there is not a significant change in the shape of the transmitted spectra for water and for this particular type of breast. Therefore, there may not be a significant difference in subject contrast for the water or for the breast regardless of which filter is used. However, the radiation exposure to the skin of the breast would be less with the aluminum filter.

The 0.5 mm aluminum filter was commonly used for Xeroradiography until the emphasis on dose reduction. As more aluminum filtration is added, radiation exposure to the breast surface is reduced, but subject contrast is also reduced. If the Xerox receptor is used, the subject contrast may not have to be as high due to edge enhancement. Therefore, the hardened beam may still result in acceptable contrast. However, this approach should be used cautiously, since, at some point, there will be a critical loss of subject contrast resulting from excessive beam hardening. It is still debatable as to what the total beam filtration should be. This depends on the radiologist's attitude regarding image contrast and dose.

In this context it should be noted that with dense breasts the transmitted spectra look quite similar regardless of whether a molybdenum or aluminum filter is used. This is, of course, a function of the absorptive capacity of the subject tissue and tends to offset the contrast advantage gained by use of the molybdenum filter.

Another factor relating to the x-ray tube is the effect of geometric unshaprness. This is determined by the size, the shape, and the intensity distribution of the focal spot in combination with the focal spot-to-object and object-to-recording system distances (7). This effect is illustrated in Figure 3. On the left is the geometrical configuration for imaging a 5 cm thick breast and on the right the modulation transfer functions (MTF) of geometric unsharpness corresponding to two extreme image planes of the breast, A and B. Also shown is the MTF of a screen-film system designed for mammography. In Plane "B" geometric unsharpness is not a limiting factor in the resolution capability of the system as it has better MTF characteristics than the image receptor. It should also be noted that scatter from composition density and thickness of the breast reduces contrast and, therefore, image quality. These factors become more important with progressively unfavorable geometric conditions.

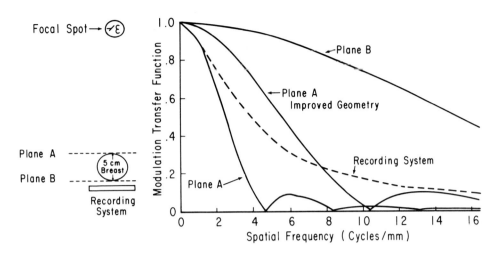

Fig. 3. Illustration of the effect of geometric unsharpness. On the left a
diagram illustrating the geometric setup for imaging a 5 cm thick breast.
On the right are MTF's of geometric unsharpness corresponding to Plane A,
Plane B, and Plane A with improved geometry. Also shown is the MTF of the
screen-film system designed for mammography.

Greater resolution of detail in Plane "A" of the breast can be achieved by
increasing the focal spot-to-object distance. The effect will be to decrease
the geometric unsharpness of the system to a point which exceeds the MTF of the
image receptor. Full benefit of the resolution capability of the receptor can
then be obtained. One wonders how frequently this situation is unrecognized in
mammography.

The modulation transfer function of geometric unsharpness based on line
spread function measurements of the focal spot is rather difficult to evaluate
and requires the use of a lead or platinum jaw slit apparatus, an x-ray sen-
sitometer, a microdensitometer, and a computer. However, we believe it is important to measure the focal spot size and not to rely on the manufacturer's
nominal dimensions. We have used a simple technique to evaluate geometric unsharpness for mammographic units. For this measurement a star resolution test
object was used (8). For most mammographic units, including the ones discussed
in Figures 4, 5, 6, and 7, the star technique will provide an accurate measurement of the equivalent focal spot size (9). With this measurement the limit of
geometric resolution for any plane within the breast can be easily calculated.

Figure 4 shows the geometric configuration employed with an overhead
tungsten-target tube used several years ago in our department for nonscreen
film mammography. The nominal dimension of the focal spot provided by the manufacturer was 2 mm. The measured focal spot, using the star technique, was 3.2
mm. The limit of resolution is indicated for 1 cm, 3 cm, and 6 cm object-to-
recording system distances. Similar schematics are provided for various dedicated mammographic units in Figures 5, 6, and 7. In reviewing these it should
be kept in mind that nonscreen films have resolution capabilities which exceed
40 cycles/mm. Several other recording systems, including Lo-dose/2, Min-R,
Xerox, and Xonics, have resolution capabilities of at least 12 cycles/mm. The
limit of resolution with this overhead tungsten-target tube was quite low.
Before dedicated mammographic units became available, compression was not as
refined nor as widely used as it is today. In some cases the breast thickness

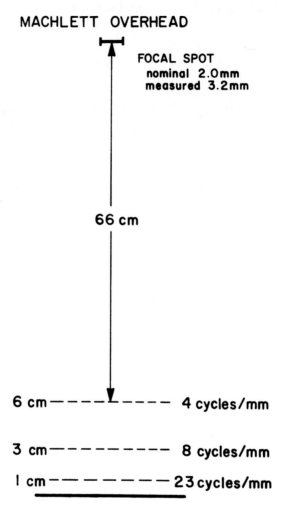

Fig. 4. Geometric configuration for the Machlett overhead tungsten target tube. The nominal focal spot
size provided by the manufacturer and the measured
equivalent focal spot sizes are shown. The limit of
resolution is indicated for 1 cm, 3 cm, and 6 cm
object-to-recording system distances. (Similar data
is provided for Figures 5, 6, and 7)

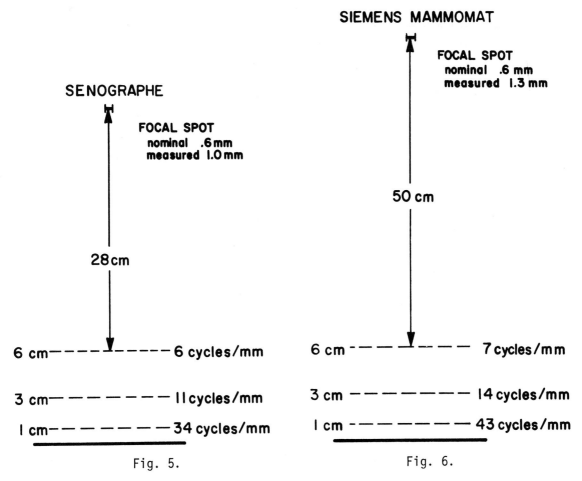

Fig. 5.   Fig. 6.

Geometric configuration for the CGR Senographe (Figure 5) and the Siemens Mammomat (Figure 6) dedicated mammographic units.

may have been greater than 6 cm with a corresponding decrease in resolution.
Additionally, for mediolateral projections in which the breast was position with
underlying sponges, the object-to-recording system distance was increased with
a further degradation of geometric resolution. Obviously, the resolution capability of nonscreen film was not being fully utilized. In fact, the capabilities of Min-R, Lo-dose/2, Xerox, and Xonics cannot be fully utilized with this
geometric relationship and focal spot size.

Figures 5 and 6 show the geometric setup for two dedicated mammographic
units, the CGR Senographe and the Siemens Mammomat. The nominal focal spot for
the Senographe is 0.6 mm and the measured focal spot using the star is 1.0 mm.
The limit of resolution at the three planes are 34, 11, and 6 cycles/mm. The
nominal focal spot for the Mammomat is 0.6 mm, and the measured size using the
star is 1.3 mm. The limits of resolution at the three planes are 43, 14, and
7 cycles/mm.

Figure 7 shows the RSI magnification technique. We have evaluated several
magnification units at M. D. Anderson (10). One of our primary concerns has

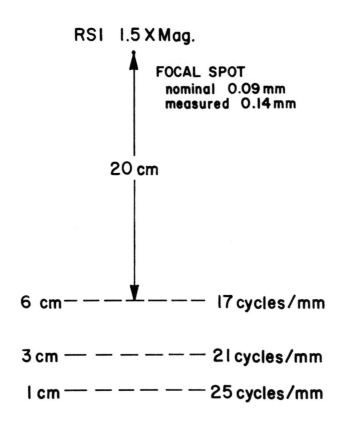

RSI 1.5 X Mag.

FOCAL SPOT
nominal 0.09 mm
measured 0.14 mm

20 cm

6 cm — — — — — — 17 cycles/mm

3 cm — — — — — — 21 cycles/mm

1 cm — — — — — — 25 cycles/mm

Fig. 7. Geometric configuration for the Radiologic Sciences,
Inc. (RSI) magnification mammographic unit.

been the unit maintain its geometric resolution so that the magnification is
used effectively. The nominal dimension of the focal spot is .09 millimeter
and the measured focal spot .14 millimeter. The limit of resolution corresponding to the 3 breast planes are 25, 21, and 17 cycles/mm. Therefore, with the
present mammographic screen-film combinations or the Xeroradiography system,
geometric unsharpness will not be a limiting factor for this magnification
technique.

During the past few years several studies have indicated that the effect
of geometric unsharpness is a significant limiting factor in obtaining maximum
resolution of the breast image (7). However, this remains a defect in many of
the dedicated mammographic units presently available. It is highly unlikely
that the effect of geometric unsharpness was less significant with conventional
tubes due to the large focal spot sizes often employed and the lack of effective compression. While the present dedicated units are somewhat better in this
regard, many units could be improved to insure that the image recording systems
are the limiting factor in resolution and not geometric unsharpness.

Table 2. Developments in mammographic recording systems

DATE	SYSTEM
1950's - Present	Non-Screen Industrial Film (Manual or industrial automatic processing)
1970	RP/M Non-screen Film for Mammography (90 second automatic processing)
1971	Xeroradiography (low kVp, minimal beam filtration)
1972	DuPont Lo-dose Screen-Film System
1976	DuPont Lo-dose/2 Screen-Film System Kodak Min-R Screen-Film System
	Xerox program to increase filtration with higher kVp
1977	Xonics Electron Radiography

MAMMOGRAPHIC RECORDING SYSTEMS

Table 2 lists some historic developments in mammographic recording systems. The nonscreen industrial-type film was used for many years for mammography (11). In 1971, Xeroradiography became available (12). Until this time little attention was paid to dose reduction techniques. Attention was primarily directed to the use of a recording system which could provide a mammogram of high resolution, low noise, and high contrast. In 1972, the first screen-film combination designed for mammography, the DuPont Lo-dose system, became available (13). Shortly thereafter the mammography radiation dose controversy began. In 1976, the DuPont Lo-dose/2 and the Kodak Min-R screen-film systems were introduced. These systems are faster than the Lo-dose system by approximately a factor of 2. Also, in 1976, the Xerox Corporation introduced the option of increasing tube filtration to reduce radiation exposure to the breast. This essentially consisted of modification of the Xerox processing unit so that higher filtration techniques, which sometimes require higher kVp as well, could be used with maintenance of adequate contrast. In 1977, the Xonics electron radiography system became available (14).

Some basic characteristics of the various mammographic recording systems are discussed below. Details of the physical characteristics of these recording systems will be discussed by other authors in this volume.

NONSCREEN FILMS

Some advantages of nonscreen films compared to screen-film systems include: 1) lower noise, 2) higher resolution, 3) higher film contrast at higher film density, and 4) the capability of using a two-film pack system (two films of two different sensitivities). Disadvantages compared to screen-film systems include; 1) higher radiation exposure (7-30x), 2) longer exposure times often with resultant motion unsharpness, 3) lower film contrast at lower film density, and 4) manual or industrial type processing.

SCREEN-FILM SYSTEMS FOR MAMMOGRAPHY

Advantages of screen-film systems compared to nonscreen film include: 1) lower radiation exposure, 2) higher film contrast at low film density, 3) high speed allowing short exposure times, and reduced scatter through the use of grids (15), 4) automatic 90 second film processing, and 5) use of other methods to improve image quality such as magnification (10,16). Disadvantages compared to nonscreen film include: 1) lower resolution, 2) higher noise, 3) reciprocity law failure at long exposure times, and 4) artifacts from the screen.

One factor often overlooked in mammography is the effect of reciprocity law failure when screen-film systems are used (17,18). The reciprocity law states that it is immaterial whether a high exposure over a short time interval or a low exposure over a long time interval is used, as long as the total exposure is the same. Film exposed directly to x-rays obeys this rule, but film exposed to light from an intensifying screen does not (19). A simple experiment was performed which illustrates the practical importance of this problem. (Figure 8). The Kodak Pathe Mammography Test object was used. The mammography chamber (20) was placed over the top of the phantom with the screen-

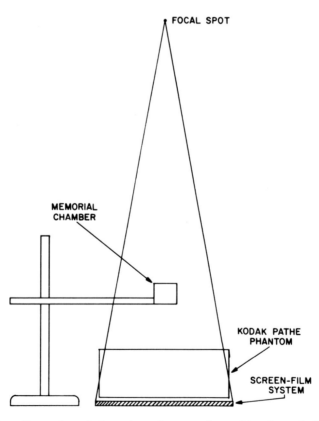

Fig. 8.   Experimental setup for reciprocity law failure measurements.

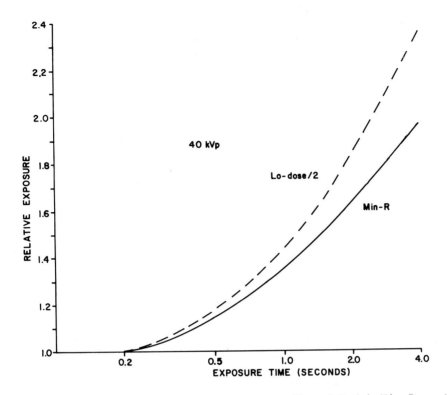

Fig. 9. Relative speeds for DuPont Lo-dose/2 and Kodak Min-R systems versus exposure time.

film system below the phantom. The receptor was exposed to a density of 1.2 using a 0.2 second exposure time. The corresponding exposure in roentgens was recorded. The exposure time was changed to 0.5 seconds, 1.0, 2, and 4 seconds and the corresponding exposure in roentgens recorded. Results are shown in Figure 9 for the Kodak Min-R and DuPont Lo-dose/2 systems.

The radiation exposure dose necessary to produce a specific density increased quite significantly as the exposure time increased. For example, the radiation exposure increases by approximately a factor of 2 when an exposure time of 4 seconds is used. Therefore, it is most important to use short exposure times. This is of practical importance in magnification mammography where exposure times of up to 4 seconds are sometimes necessary for screen-film systems. Likewise, this may be important when grids are used and longer exposure times required. Reciprocity law failure varies for different exposure times and for different films.

XERORADIOGRAPHY

It is difficult to compare physical factors as resolution, contrast, and noise for the Xeroradiographic system with screen-film and film systems. The advantages of Xeroradiography are well known and include wide latitude and increased small area contrast as a result of the edge enhancement effect. However, these do not have exact counterparts in film systems.

Also, as pointed out previously, even though subject contrast may not have to be as high for Xeroradiography due to its edge enhancement, it is most important that contrast is not reduced by too much filtration or by excessively high kVp settings. Both may result in loss of diagnostic detail.

CONCLUSIONS

Several conclusions can be drawn by comparison of the image quality obtained a few years ago with high dose techniques and that achieved with current low dose recording systems and techniques.

Tungsten targets were used prior to the introduction of dedicated mammographic units with molybdenum target tubes. With tungsten target tubes, subject contrast is lower for film mammography. The use of the molybdenum target provides increased subject contrast. The resolution capability of nonscreen film was seldom fully utilized, since geometric unsharpness was the limiting resolution factor.

Nonscreen films were often overexposed and bright-lighted to take full advantage of the high contrast. The primary advantage of nonscreen film is the lower noise compared to screen-film systems. Therefore, if a) subject contrast is good, b) photographic density range is such that film contrast is high, and c) the effects of geometric unsharpness and motion unsharpness are minimal, it is technically possible to obtain better image quality using nonscreen film than with screen-film or Xeroradiographic systems.

For screen-film systems the resolution is lower and the noise level is higher than in nonscreen film. However, lower resolution is not critical if geometric unsharpness is the limiting factor. Improvement in image quality can be accomplished by optimizing other factors including: 1) geometric unsharpness by using longer focal spot-to-skin distances, 2) short exposure times to reduce motion unsharpness and avoid additional exposure due to reciprocity law failure, 3) lower kVp techniques, 4) use of grids to reduce scatter, and 5) selected application of magnification techniques.

For Xeroradiography wide latitude and edge enhancement offer technical advantages that make Xeroradiographs easier to evaluate. However, it is important to avoid excessive filtration of the beam or excessively high kilovoltages which could result in reduced subject contrast. It is also important, as with screen-film or film systems, that geometric unsharpness not be the limiting factor in resolution.

In summary, there are technical advantages and disadvantages for both the higher and lower dose techniques. On the basis of physical measurements it is difficult to determine which system or technique is best. However, by evaluating the factors which affect image quality and by optimizing limiting factors, image quality can be and has been improved. This improvement may be obtained with lower dose techniques if both equipment and recording system factors are considered for the total mammographic imaging system and properly optimized.

REFERENCES

1. Bailar, J.C.: Mammography: A contrary view. Am Intern Med 84:77-84, January, 1976
2. Bailar, J.C.: Screening for early breast cancer: pros and cons. Cancer 39: 2783-2795, 1977.
3. Haus, A.G., Doi, K., Metz, C.E., and Bernstein, J.: Image quality in mammography. Radiology 125:77-85, October, 1977

4. Gershon-Cohen, J., Hermel, M.B., and Birsner, J.W.: Advances in mammographic technique. Am J Roentgenol 108:424-427, February, 1970

5. Haus, A.G., Metz, C.E., Doi, K., and Bernstein, J.: Determination of x-ray spectra incident on and transmitted through breast tissue. Radiology 124:511-513, August, 1977

6. Haus, A.G., Metz, C.E., Chiles, J.T., and Rossmann, K.: The effect of x-ray spectra from molybdenum and tungsten target tubes on image quality in mammography. Radiology 118:705-709, March, 1976

7. Haus, A.G.: The effect of geometric unsharpness in mammography and Xeroradiography. Breast Carcinoma, The Radiologists Expanding Role, Edited by W. Logan, J. Wiley and Sons, 605 Third Avenue, New York, New York:93-108, 1977

8. Haus, A.G., Cowart, R.W., Dodd, G.D., Bencomo, J., and Paulus, D.: A method of evaluating and minimizing geometric unsharpness for mammographic x-ray units. Radiology 128:775-778, September, 1978

9. Braun, M.: X-ray tube performance characteristics and their effect on radiologic image quality. Society of Photo-Optical Instrumentation Engineers. Proceedings (Recent and Future Trends in Medical Imaging) Vol. 152:94-103, 1978

10. Haus, A.G., Paulus, D.D., Dodd, G.D., and Bencomo, J.: Evaluation of magnification mammography. Society of Photo-Optical Instrumentation Engineers. Proceedings (Recent and Future Trends in Medical Imaging) Vol. 152:85-92, 1978

11. Egan, R.L.: Mammographic image quality and exposure levels using conventional generators and type M film. Application of Optical Instrumentation in Medicine IV:393-397, 1976

12. Wolfe, J.N.: Developments in mammography. Am J Obstet Gynecol Vol. 124 No.3:312-323, February, 1976

13. Weiss, J.P., and Wayrynen, R.E.: Imaging system for low-dose mammography. J App Phot Eng Vol.2, No.1:7-10, Winter, 1976

14. Muntz, E.P., Lewis, J., Azzarelli, T., et al: On the characteristics of electron radiographic images in diagnostic radiology. SPIE Proceedings 56, 1975

15. Friedrich, M., and Weskamp, P.: New modalities in mammographic imaging: comparision of grid and magnification techniques. Medicamundi Vol. 23:1-16, 1978

16. Sickles, E.A., Doi, K., and Genant, H.K.: Magnification film mammography: image quality and clinical studies. Radiology 125:69-76, October, 1977

17. Arnold, B.A., Eisenberg, H., and Bjarngard, B.E.: Measurement of reciprocity law failure in green sensitive x-ray films. Radiology 126:493-498, February, 1978

18. Bencomo, J., and Haus, A.G.: The effect of reciprocity law failure when determining the characteristic curve for screen-film systems (abstract) Medical Physics 5 (4):322-323, July/August, 1978

19. Mees, C.E.K., and James, J.T.: The theory of the photographic process. New York:MacMillan, 1966

20. Rothenberg, L.A., Kirch, R.L.A., and Snyder, R.E.: Patient exposure from film and Xeroradiographic mammographic techniques. Radiology 117:701-703, December, 1975

INTENSIFYING SCREEN AND ELECTROSTATIC IMAGING IN MAMMOGRAPHY: INFORMATION AND DISPLAY PARAMETERS

Robert F. Wagner, Ph.D.
Medical Physics Branch
Division of Electronic Products
Bureau of Radiological Health, FDA,
Rockville, MD 20857

E. Phillip Muntz, Ph.D.
Departments of Aerospace Engineering and Radiology
University of Southern California
Los Angeles, CA 90007

I. INTRODUCTION

The purpose of this paper is to present classical image parameter measurements on an intensifying screen/film mammography system, the Kodak Min-R system, and the same measurements on an electrostatic mammography system, the Xonics electron radiographic (XERG) system.* These measurements will be interpreted from two points of view: (1) How much information is recorded by the system? (2) How is the information displayed by the system? This distinction and its implementation have been emphasized in the recent literature (1,2,3,4) and we believe that the mammographic context provides a practical demonstration of the need for the two points of view.

The imaging measurements are: (1) the system gray-scale and speed characteristics, summarized in the density (D) versus exposure (E or log E) dependence; (2) the system modulation transfer function (MTF), a description of image fidelity and sharpness; and (3) the system noise characteristics, summarized in the noise power or Wiener spectrum (W_D) of the density fluctuations.

II. IMAGING MEASUREMENTS

(1) DENSITY VERSUS EXPOSURE CHARACTERISTIC CURVES

The large area exposure characteristic for the XERG system is shown in Figure 1. The system is linear with an x-intercept of 1 to 2 mR, corresponding to a bias voltage of 10 volts (earlier work shows that the system is linear up to densities higher than 2.5 optical density units) (5). The measured points are · replotted in Figure 2 together with the corresponding results for the Min-R system, for which we have data over a wider range of exposures in this study. Both systems required about 20 mR at the cassette to achieve a density of 1.0. The beam quality used for the Min-R system corresponds to a spectrum used in the paper by Jennings et al. (6): W anode tube at 30 kVp, 0.002" Pd filter, (at this point HVL = 0.72 mm Al, $\bar{E}$ = 21 keV), through 5 cm lucite phantom (at cassette HVL = 0.94 mm Al, $\bar{E}$ = 22.4 keV). The beam quality used _for the XERG measurements is characterized by: W anode, Al filtered beam with $\bar{E}$ = 20.5 keV.

---

*The mention of commercial products herein is not to be construed as either an actual or implied endorsement of such products by the Department of Health, Education and Welfare.

The slope of the D versus log Exposure curve at a given operating point is referred to as the point gamma (7), $\dot{\gamma}$. At a density of 1.0 a value of $\dot{\gamma} = 2.1 \pm 0.1$ was found for the Min-R system. The value for the XERG system can be calculated with high accuracy from Figure 1 using the scaling relation

$$\dot{\gamma} = g\, E/\log_{10} e \qquad\qquad (1)$$

between $\dot{\gamma}$ and g, the slope of the linear D versus E characteristic, and at an operating point corresponding to exposure E. At D = 1.0 a value of $\dot{\gamma} = 2.3$ is obtained for the XERG system. Eq. (1) indicates that this value continues to increase as a function of exposure while g is constant. The XERG system may be varied to provide significantly different γ's or process speed, by changing conditions in the processor. The values obtained here are fairly typical but by no means unique. (For further discussion about the complexities of electrostatic image development in radiography the reader is referred to Muntz et al. (5). For the range of conditions usually found in XERG mammography, reference should also be made to the article by Kaegi (8) in this proceedings.)

(2) MODULATION TRANSFER FUNCTION

The detail contrast transfer characteristic used in this study is the modulation transfer function (MTF), a measure in the spatial frequency domain. This can be obtained from scans of images of bar patterns, or from scans of slit images or edge images (9). The slit method has been preferred over the edge technique for screen-film systems since the edge technique requires differentiation and this intrinsically enhances high frequency noise. Both methods are sensitive to alignment of the test target and the tube focus.

The edge scan method was used for determining the MTF of the XERG system simply because edge images were available. In Figure 3 we give the result of averaging ten parallel scans across an XERG edge using the PDS microdensitometer (0.11 N.A., 15 μm x 600 μm post-slit). The ordinate is the specular density corresponding to the microdensitometer optics and geometry. It is higher than the more commonly used diffuse density by the Callier coefficient, Q. The value of Q ranged from 1.10 to 1.20 over the range of densities in the scan (Q values for x-ray and photographic film in this range are close to 1.4). This variation of less than 10 percent is neglected in our analysis, and is indeed negligible in the context of further simplifications and errors discussed below.

After experimenting with numerical techniques for smoothing and differentiating edge scans, it was determined that smoothing by eye and simple differentiation of successive parabolic three point sections gave the most repeatable estimates of the line spread function (LSF) and its Fourier transform, the MTF. The resulting MTF for the XERG system is given in Figure 4. With the conventional normalization to unity at zero spatial frequency (not shown in logarithmic coordinates), the system MTF takes on values greater than 2 in the mid-frequency range between 0.5 mm^{-1} and 1.5 mm^{-1}, where the eye has its maximum sensitivity at normal viewing distances (0.5 m) and normal radiographic display luminances (10). At frequencies beyond 4 mm^{-1} the results are noisy and uncertainties regarding the edge alignment remain.

Both edge and slit techniques for screen-film MTF determination are undergoing refinement and error analysis in the BRH laboratories. We depend, at present, therefore, on the Kodak measurement of the MTF for the Min-R system given in the Kodak Min-R brochure. It is also shown in Figure 4. Contrast degradation is seen to be negligible below 1 mm^{-1}, and the MTF fall-off is quite slow compared to that of conventional screen-film characteristics.

(3) SPECTRUM OF DENSITY FLUCTUATIONS

The density fluctuations will be characterized by their noise power (Wiener) spectrum. For the XERG system the region just beyond the high density side of the edge measured for Figure 3 was measured by the techniques of Ref. (11) (P.D.S. microdensitometer, 0.11 N.A., 15μm x 1200 μm post-slit). This region had a diffuse density of 0.96 - 0.98 (specular or instrument density = 1.16). The resulting measured noise power spectrum W_D is shown in Figure 5: the measured results are normalized to diffuse density for this figure by multiplying the measured values by $1/Q^2$. The contribution to density fluctuations from the film and its processing alone are shown dashed. This result was obtained from measurements on a sample obtained by applying to the image receptor a uniform charge distribution with a corona discharge and then processing the receptor in a normal development cycle to a density of 0.98 ± 0.02.

The density fluctuations for the Min-R system were obtained in like manner from films exposed with the beam quality of Sec. II (1) to a density of 1.0 ± 0.02. The resulting spectrum is also shown in Figure 5, solid curve, together with results for Min-R film flashed with green light and normally developed to the same density, dashed curve. Again the results are normalized to diffuse density (Q = 1.4).

The spectrum for the XERG system is everywhere higher than that for the Min-R system. Both systems have about the same noise bandwidth, and strikingly similar shapes. Finally, at the lowest spatial frequencies there are strong contributions to both spectra from the film and its processing alone.

All the above noise measurements have a precision better than 10 percent and a reproducibility of about 10 percent for the solid curves, and dashed curves above 1 mm^{-1}, and 15 - 20 percent for the dashed curves in the lowest frequencies.

III. ANALYSIS

The fundamental limitation to image information content was identified by many investigators in the 1940's and 1950's to be the number of quanta effectively used to form the image (Ref. 12 traces the development of this work). The word "effectively" refers to the fact that the actual noise limiting the image information content may be greater than the noise associated with the exposure quanta. This leads to the concept of noise equivalent quanta (NEQ), the number of quanta inferred from a noise measurement as being effective in forming the image (12,13). It is generally lower than the density of exposure quanta, due to less than 100 percent absorption of exposure quanta, and additional sources of noise in the detector, e.g., a variable brightness gain in a phosphor due to optical path differences for light from different absorption depths, or local variations in K-fluorescence escape. The NEQ value is obtained from a measurement of the density fluctuations by scaling this measurement to the exposure axis. If we take out the film noise component for separate analysis the scaling becomes

$$W_D(f) = \frac{(\log_{10} e)^2 \gamma^2}{NEQ_x} MTF^2(f) + W_D(FILM) \qquad (2)$$

The reader might be tempted to identify this formula with the model used by Rossmann (14), Lubberts (15) and others for quantum mottle and its transfer to film. It is used here, however, not as a model but as the appropriate scaling law from density fluctuations to equivalent x-ray exposure fluctuations. (13)

Based on the reproducibility of the measurements and previous experience we will apply Eq. (2) to the noise measurements at 1 mm^{-1}. The difference of the XERG noise from its film noise at this value is approximately 15 μm^2. Values of the point gamma at density 1.0, and the MTF at 1 mm^{-1} for this system are given in Table I and are used in the first term of Eq. (2) to obtain a value of NEQ$_x$ of 3.4 x 10^5 /mm^2 at this operating condition. Similarly for the Min-R system we read from Figure 5 a difference between the screen-film noise and film noise alone a value of approximately 2 μm^2 at 1 mm^{-1}. Substitution into the first term of Eq. (2) yields an NEQ$_x$ value here of 3.8 x 10^5/mm^2. Based on the errors stated above the difference in the NEQ$_x$ values for the two systems is not significant.

Both the Min-R system and the XERG system required about 20 mR exposure to achieve a film density of 1.0. For the beam quality incident upon the cassette this represents about 1.25 x 10^6 quanta/mm^2 for the Min-R beam (6), and slightly less than this value for the XERG beam. Discounting cassette absorption, it is estimated that both image receptors extract about 50 percent of the photons in the incident beam. This should yield about 6 x 10^5 quanta/mm^2, a value 50 percent in excess of the measured NEQ value. This is an excess of almost 2 sigmas based on the errors in W_D and γ given above and suggests a search for additional noise sources in these systems.

Plus-X film was used with the Min-R screen in additional slower (i.e., higher) exposures to attempt to separate the quantum noise from possible structure noise. It was concluded that the variability of the low frequency noise in the film processed after exposure with light was in the same order as the effect being investigated. The question of screen structure noise therefore remains open. (If such noise is numerically significant it would probably remain important only for the rigorous quantification of information; it would not be clinically visible.)

The remaining source of discrepancy is the possibility of a broad pulse height distribution for the screen light in the Min-R case and variable charge generation and collection in the XERG case, i.e., intrinsic gain fluctuations. Work proceeds in at least three institutions on the former question (16,17,18) and at least in one institution on the latter (19). It is too early to assess the significance of this work to the discrepancy noted here.

We note that our application of eq. (2) to the XERG system assumes that the MTF measured using the large contrast edge shown in Figure 3 remains the same for the very small contrast changes found in the image noise. Such an assumption is not unreasonable, yet not established. Muntz has shown that a sufficient condition is that the toner particles follow the electro-static field lines (5). Thourson (20) has reported that the peak-to-peak contrast at a step edge is asymptotically linear for low voltage contrasts with the xeroradiographic system. The development process for this latter system is not unlike that of the XERG system.

Since the step contrast and possibly the peak-to-peak contrast at a step might be proportional to voltage contrast, the assumption of a contrast independent MTF as used here is not unreasonable. The assumption will have to be tested by studying lower contrast edges.

IV. CONCLUSIONS

The Min-R intensifying screen-film system and the XERG electrostatic imaging system yield about the same number of noise equivalent quanta (NEQ$_x$) in the image according to the measurements and scaling law given above (we have given here only an indication of the plausibility of equal low frequency information density, not a proof). The noise measurements also indicate that both systems have about the same bandwidth limitation. Their exposure requirements are similar (at the cassette). We conclude that there is limited evidence that the two systems have the same information/radiation efficiency.

The more difficult aspect of imaging performance to quantify is the ultimate display. The measurements indicate that the XERG system has both a higher large area, or low frequency, display contrast and a higher mid-frequency display contrast near the maximum of visual sensitivity. The high frequency contrast transfer was not measured accurately enough to make further conclusions, but the noise transfer characteristics indicate that the systems are comparable in this region.

The ultimate significance of these results needs to be tested subjectively. For example, high intensity illumination or some reduction in subject contrast is required with the XERG system in order to achieve the same large area latitude as the Min-R system. The edge enhancement of the former makes up somewhat for this latitude constraint, however.

We conclude that further progress in mammography requires knowledge of whether its tasks are information limited, display limited, or both. If mammography is display limited, the objective measurements indicate that the XERG system offers an advantage through higher display contrasts in low and mid-frequency ranges.

If mammography is information limited, both systems will have to improve by either:

(1) improving on detection efficiency;
(2) coping with image scatter;
(3) employing more optimal x-ray spectra.

If mammography is not information limited, faster systems could be used. These questions are explored by others elsewhere in this conference.

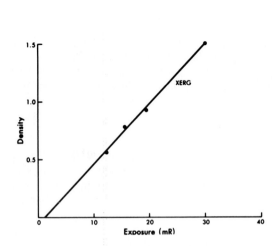

Fig. 1. Density versus Exposure for XERG system as used in this study.

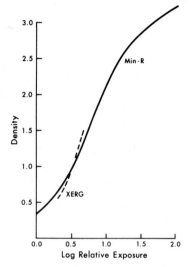

Fig. 2. Density versus log Exposure for XERG and Min-R systems as used in this study.

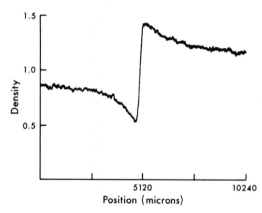

Fig. 3. Average of ten traces of XERG edge.

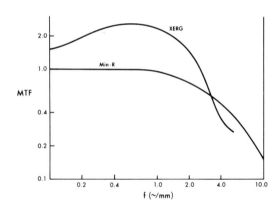

Fig. 4. Modulation transfer function (MTF) for XERG and Min-R systems.

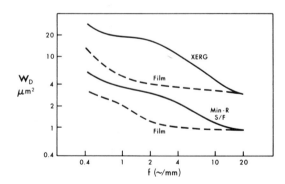

Fig. 5. Noise power (Wiener) spectra W_D for XERG and Min-R systems exposed with x rays (solid) and with uniform charge or light distributions (dashed).

	$\dot{\gamma}$	MTF(1/mm)	n	q
Min-R	2.1	0.95	$3.8 \times 10^5/mm^2$	$>10^6/mm^2$
XERG	2.3	2.25	3.4	"

Table I. Summary imaging parameters for Min-R and XERG systems.

164

REFERENCES

1. Motz, J.W., and M. Danos.   Image information content and patient exposure. Med Phys 5:8-22 (1978).

2. Muntz, E.P., M. Welkowsky, E. Kaegi, L. Morsell, E. Wilkinson, G. Jacobson. Optimization of electrostatic imaging system for minimum patient dose or minimum exposure in mammography. Radiology 127, 517-523 (1978).

3. Wagner, R.F. Decision theory and the detail signal-to-noise ratio of Otto Schade. Photog Sci & Engr 22: 41-46 (1978).

4. Wagner, R.F., D.G. Brown and M.S. Pastel. The application of information theory to the assessment of computed tomography. Med Phys (to be published).

5. Muntz, E.P., J. Lewis, T. Azzarelli, M. Welkowsky, A.L. Morsell, E. Kaegi and G. Jacobson. On the characteristics of electron radiographic images in diagnostic radiology. In Medical x-ray photo-optical systems evaluation, Proceedings of a symposium, Ed. by K.E. Weaver, R.F. Wagner, and D.J. Goodenough. (SPIE Proceedings 56, or HEW publ (FDA) 76-8020, US GPO, Washington, DC 1975-76) pp. 45-53.

6. Jennings et al. This conference, and private communication.

7. Wagner R.F. Toward a unified view of radiological imaging systems. Part II: Noisy Images. Med Phys 4:279-296 (1977).

8. Kaegi, E. Ths conference.

9. Doi K. and K. Rossmann. Measurements of optical and noise properties of screen-film systems in radiography. In Medical x-ray photo-optical systems evaluation. See Ref. 5.

10. DeBelder, M., R. Bollen & R. Duville. A new approach to the evaluation of radiographic systems. J. Photog. Sci. 19:126 (1971).

11. Wagner, R.F. Fast fourier digital quantum mottle analysis with application to rare-earth intensifying screen systems. Med Phys 4:157-162 (1977).

12. Dainty, J.C. and R. Shaw. Image Science (Academic Press, New York, 1974).

13. Shaw, R. Some fundam ental properties of xeroradiographic images. Proc SPIE 70:359-363 (1975).

14. Rossmann, K. Recording of x-ray quantum fluctuations in radiographs. J. Opt. Soc. Am 52,1162-1164 (1962).

15. Lubberts, G. Random noise produced by x-ray fluorescent screens. J Opt Soc Am 58:1475-1483 (1968).

16. Kingsley, J.D. General Electric Corporate R & D (private communication).

17. Dick, C. National Bureau of Standards (private communication).

18. Rohrig, H. University of Arizona (private communication).

19. Korn, D.M. Influence of random fluctuations in charge transport upon image quality in electroradiography. J of Appl Photog Engr 4:48-51 (1978).

20. Thourson, T.L. Xeroradiography. In Medical x-ray photo-optical systems evaluation. See Ref. 5.

OBSERVED DETECTOR CHARACTERISTICS IN MAMMOGRAPHY: SUGGESTIONS FOR FURTHER STUDIES

Kunio Doi, Ph.D., and Gunnila Holje, M.Sc.

Kurt Rossmann Laboratories for Radiologic Image Research,
Department of Radiology, The University of Chicago,
and The Franklin McLean Memorial Research Institute
(operated by The University of Chicago for the
U.S. Department of Energy under Contract No. EY-76-02-0069),
Chicago, Illinois 60637

Patient exposure in mammography must be minimized without sacrifice of the diagnostic quality of mammograms. The choice of an appropriate recording or detector system with which this goal can be achieved in mammography is therefore very important, since the speed of the system is directly related to the patient exposure and since its imaging properties influence the diagnosis significantly. Although a number of different recording systems have been used in mammography, few physical evaluations of these systems have been reported in the literature.

The basic physical detector characteristics in mammography include speed, contrast, resolution, and noise, as shown in Table 1. The speed of a recording

Table 1. Observed detector characteristics in mammography

(1) Basic physical detector characteristics:

    Speed

    Contrast

    Resolution

    Noise

(2) Other related applied detector characteristics:

    Patient exposure

    Detectability or visibility

(3) Diagnostic accuracy

system has frequently been evaluated in terms of the relative speed, which depends on many parameters including beam quality and the test object used. An absolute number for the speed, such as the reciprocal of the exposure, or the reciprocal roentgen, that produces a certain film density for a given beam quality, should be more thoroughly investigated. This approach will provide a closer relationship between the speed and patient exposure or absorbed dose in the breast.

The contrast of the mammographic recording system has been evaluated by determination of the average gradient or of the gradient derived from the H & D curve. The average gradient is a useful concept and a simple means of representing the "average" property of the contrast reproduction capability for the radiographic system. It may be misleading, however, because the shapes of the H & D curves of different mammographic systems vary a great deal, and thus their average behavior does not always represent the small density difference that occurs in microcalcifications at high film densities. For example, for direct x-ray films, the average gradients are generally lower than those of screen-film systems, whereas the gradients at high densities are greater than those of screen-film systems.

The resolution property has been evaluated in terms of the modulation transfer function or line spread function of the recording system. The technique and procedure of the measurements have become well established in the conventional diagnostic energy range, which is higher than that used in mammography. Thus, translation of the technique to mammographic energies is needed. This involves not only the use of a mammographic beam quality, but also the analysis of fundamental imaging processes that occur in the mammographic system. For example, it is not known at present whether the mammographic screen-film system is linear or not. The contribution of the direct x-ray image relative to the image formed by the screen light has not been investigated in detail; the linearlity of the mammographic screen-film system may be influenced significantly by the presence of the direct x-ray image.

The noise of mammographic systems has been evaluated by use of the Wiener spectra. It has been assumed in some cases that the noise in mammographic systems is due to quantum mottle. According to our experience, however, structure mottle and artifacts from the processor contribute significantly to noise patterns which appear in mammographic screen-film systems. Therefore, a simple estimate of the number of x-ray quanta absorbed in these systems is not a reliable indicator of mammographic noise. Instead, measurements of the resulting images for a uniform x-ray exposure are necessary for the determination and characterization of noise.

Other related applied detector characteristics include patient exposure or absorbed dose, which is related to the speed, and detectability or visibility of a given object, which is related to contrast, resolution, and noise in a complicated way. These applied detector characteristics, which have been determined with phantoms and directly with patients, closely reflect the clinical situation in some instances. No single phantom or patient, however, can adequately represent the complicated clinical variations encountered in diagnostic radiology.

We believe that diagnostic accuracy is related to both the basic physical characteristics and the applied characteristics of the detector. Ultimately, the study of detector characteristics is expected to lead to the improvement of diagnostic accuracy. Such improvement should be determined by means of the statistical analysis of many mammographic examinations.

When we were preparing this paper, Dr. Philip Muntz asked us to give a critical review of this matter by comparing published data. However, we found that very few systematic experimental data had been published, except for some abstracts of papers presented and some sporadic data from The University of Chicago and from manufacturers concerning mammographic recording systems. A

A COMPARISON OF DIRECT FILM MAMMOGRAPHY
WITH SCREEN FILM MAMMOGRAPHY

M. Friedrich and P. Weskamp

The need for a lower dose in mammography is being more and more widely accepted also in Europe, and the times of high-dose mammography seem almost to have passed. Whereas the adepts of dose considerations are proclaiming the end of high-dose mammography, a respectable minority of radiologists, at least in Germany, feel some serious concern about the diagnostic quality of low-dose techniques in mammography. In this respect, one question is of outstanding clinical importance: how many early and clinically occult carcinomas are missed using low-dose systems compared with high-resolution mammography? To our knowledge, little information on the diagnostic significance of fine detail in mammograms is available as yet. Irrefutable comparative series are scarce and offer no clear-cut decision. According to some newer German publications, tiny microcalcifications and/or fine fibrous septa are the unique or prevailing signs of malignancy in some 10 to 20 percent of clinically occult carcinomas. In our own evaluation of 29 cases out of a series of some 70 occult carcinomas from the breast cancer screening program of Hamburg, directed by Professor Frischbier, 18 were detected only by microcalcifications. Three of them showed only small calcific particles well below 500 μ in diameter, whose detectability by low-dose techniques seemed at least questionable in this retrospective study. Out of the other 11 cases, 2 carcinomas were seen exclusively by some faint fibrous septa,which are even more critical in detection with silver-halide-poor, low-contrast systems. This figure, 5 out of 29, is in exact accordance with the published data. We are certainly aware of the various critical points of such a retrospective study.

In view of this uncertain situation, 2 years ago we tried to get a survey of opinion on diagnostic image quality among the competent mammography experts. From a realistic breast phantom (Fig. 1 and 2) mammograms on various image recording systems were made and sent to 12 German and 1 Swedish mammography experts. Fig. 3 and 4 show the tissue composition of the phantom and the microcalcifications of different sizes (100 - 1000 μ) and densities (CaCl, high contrast, OH-apatite, low contrast) localized in wire loops, which form the basis of the quality assessment. The mammograms were to be classified into two main quality categories: those acceptable and those to be discarded (Fig. 5). As can be seen, the by now classic non-screen silver-halide-rich, long processing films were judged acceptable with respect both to visualization of microcalcification and to image contrast, whereas all film-screen combinations offered for mammography by that time were at least partially discarded. They were throughout unable to delineate finest microcalcifications regarded as essential in the diagnosis of occult breast carcinoma. Also discarded in this blind study were all rapid-processing non-screen films still widely in use for mammography in Germany. The grid mammogram was judged unanimously as outstanding both in detail rendition and general image contrast with this 6 cm thick breast phantom.

On the background of this result, we began to analyze the different factors influencing image quality of low-dose mammography systems and to trace their apparent deficiencies.

Certainly in view of its high quality, but not with respect to radiation detection efficiency, the double-emulsion silver-halide-rich, long-processing non-screen film of low granularity has been considered for years as an ideal mammographic image recording system. Its poor quantum efficiency, at least in terms of quantum absorption efficiency (about 10%) in comparison with film screen systems (about 70%), is obvious.

What possibilities to increase film sensitivity exist?

1. An even thicker coating of films would yield a film with prolonged processing time and necessitate tank development. The gain in sensitivity would be very limited anyway.

2. Sensitization of the emulsion layer at the expense of low granularity. This yields a speed factor of 2 to 3 times (for instance, Mammoray M 4 or Kodirex). The quality is, of course, lowered.

3. Use of film-screen combinations. This provides sufficient sensitivity gain, but questionable film quality in mammography.

In our opinion, the commercially available low-dose systems suffer two major deficiencies, besides the unsolved problem of annoying screen artifacts: 1. poor or insufficient contrast with a narrow optimum gradient working range and 2. poor resolving power.

Poor contrast (Fig. 6)

The Min R- and Lo-Dose Systems are single-emulsion, rapid-processing, silver-halide-poor films of low inherent contrast, the 3M Alpha M System offers a somewhat better contrast. The Lo-Dose Duplex System (low-dose RP System) and the Agfa RP 3 MR 50 System have double-coated films, which offer slightly better general image contrast but have other drawbacks. The contrast characteristics of these low-contrast single-emulsion systems were conceived to cover an overall exposure range between skin line and the prepectoral region of 1.4 within a density range between zero plus fog and density 3.0. With good breast compression up to the prepectoral region and neglecting the skin line, whose visualization in mammography is not essential in our opinion, we assume an overall exposure range in the mammogram of delta-log E = 1.0 - 1.1. The contrast characteristics of a panchromatic, silver-halide-rich, high-contrast, double-emulsion film on a screen, as shown with curve 5 and 6 in Fig. 6, are achieved by none of the commercially available film-screen combinations.

Resolving power (Figures 7 - 12)

There are 2 (un-)sharpness components in film-screen combinations: screen unsharpness and film unsharpness. The latter is insignificant and need not be dealt with here.

Figure 7 shows edge traces, actually a sum of 45 single recordings superimposed on each other by the computer to minimize film granularity. Out of the screens tested the MR 50 screen is the sharpest, the Min R screen, the Lo-Dose 1, the 3M Alpha M screen are more or less equal and the Lo-Dose 2 screen clearly is the worst. (Fig. 8). Removing the protective coating from the screen, the MR 50 screen becomes even sharper, it is, to our knowledge, unsurpassed by any other screen at present.

As mentioned, the resulting sharpness of the film-screen combination is a density-dependent composition of screen and film sharpness. Thus the compound sharpness is determined by the ratio of the direct X-ray exposure and screen-light exposure of the film. (Fig. 9). In commercial film-screen systems, the spectral sensitivity of the film is matched to the screen-light emission spectrum as to yield maximum system speed. The film is exposed up to 95% by screen light, thus transferring almost the complete screen unsharpness to the image. We offer a different approach to high resolution film-screen systems for mammography. Combining a double-coated, relatively X-ray sensitive, panchromatic film with good optical shielding between both emulsion layers, a film-screen combination with higher film modulation component is obtained (see curve 1 - 3 and 5 - 8). The 20% of residual film modulation of the total film density, for instance in the system NDT 75 MR 50, add just the amount of sharpness to image finest high-contrast detail (compare the detail mammograms of Figures 14 a - d). It is essential that the optical shielding between both emulsion layers be complete, at least in the density range up to D = 4. (Fig. 12). Otherwise cross-over exposure of the off-screen will occur, adding a strong unsharpness component to the image and degrading the resolution to that of a single-coated system or even worsening it. In Figure 12, the density-dependent percentages of direct X-ray exposure and cross-over exposure of the off-screen emulsion layer in the Duplex Lo-Dose System and the Agfa System Mammoray RP 3 MR 50 is depicted.

Before giving some practical examples of the critical detail rendition in mammograms, the time-sensitometric data of some of the systems investigated by us are given in Figure 13. As to speed, the film-screen systems for mammography can be classified into 2 main categories: the high-resolution,medium-speed systems with a speed factor of about 4 to 5 compared to non-screen industrial X-ray film and the high-speed, low-resolution systems offering a speed factor of 7 to 12, depending on the respective mean density compared.

Figures 14 a to d give practical examples of detail rendition by some representative film-screen systems and the industrial X-ray film.

Image noise (Figures 15 - 18)

Up to now I deliberately left out of consideration one of the most important image factors in low-dose radiographic imaging techniques: image noise. Exact noise measurements, especially with double-emulsion film-screen systems, are rather time-consuming and problematic in any case both in theory and in practice. With film-screen combinations, it is generally sufficient to consider two noise components: film granularity and quantum noise. These components are mainly characterized by their different frequency content and can therefore be distinguished and quantified in a plot of the noise energy frequency distribution known as the power- or Wiener spectrum. (Fig. 15). Generally high-speed, high-resolution and high-contrast film-screen systems or, for instance, the electroradiographic imaging system are, because of their sharpness and high contrast, good examples of apparent visibility of quantum mottle and consequent image quality degradation. With the low-contrast film-screen combinations for mammography and especially in the mammographic energy range,assuming a K-edge filtered molybdenum

spectrum, quantum mottle is considerably less than in normal diagnostic radiology. Especially in the low-contrast single-coated
systems currently on the market, we have to scrutinize the mottle;
it may be of some importance, however, with the high-contrast film-
screen systems advocated by us. Thus in first approximation, it
may be legitimate to assume a nearly uniform frequency distribution
of the noise energy in film-screen combinations for mammography.
Another current measurement of image noise, more exactly speaking,
the mean noise amplitude in a certain frequency band of the spectrum, is the rms granularity, which equals the standard deviation
of film density fluctuations measured with a circular scanning
area. With a uniform noise frequency distribution, these reciprocal values of the standard deviation of density fluctuations and
the corresponding sampling area are linked together by a constant,
the so-called Selwyn granularity constant, which is valid over a
wide range of sampling areas. With radiographic films, however,
and their different granular structure, the Selwyn relationship no
longer holds; thus for different sampling areas, the standard
deviation has to be determined individually. Depending on the different theoretical models of signal detection by the human eye, to
each line frequency out of the object frequency spectrum, an individual pass band of noise energy can be formed, which interferes
with the signal detection. The two models discussed in the literature are the more optimistic Rose-model (1) assuming a functional
sampling area or aperture diameter of the eye the same size as the
signal to be detected, and the more pessimistic approach according
to Morgan (2) calculating the signal detection probability according to the modulation transfer function of the visual system
with its well-defined peak sensitivity at line frequency 1 with
normal viewing distance. In all our calculations, we follow
Morgan's approach, assuming a perfect signal transfer through the
modulation transfer function of the eye for each individual detail
size and measuring and calculating the individual noise amplitude
within a noise equivalent pass band corresponding to the MTF of the
respective viewing conditions. Thus in Fig. 16 the increase of
noise amplitude filtered out by the noise equivalent pass bands
corresponding to the different detail diameters associated with
each line frequency resp. object diameter is shown. According to
some recent investigations (3 - 5) the noise equivalent pass band
of the eye seems to be much narrower than the square of the MTF of
the eye used by us. Thus in our signal-to-noise calculations the
noise amplitude is probably overestimated. On the other hand,
noise energy varies with film density. (compare Fig. 17). Thus to
each signal diameter respective object line frequency on one axis
and to the different film densities respective exposure levels on
the second axis a corresponding noise amplitude filtered out of
the spectrum with the corresponding noise equivalent pass band can
be calculated and a frequency- and density-dependent noise matrix
be formed. (Fig. 18).

Image Quality Concept
    In a similar way, the film-gradient matrix and the MTF ma-
trix can be generated (Figures 19,20). Forming the term of the
linear signal-to-noise ratio multiplying the gradient by the MTF
factor and dividing by the noise amplitude, out of these three
matrices the signal-to-noise matrix can be calculated. (Fig. 21).
The absolute values in this crude matrix are, of course, meaning-
less, because the signal amplitude offered to the image-recording
system, that is to say, the radiographic contrast delta-log E was
not included. For relative comparisons of the image-recording

systems, the delta-log E of an individual detail, e.g. a micro-calcification, need not be known, because the matrix can be normalized by comparison of the different practical phantom mammograms. We normalize the matrix in such a way that at the detail frequency resp. detail diameter with borderline visibility of the detail in the mammogram we set the value of the matrix to 2. (Fig. 21). Thus we get a perceptibility matrix which has immediate perceptual evidence. It allows us to predict visibility of such a detail with the same radiation contrast on a new imaging system once its imaging factors are known. Applying the concepts of information theory on radiographic imaging systems, we can form the logarithm to the basis of 2 of the signal-to-noise matrix and get some measure of "information quality" for the different detail sizes at different film densities. This information quality matrix gives to each detail size resp. line frequency and film density the number of just perceivable exposure levels. (Fig. 22). As can be seen, these are highest at the gradient maximum and for the lowest spatial frequencies, i.e. large areas in the image. With decreasing detail diameter, information quality in the image decreases rapidly to the point where the information quality index underpasses the perceptibility borderline defined at a numerical value of 1 bit = $_2lg^2$. This is the smallest information unit allowing a clear decision on the existence of the detail on the radiograph. However, with a normal mammographic radiation quality, visualization of large area contrast has never been critical in film-screen-mammography contrary to details of line frequency 2 to 5 line-pairs/mm. To take this into account, one can introduce a new weighting function for the frequency scale, the most common in terms of information theory being the so-called unit area information density. This defines the number of details, e.g. a cluster of microcalcifications which can be visualized independently of each other on a certain unit area, for instance 1 sq. cm. (Fig. 23). Out of the information quality matrix and this unit area information density matrix, the so-called "information capacity matrix" can be generated. (Fig. 24). As can be seen, according to this concept, the information content transmitted in the range of low object frequencies, i.e. large areas in the mammogram, would be very small, although the information quality is highest. As we all know from the experience with Xero-mammography, large-area contrast is of equal diagnostic significance as detail rendition. Therefore the concept of information capacity of an image recording system, as defined here and used commonly for technical purposes, is not appropriate for a general comprehensive radiographic image quality assessment. The most suitable image quality measure for quantitative comparison is the normalized signal-to-noise matrix because of its linear image quality scale in contrast to the matrices derived from it (image quality matrix and information capacity matrix). We calculated the normalized signal-to-noise matrix of 18 film-mammographic image recording systems, assuming a total focus-to-film distance of 45 cm with the non-screen films and 70 cm for the film-screen combinations. We took 3 cm as a mean object-to-film distance. As mentioned above, the numerical value of 2 in the normalized signal-to-noise matrix corresponds to borderline perceptibility. Thus, to get a measure of the diagnostically significant information, we have to take into account only values equal to or greater than 2. In order to reduce the three-dimensional matrix to a two-dimensional plot of signal-to-noise ratio vs spatial frequency resp. detail diameter, we integrated over a density range of the film corresponding to an exposure range of delta-log E = 1. Fig. 25 shows these density-integrated signal-to-noise ratios of some representative film systems as a function of spatial frequency resp. detail diameter. From a diagnostic point of view, 2 frequency ranges have to be considered: from 0 frequency to 1 lp/mm corresponding to the large area contrast of the image and the frequency range from 1 to 5 lp/mm corresponding to the detail rendition on the image. As can be seen, most of the single-coated film-screen systems are in reality low-contrast systems compared with an adequately exposed high-contrast double-coated mammographic film. They offer a small advantage in contrast only in the lower film density range, where contrast with industrial film is poor. In the line-frequency range of 1 to 5 lp/mm (Fig. 25) the superior quality of the industrial film over single-coated high-speed film combinations is obvious. It is extremely remarkable, however, that the medium-speed film-screen systems advocated by us for mammography, composed of a panchromatic high-contrast industrial film on a high-resolution screen offer the same image quality as industrial film in the frequency range of 1 to 5 lp/mm.

Image quality and dose (Figures 26 - 27)

Although we feel that a certain image quality is absolutely necessary from a diagnostic point of view, another aspect of equal importance in mammography is the dose. In view of the uncertainties and difficulties in defining the image quality necessary for an exact diagnosis in mammography, it is tempting to define as an optimization criterion the relation between image quality as measured here by the signal-to-noise ratio and the corresponding dose. Unfortunately, this is not possible, because some film-screen systems with excellent relation of signal-to-noise ratio to dose offer poor and insufficient image quality on an absolute scale. Therefore we feel that the scope of image quality vs dose considerations is limited. Fig. 26 shows a plot of the density-integrated signal-to-noise ratios in the frequency range of 0 to 1 lp/mm in relation to dose. The slope of the regression lines can be regarded as a measure of the film system's efficiency to transform dose into image information as defined here. In the calculation of the regression lines, we assumed that 0 dose yields 0 perceptibility corresponding to a numerical value of 2 in the normalized signal-to-noise matrix and to a value of 0 in the modified net-perceptibility signal-to-noise matrix. For evaluation the frequency ranges of large area contrast and detail rendition must be separately discussed. Regarding large-area contrast, the silver-halide-rich, high-contrast industrial films both with and without screen yield an equally high contrast. (a,b,c,l,i). The rapid processing non-screen films as well as the single-coated high-speed film-screen systems (d-f,r,q) afford a slightly better image contrast compared with the single-coated systems. Under the aspect of dose efficiency, that is to say the slope of the corresponding regression lines, it is obvious that the rapid-processing low-contrast double-coated non-screen films are by far the worst and should be discounted for mammography. Dose efficiency of the commercial single-coated high-speed low-dose mammographic film-screen systems is higher than that of the industrial film (m,n,p,o). The highest dose efficiency in terms of large-area contrast is achieved, however, by the double-coated high-speed systems (r,q) with medium contrast on an absolute scale and, above all, by the medium-speed high-contrast film-screen systems composed of a light-sensitive industrial film on a high-resolution screen (i,k,l).

In the frequency range of detail rendition, that is to say from 1 to 5 lp/mm (Fig. 27), it is remarkable that dose-efficiency of the high-speed both single- and double-coated rapid processing film-screen systems is basically the same as for the non-screen low-granularity high-contrast industrial films as well as the sensitized high-granularity high-contrast non-screen films (g,h). The inacceptably bad dose-efficiency concerning detail rendition of the rapid processing non-screen films used for mammography should be noticed as well as the excellent dose-efficiency of the medium-speed high-contrast high-resolution film-screen systems advocated by us (i,k,l).

Conclusions

1. In terms of large-area or general image contrast, detail rendition and dose efficiency, the commercially available single-emulsion high-speed film-screen systems for mammography cannot be considered as optimized. Mid-speed film-screen systems composed of a high-resolution screen and a high-contrast double-coated low-granularity industrial film of limited light sensitivity yield better results under the compound aspect of general image contrast, detail rendition and dose efficiency.

2. On an absolute quality scale, the commercial low-dose, low-contrast rapid-processing film-screen systems are critical in the visualization of fine mammographic detail considered essential in the diagnosis of occult breast carcinoma. This fact casts a critical light on the limitations of dose-efficiency considerations in practice.

3. There are strong indications that fine-detail rendition is needed in the mammogram for the diagnosis of early breast carcinoma. According to a retrospective study of some 30 clinical occult carcinomas, it seems justified to assume that at least 10% of early carcinomas are missed with these low-dose poor-resolution systems. With inappropriate mammographic equipment, this rate may even be higher.

4. High-resolution film-screen systems advocated by us with a dose-reduction factor of about 5 yield excellent and impeccable image quality provided artifacts from the film can be kept reasonably low.

5. The presented image quality model which essentially is not new reflects the diagnostically significant performance data of mammographic film systems in an excellent way and gives many hints to the manufacturer where to improve quality.

6. Artifacts on film-screen mammograms can be kept reasonably low only with careful handling of all components, which cannot be the case in practice. We have seen film-screen mammograms dotted all over with hundreds of dust particles. In such a mammogram it will be extremely difficult even for a well-trained observer to detect low-contrast details, though they are visualized by the film system. Therefore we urgently advocate an automatic film handling, e.g. a closed daylight system for mammography warranting clean, rapid and simple handling of all system components.

References

1. Rose, A.: The Sensitivity Performance of the Human Eye on an
    Absolute Scale.
    J. Opt. Soc. Am. 38 (1948) 196 - 208.

2. Morgan, R.H.: Visual Perception in Fluoroscopy and Radio-
    graphy.
    Radiology 86 (1966) 403 - 416.

3. Blakemore, C., Nachmias, J., and Sutton, P.: The Perceived
    Spatial Frequency Shift: Evidence for Frequency-Selective
    Neurones in the Human Brain.
    J. Physiol. 210 (1970) 727 - 750.

4. Schnitzler, A.D.: Theory of Spatial-Frequency Filtering by
    the Human Visual System. I. Performance Limited by Quantum
    Noise.
    J. Opt. Soc. Am. 66 (1976) 608 - 625.

5. Stecher, S., Sigel, C. and Lange, R.V.: Spatial Frequency
    Channels in Human Vision and the Threshold for Adaptation.
    Vision Res. 13 (1973) 1691 - 1700.

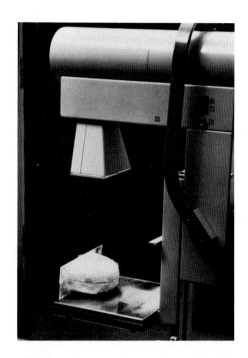

Figure 1.   Breast Phantom in Use

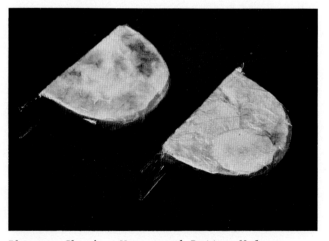

Figure 2.   Breast Phantom Showing Upper and Bottom Halves

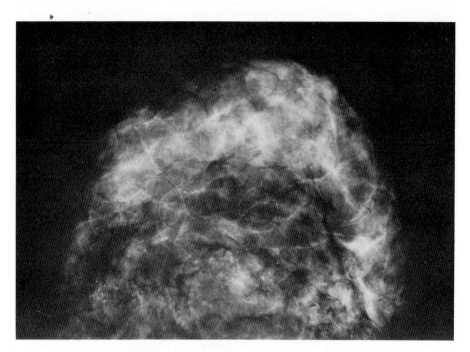

Figure 3. Radiograph of Breast Phantom.

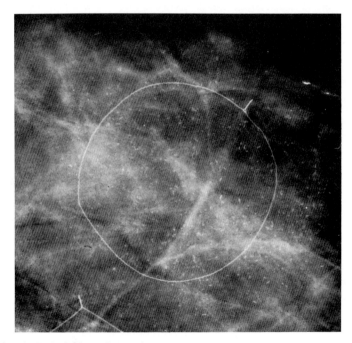

Figure 4. Typical Calcifications in Breast Phantom.

FILM–SYSTEM,HERSTELLER	AUFNAHMEBEDINGUNGEN	ABBILDUNGSQUALITÄT FÜR			
		MIKROKALK		BINDEGEWEBSSTRUKTUREN	
		G U T	MANGELHAFT	G U T	MANGELHAFT
CRONEX 75m,DUPONT	31 kV,Mo–Anode,FFA:45 cm	xxxxxxxxxx	oo	xxxxxxxx	oooo
DEFINIX MEDICAL,KODAK	„ „ „	xxxxxxxxxxx	o	xxxxxxxxx	ooo
MAMMORAY T3,AGFA–GEV.	„ „ „	xxxxxxxxxxx	o	xxxxxxxxxx	oo
MAMMORAY M4,AGFA–GEV.	„ „ „	xxxxxxxx	oooo	xxxxxxxxxx	oo
PE 4006,KODAK	„ „ „	xx	oooooooooo	xxxx	ooooooo
MAMMORAY RP3,AGFA–GEV.	„ „ „	x	ooooooooooo	x	ooooooooooo
TYPE S,Fa. 3 M	„ „ „	xxx	ooooooooo	xxxx	ooooooo
LO–DOSE SYSTEM,DUPONT	„ „ FFA:60 cm	xxx	ooooooooo	xxxxxxx	ooooo
MIN R SYSTEM,KODAK	„ „ „	xxx	ooooooooo	xxxxx	ooooooo
RP 3/MR 50,AGFA–GEV.	„ „ „	xx	oooooooooo	xxxx	ooooooo
CRONEX 75m/DETAIL,DUPONT	„ „ „	xxxxxxx	ooooo	xxxxxxxxxx	oo
CRONEX 75m/DETAIL/RASTER	„ „ (Raster),,	xxxxxxxxxxxx		xxxxxxxxxxxx	
RPS NORMAL FILM,KODAK	„ „ FFA:45 cm	x	ooooooooooo	x	ooooooooooo
CRONEX 75m,DUPONT	50 kV, „ „	xxxxx	ooooooo		oooooooooooo
CRONEX 75m,DUPONT	35 kV,Wo–Anode,FFA:70 cm 2 mm Al	xxxx	oooooooo		oooooooooooo

Figure 5. Results of Evaluation by Radiologists of Mammography Detectors. Categories Include Good and Unacceptable Visibilty of Microcalcifications and Tissue Structure.

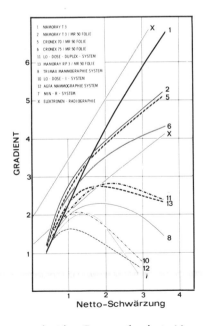

Figure 6. Slope of Characteristic Curve (point λ) versus Net Density.

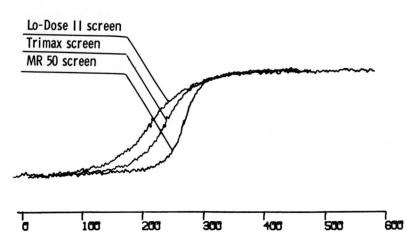

Figure 7. Microdensitometer Trace of Edge Images for Three Detector Systems.

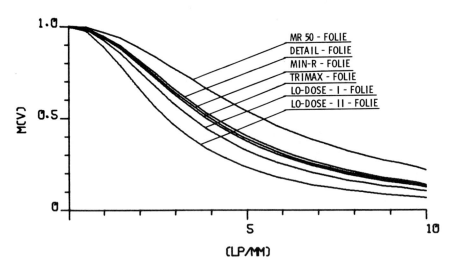

Figure 8. MTF'S for Six Film-Screen Detector Systems.

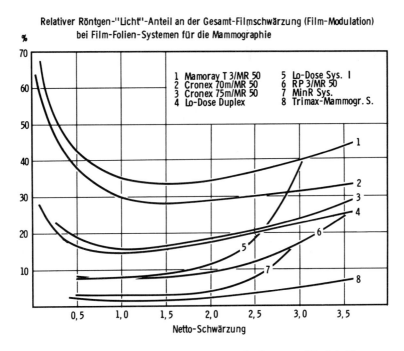

Figure 9. Ratio of Direct X-ray Exposure and Screen Light Exposure for Film-Screen Systems as a Function of Net Density.

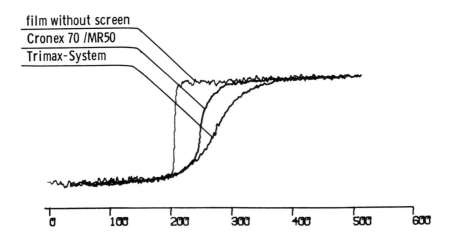

Figure 10. Edge Trace of Images.

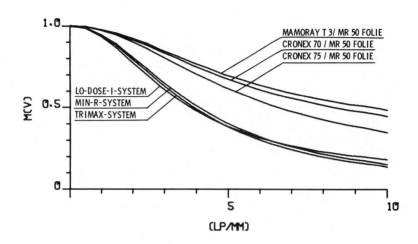

Figure 11. MTF'S of Indicated Detector Systems

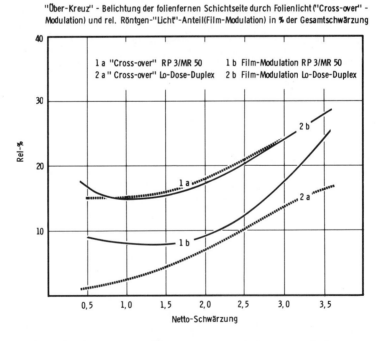

Figure 12. Ratio of Direct X-ray Exposure and Screen Light Exposure from Cross-Over in Double Emulsion Film Screen Systems.

Zeitsensitometrischer Empfindlichkeitsvergleich

Film-Netto- System Schwärzung	1,0	1,5	2,0
Mamoray T 3	1,0	1,0	1,0
Mamoray M 4	2,2	2,3	2,4
Mamoray T 3/MR 50	3,0	3,0	3,0
Kodirex	3,6	3,3	3,7
Cronex 70m/MR 50	4,1	3,8	4,2
Cronex 75m/Detail	4,0	4,2	4,1
Trimax-Mammogr.-S	4,0	3,0	2,0
Agfa-Gev. Sys. (einstg)	6,7	5,5	3,4
Lo-Dose Sys. I	7,8	5,8	5,2
Lo-Dose Duplex Sys.	7,9	6,2	6,2
Cronex 75m/MR 50	8,1	6,8	6,9
MinR-Sys.	9,3	6,8	5,8
RP 3/MR 50	11,3	8,5	8,0

Figure 13. Relative Exposure Times Normalized to Mamoray T3 as a Function
of System and Density.

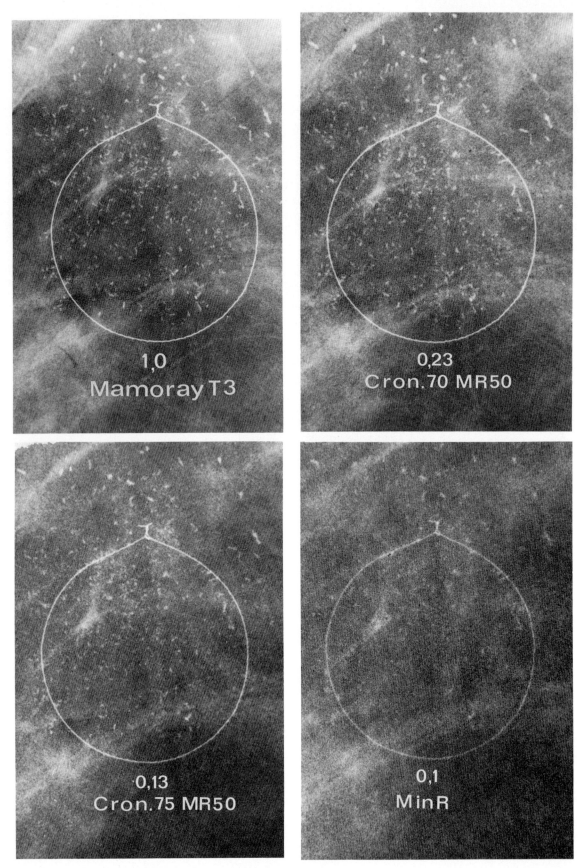

Figure 14. Examples of Detail Rendition.

186

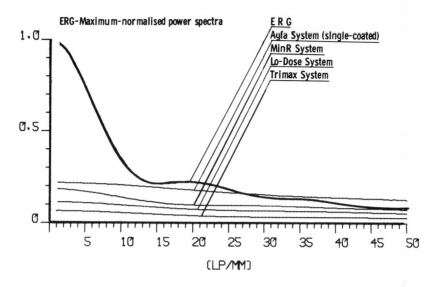

Figure 15. Noise Power Spectra of Mammography Systems.

Assumed noise-equivalent passbands (MTF^2) of the visual system in XERG - Mammography
MTF of the visual system according to de PALMA and LOWRY
Viewing conditions according to MORGAN:

1. 1,8 x magnification, corresp. 1 lp/mm resp. 500 micron detail diameter
2. 5,4 x   "   "   3 lp/mm "   166 micron detail diameter
3. 9,0 x   "   "   5 lp/mm "   100 micron detail diameter
4. 18 x   "   "   10 lp/mm "   50 micron detail diameter

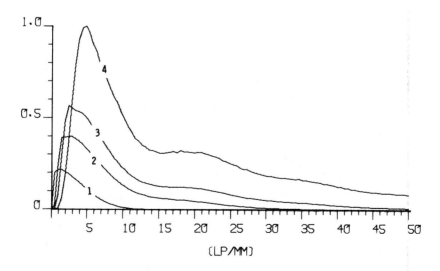

Figure 16.(a)   Noise Filtered by Passband of Eye for Obversation of Different
                Detail Diameters.

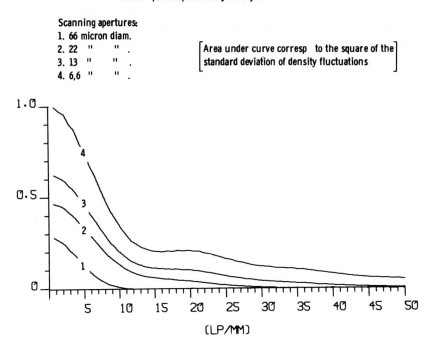

Noise-equivalent passbands (MTF^2) of circular scanning aperture in rms-granularity measurements
XERG - power spectrum , density : 1

Scanning apertures:
1. 66 micron diam.
2. 22 "   " .
3. 13 "   " .
4. 6,6 "   " .

[Area under curve corresp to the square of the standard deviation of density fluctuations]

(LP/MM)

Figure 16.(b) Noise Filtered by Circular Scanning Apertures.

1) rms granularity vs. density ($= \sigma_d = f(d)$)
2) rms granularity vs. detail diameter resp. lp/mm =($= \sigma_d = f(v)$)

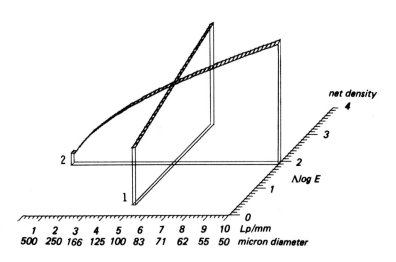

net density

Δlog E

1 2 3 4 5 6 7 8 9 10 Lp/mm
500 250 166 125 100 83 71 62 55 50 micron diameter

Figure 17. Noise (Vertical Scale) vs Density and Noise vs Detail Size.

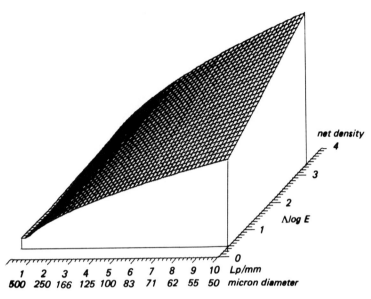

noise matrix of total system $= \sigma_d = f(v, d)$

Figure 18.   Noise Matrix of a System.

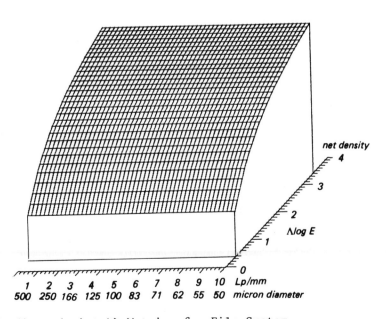

gradient matrix of total system

Figure 19. Gradient (point λ) Matrix of a Film System.

total system MTF = f(v, d)

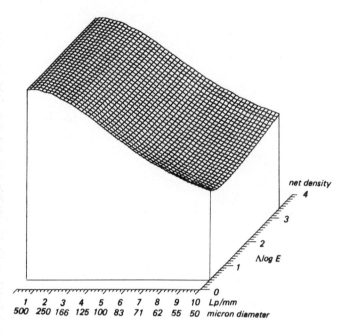

Figure 20.   MTF Matrix for a Film System.

normalised signal / noise matrix, S/N $\geqslant$ 2.

$$S_{/N} = \frac{\gamma(d)\ M(v,d)\,\Delta \log E}{\sigma_d\,(v,d)}$$

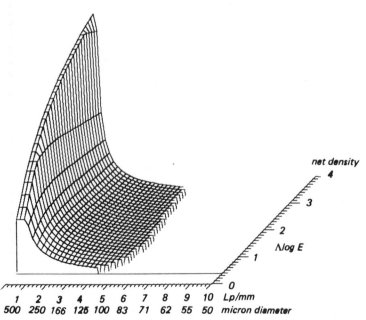

Figure 21.   Signal to Noise Ratio Matrix from Figures 17, 18, 19.

information quality matrix ($\geqslant$ 1 bit) $^2\log {}^S\!/_N - 1$

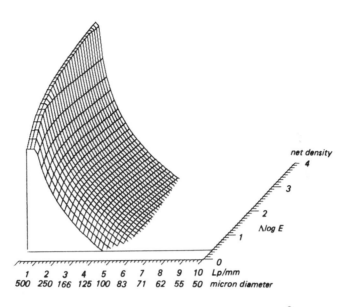

Figure 22.   Information Content Normalized to 1 bit $\equiv {}^2\log 2$.

unit information density matrix (bit/cm^2) $4 v^2 . a$

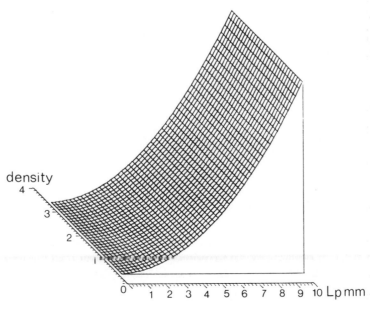

Figure 23.   Unit Information Density Matrix (See Text).

191

information capacity matrix (bit/cm^2) $4 v^2 a$ (^{2}log $^S/_N$ $- 1$)

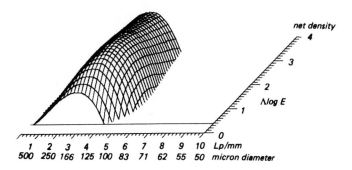

Figure 24.   Information Capacity Matrix of a System.

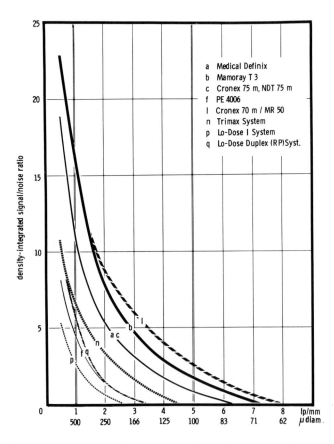

Figure 25.   Density Integrated Signal to Noise Ratio vs Frequency.

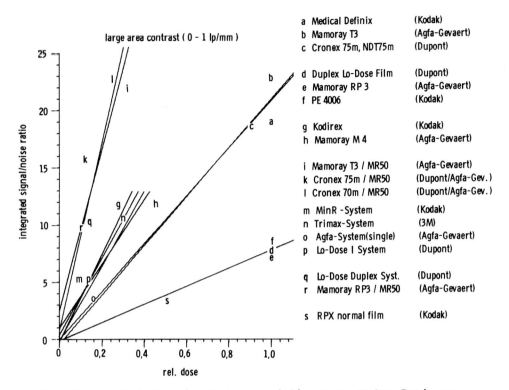

large area contrast (0 - 1 lp/mm)

a	Medical Definix	(Kodak)
b	Mamoray T3	(Agfa-Gevaert)
c	Cronex 75m, NDT75m	(Dupont)
d	Duplex Lo-Dose Film	(Dupont)
e	Mamoray RP 3	(Agfa-Gevaert)
f	PE 4006	(Kodak)
g	Kodirex	(Kodak)
h	Mamoray M 4	(Agfa-Gevaert)
i	Mamoray T3 / MR50	(Agfa-Gevaert)
k	Cronex 75m / MR50	(Dupont/Agfa-Gev.)
l	Cronex 70m / MR50	(Dupont/Agfa-Gev.)
m	MinR -System	(Kodak)
n	Trimax-System	(3M)
o	Agfa-System(single)	(Agfa-Gevaert)
p	Lo-Dose I System	(Dupont)
q	Lo-Dose Duplex Syst.	(Dupont)
r	Mamoray RP3 / MR50	(Agfa-Gevaert)
s	RPX normal film	(Kodak)

Figure 26.   Integrated, Density Integrated Signal to Noise Ratio vs Relative Dose for Details.

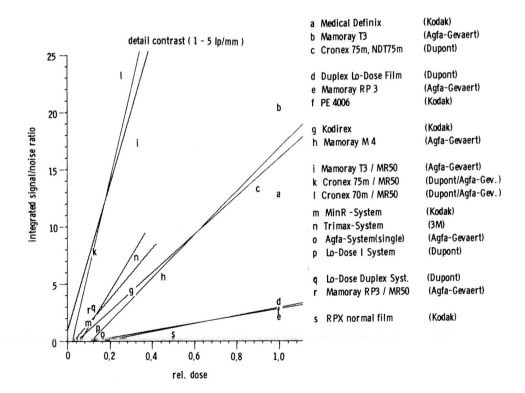

detail contrast (1 - 5 lp/mm)

a	Medical Definix	(Kodak)
b	Mamoray T3	(Agfa-Gevaert)
c	Cronex 75m, NDT75m	(Dupont)
d	Duplex Lo-Dose Film	(Dupont)
e	Mamoray RP 3	(Agfa-Gevaert)
f	PE 4006	(Kodak)
g	Kodirex	(Kodak)
h	Mamoray M 4	(Agfa-Gevaert)
i	Mamoray T3 / MR50	(Agfa-Gevaert)
k	Cronex 75m / MR50	(Dupont/Agfa-Gev.)
l	Cronex 70m / MR50	(Dupont/Agfa-Gev.)
m	MinR -System	(Kodak)
n	Trimax-System	(3M)
o	Agfa-System(single)	(Agfa-Gevaert)
p	Lo-Dose I System	(Dupont)
q	Lo-Dose Duplex Syst.	(Dupont)
r	Mamoray RP3 / MR50	(Agfa-Gevaert)
s	RPX normal film	(Kodak)

FOCAL SPOTS IN THE FUTURE OF MAMMOGRAPHY

By
Martin Braun, Ph.D.
Radiologic Sciences Inc.
Santa Clara, California
a Subsidiary of Pfizer Inc.

Mammography is changing, and the future will see more changes. One major component in this change is the x-ray focal spot. Micro-focal spots have become available allowing the application of magnification techniques with their many options, flexibility, as well as pitfalls. More than in conventional techniques, magnification requires careful optimization of the whole imaging system. Other manifestations of the ongoing change in mammographic procedures are manipulation of the beam spectrum and scatter rejecting systems.

In terms of systems parameters and components, the imaging systems can be divided into four categories, each having a major part in forming the image.

1. The OPTICAL PERFORMANCE of the system is basically described by MTF type tools applied to the stationary system (patient motionless, noise free approximation) - even if "MTF" is not explicitly utilized in the analysis. Focal spot dimensions and intensity distribution, in the following also called "source geometry", are one essential part of this first category. The other part is the optical characteristics of the image receptor; and the link between the two is the magnification factor.

2. Under ENERGY RELATIONS of the system we are including both tube loadability ("source strength") and image receptor efficiency, factors which determine exposure duration, which in turn affects optical performance via image unsharpness caused by tissue motion. The ideal system would have the energy parameters optimized within the optical parameters. A "Figure of Merit of Focal Spots" can be defined for rotating anodes, describing loadability relative to optical performance[1].

3. BACKGROUND OR SPURIOUS PHOTONS are those x-ray photons which are received by the film or image receptor, but which do not contribute in forming the image.

Scatter is the more important part of these photons. The removal of scattered photons is inter-related with the other two categories, for instance with magnification (category 1) or with increased tube load requirements when using grids or moving slit systems (category 2).

Off-focus radiation is the other important part of background photons, generated from tube internal parts, and therefore more difficult to reduce.

4. X-RAY BEAM QUALITY or the beam spectrum is determined internally of the tube by the target material and tube construction ("inherent filtration") and externally by filtration usually added intentionally. To this category of the system also belong the spectral absorption characteristics of patient and receptor.

1. CONSIDERATIONS ON OPTICAL PERFORMANCE OF FOCAL SPOTS

1.1 SYSTEMS ANALYSIS

In order to describe the optical role of the focal spot within the x-ray imaging system, tools of modern optics must be used, such as Fourier analysis and the cascading principle to synthesize systems performance. In most cases it is not necessary to use the somewhat cumbersome MTF curve analysis, a single parameter representing approximately the MTF curve for each system's component is often adequate. The cascading rule using these parameters is a convenient approximate means of checking optical performance of a system and to find an optimum:

$$B_0^2 = (B_F')^2 + (B_S')^2 + (B_V)^2 = (\frac{B_F}{M/M-1})^2 + (\frac{B_S}{M})^2 + (B_V)^2. \qquad (1)$$

The B's are measures of unsharpness ("blurs") of focal spot (B_F), screen film system (B_S) and, if included in the analysis, of tissue motion, (B_V). $B_F' = B_F(M-1)/M$ and $B_S' = B_S/M$ are focal spot and screen blur relative to the object plane. B_0 is the unsharpness of the object (tissue structure) as appearing on the film yet in a scale reduced by the magnification factor M and therefore related to the location in the breast. We will call B_0 also "Systems resolution", bearing in mind that it will mean the systems blur or unsharpness effect related to the imaged object. There is some question as to which type of parameter is best suited for the systems analysis. However, since the real world is only an approximate fit to the mathematical model (take alone the uncertainties of focal spot dimensions both in terms of inherent tolerance range as well as blooming effect), a meaningful approximation is all what is needed. For the focal spot, we propose to use the "RMS equivalent uniform focal spot size" as introduced by Doi and Rossman [2], as a measure of unsharpness and call it "Focal Spot Size (RMS)", or just "RMS size" or "Focal Spot RMS". In Ref. [1], we call this size index the "Resolving Index". Here, we also use simply focal spot "blur". The RMS size B_F is not to be confused with the "Effective size" f (also called "Equivalent Size" F_{eq}) obtained from a star pattern image according to the NEMA standard [6], although for a large class of focal spots, B_F equals F_{eq}. Unfortunately, F_{eq} fails as a performance descriptor for many micro-focus tubes with filamentary cathodes. We will discuss this phenomena later.

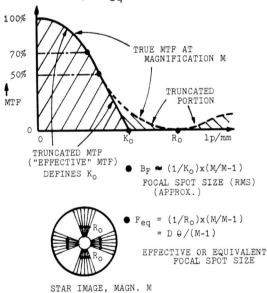

100%

70%

50%

MTF

0

TRUE MTF AT MAGNIFICATION M

TRUNCATED PORTION

K_0 R_0 lp/mm

TRUNCATED MTF ("EFFECTIVE" MTF) DEFINES K_0

● $B_F \approx (1/K_0) \times (M/M-1)$

FOCAL SPOT SIZE (RMS) (APPROX.)

● $F_{eq} = (1/R_0) \times (M/M-1)$
     $= D \theta/(M-1)$

EFFECTIVE OR EQUIVALENT FOCAL SPOT SIZE

R_0
R_0

STAR IMAGE, MAGN. M

FIG. 1
APPROXIMATE FOCAL SPOT SIZE (RMS) FROM PLOTTED MTF CURVE.

Sometimes it is of interest to do a quick analysis of a system of which the component MTF's are known, e.g. a system described in the literature. A simple approximate method to find the B's from the MTF curves is as follows:

From the focal spot MTF, the approximate value of B_F can be found by a linear extrapolation through the 70% and 50% points of the MTF curve, calculated for a magnification M, see Fig. 1 [1]. This results in a truncated MTF. Then,

$$B_F = \frac{M}{M-1} \frac{1}{K_0} \qquad (2)$$

with K_0 the frequency for the zero point of the truncated MTF. An approximate formula for the screen "blur" is

$$B_S = 0.65/(Mf_{50}) \qquad (3)$$

with f_{50} the spatial frequency corresponding to the 50% point of the screen MTF, taken relative to a location corresponding to a magnification M. See[3] for a similar formula using for B_S the effective sampling aperture or noise equivalent passband defined by Wagner et al. [5]

The screen "blur" B_S is approximately 700 μm (microns) for Lightning Plus screens, 350 μm for Par, 220 μm for Detail, 160 μm for Low-Dose, and very small for films [3], [4].

1.2 DESCRIPTION OF THREE MAMMOGRAPHIC TECHNIQUES

The three major mammographic techniques in terms of the unsharpness contributions of focal spot and image detector are:

(1) No-screen, contact: $B_S \approx 0$, $B_0 = B_F' = \dfrac{OID}{SID} B_F$ (4)

                        for $M = 1.1: B_0 \approx 10\%$ of B_F (5)

(2) Screen, contact: $B_F' \ll B_S$; for long cone: $B_0 \approx B_S$

(3) Magnification: $B_S' \approx B_F'$ or $\dfrac{1}{B_{0(opt)}} \approx \dfrac{1}{\sqrt{2}} \left(\dfrac{1}{B_F} + \dfrac{1}{B_S} \right)$ (6)

                       $M_{opt} \approx 1 + B_S/B_F$ (7)

                with $B_0(opt)$ the systems unsharpness in the optimum case.

(a) No-screen, contact
In conventional mammographic no-screen contact techniques resolution of details is entirely dependent on the focal spot, since the film has very high resolution capability, which means $B_S \approx 0$. In Figure 2 labelled "FILM ONLY", we show in terms of systems blur how sharp details in the breast appear on the film (in a noise free approximation), depending on their location in the breast. Sharpness is indeed very non-uniformly distributed, increasing linearly with distance from the film.

(b) Screen, contact
With screen-film systems, sharpness is more uniformly distributed over the depth of the breast. Figures 2 and 3 depict screen-film contact techniques, using a Min-R screen Min-R film combination, with $B_S = 0.12$ (taken from Arnold et al [7]. For the long cone technique [22] (Fig. 3), sharpness is basically determined by the screen. The focal spot must be limited to a certain size which depends on screen resolution and maximum distance to be covered.

(c) Magnification
Finally, in Fig. 4, which shows magnification techniques, sharpness is a function of both the blurring effect of the screen as well as the focal spot. If we work at or near the minimum of the curves, the system is "optimized". Often, these curves have a shape with a very extended flat minimum towards large magnifications. In this case, see Fig. 4, it is certainly not wise to optimize the system exact at the minimum. Large

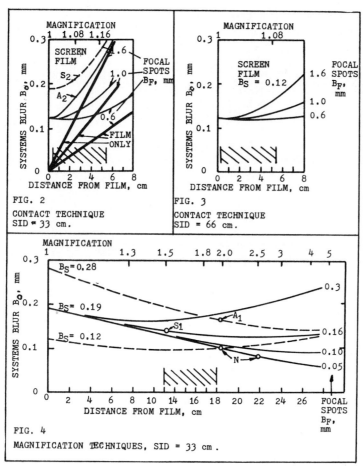

FIG. 2
CONTACT TECHNIQUE
SID = 33 cm.

FIG. 3
CONTACT TECHNIQUE
SID = 66 cm.

FIG. 4
MAGNIFICATION TECHNIQUES, SID = 33 cm.

magnifications greatly reduce systems efficiency, large SID's cause sharply reduced x-ray flux at the film. Therefore, it is often impractical to use the formula:

$$M_{opt} = 1 + (B_S/B_F)^2 \qquad (8)$$

which is derived from the cascading formula [1] by determining the mathematical minimum of the curves. At the expense of a slight loss in systems sharpness, but often large gains in the energy balance of the system, the formula:

$$M_{opt} = 1 + B_S/B_F \qquad (9)$$

is more practical, derived from setting the unsharpness contributions of both the focal spot and the screen equal with regard to the image plane.

1.3 THREE EXAMPLES OF SYSTEMS ANALYSIS

In Fig. 5 we have plotted the relations for the optimum case (6) and (7). The screen blur B_S is on the abscissa (x-axis), the focal spot blur or focal spot RMS B_F is on the ordinate (y-axis). The curves labeled B_O depict the systems resolution for optimum magnification.

The three examples are labeled A_1 and A_2, S_1 and S_2, and N. The black dots correspond to the blurs of focal spot and receptor used in each technique. The approximate values for B_F and B_S were derived from the published MTF graphs using formulas (2) and (3). Optimum magnification and systems resolution can then be read from the graph. The open circles correspond to the magnification value M actually used in the experimental techniques, and to the resulting systems resolution B_O calculated with the cascading formula (1).

(I) A_1 and A_2 are from Arnolds et al work[7]. The black dot at A_1 corresponds to a system consisting of a microfocal spot with $B_F = 0.17$ mm* and a double emulsion film - double screen combination with $B_S = 0.28$ mm (two Min-R screens, Ortho-G film). Optimum magnification would be $M_{opt} = 2.6$, with systems resolution of $B_O = 0.15$ mm from (1) or (6). In the paper, M = 2 was used, which results in $B_O = 0.16$ mm, which is only a slight loss in systems resolution, however a gain of 70% in x-ray flux at the film, if focus-object distance is kept constant. Arnold et al report that image quality was improved significantly at 3X magnification. System A_1 is also depicted in Fig. 4.
*Machlett DX-78E

198

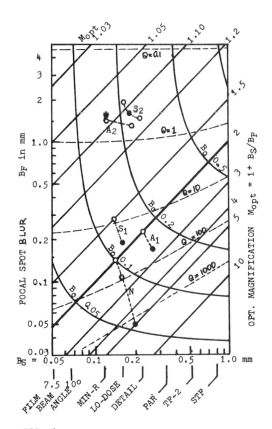

FIG. 5

FOCAL SPOT BLUR B_F, SCREEN BLUR B_S, OBJECT (SYSTEMS) BLUR B_O, AND OPTIMUM MAGNIFICATION.

$Q = M^2/B_F^{3/2} =$ RELATIVE ENERGY NEED FOR CONST. OID (ROTATING ANODE).

Arnold et al compare their magnification technique with a conventional contact technique (B_F = 1.6 mm**, B_S = 0.12 mm, Min-R - Min-R system), see A_2 in Fig. 5 (also in Fig. 2). The resulting systems resolution is B_O = 0.16 and 0.24 mm for magnification values M = 1.08 and 1.16. With M = 1.16 and film-only, B_O = 0.22 mm.

(II) S_1 and S_2 are from Sickles et al[8] work. The black dot at S_1 corresponds to a micro focal spot*** with B_F = 0.16 mm and a single screen, single emulsion recording system with B_S = 0.19 mm (Lo-Dose systems). Optimum magnification would be $M_{opt} \approx 2.2$, with systems resolution B_O = 0.14 mm - again, only a slight loss in systems resolution compared to the "optimum" system (see also Fig. 4, point S_1). For comparison, a contact technique was used, with the same recording system, but with a focal spot of B_F = 1.6 mm**(S_2 in Fig. 5). Resulting systems blurs: B_O = 0.21 mm for M = 1.08, and B_O = 0.27 mm for M = 1.16, which is twice the unsharpness resulting from the magnification technique (see also Fig. 2, curve S_2).

(III) It is interesting to analyze a 50 micron (B_F = 0.05 mm) focal spot system (see points labeled "N" in Fig. 5) combined with a system with B_S = 0.19 mm (e.g. Lo-Dose). Optimum magnification would have to be M_{opt} = 5. Systems resolution obtained under this condition is B_O = 0.060 mm = 60 μm. Objects this small require extreme object contrast to be detectable. Arnold et al[9] report that calcifications smaller than 300 μm have too small a contrast rendition to be detectable. Also, with M = 5, our hypothetical system would need an x-ray tube with a loadability most likely exceeding those presently available, even if source-recorder distance is shortened. If we reduce magnification to M = 2.5, systems resolution becomes B_O = 0.085 mm, still very high. At M = 2, B_O = 0.10 mm = 100 μm (see also Fig. 4, points N). As Fig. 4 shows, use of a 0.1 mm = 100 μm focal spot results in basically the same resolution at M = 2.

1.4 FOCAL SPOT CHARACTERIZATION

In formula (2), we have given a simple recipe on how to obtain the focal spot RMS size B_F from an MTF curve. The exact method is given in Ref. (2) or (1). But what if we do not have the means to measure line spread function and to calculate the MTF or the RMS size? We have dealt with this question to some extent in Ref. (1).

**CGR Senographe
***RSI MFT-1

We like to repeat here the following:

(1) The geometrical size - measured by pinhole or slit method - is usually not identical to the Focal Spot RMS size or unsharpness parameter B_F. There are also great uncertainties in terms of focal spot boundaries determining the focal spot dimensions, see Fig. 6 for a visualization of some of the problems.

TODATE, MOST FOCAL SPOTS HAVE <u>DOUBLE BAND</u> DISTRIBUTION

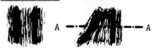

PINHOLE RADIOGRAMS

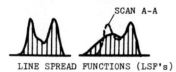

LINE SPREAD FUNCTIONS (LSF's)

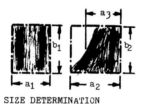

SIZE DETERMINATION
AMBIGUOUS

FIG. 6
TYPICAL FOCAL SPOTS
AMBIGUOUS SIZE DETERMINATION.

(2) The "effective" size - measured by a resolution pattern [6] - can be used for a large class of focal spots. This class of focal spots may be defined by the requirement that the blur regions of the star pattern image are easily identifiable as a band followed by regions of "spurious resolution" towards higher line pair frequencies. This behavior of the pattern image indicates sharp MTF minima. Then, for this class of focal spots, the RMS size B_F equals to a good approximation the "effective" focal spot according to the NEMA[6] prescription (now often called "equivalent" focal spot).

(3) The determination of the RMS size B_F of focal spots which do not have well defined blur regions of the star pattern image is difficult. This is often the case for micro focus tubes with a filament cathode. The upper part of Figure 7 shows an example of a micro focal spot of a commercially available x-ray tube with filament cathode. For this tube, in one special direction,
the geometrical size is 780 μm
the effective size (by star) is 140 μm
an exceedingly large difference between the two size values. For this focal spot, the calculated RMS size equals B_F = 340 μm.

We found a curious behavior for many - conventional and irregular - focal spots in that the geometric mean of the two numbers, - the size derived from slit pictures (or somewhat overexposed pinhole pictures) and the size derived from star pattern images, - comes out very close to the RMS size B_F; see Fig. 7. Certainly, this rule of thumb must be used with caution.

It is very safe to say that the focal spot RMS Size B_F can never be smaller than the size derived from the star pattern method. In other words, the star pattern "size" describes the "best" case, the real focal spot can only be equal or worse.

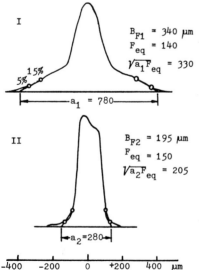

FIG. 7
LSFs OF TWO EXPERIMENTAL FOCAL SPOTS.

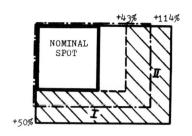

FIG. 8

NEMA FOCAL SPOT TOLERANCES
FOR FOCAL SPOTS < 0.8 mm NOM.

(5) A remark to the present focal spot standard regarding the pinhole method; see Fig. 8: According to the tolerance limits specified in the standard, the actual focal spot boundaries I and II must be in the shaded area. In the length direction, the focal spot <u>must</u> be at least 43% larger than the nominal size, and is still within the tolerance limits if being up to 114% larger! However, as said before, the pinhole dimensions - whether "Nominal" or actual - might not have a very close relation to the RMS size B_F anyway.

1.5 ELECTRON BEAM FOCUSING

At present, two technologies are employed in x-ray tube electron guns.

(a) Conventional Filament Gun (fig. 9)

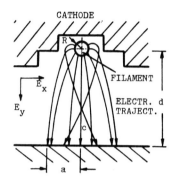

FIG. 9

CONVENTIONAL CATHODE AND
ELECTRON TRAJECTORIES.

In a conventional x-ray tube the electrons are emitted from a filament surface into all directions and then pulled down towards the anode by the high electric field, see Fig. 9. The impact pattern of of the electrons on the anode is rather unpredictable (Fig. 6). Also, "blooming" of the focal spot with increased tube current is very common. In microfocus tubes, very small clearances are required between the fragile, small filament and the surrounding cathode head.

This makes focal spot size control very difficult and requires a larger manufacturing tolerance range. Minute filament warpage has a large effect on focusing, and can even lead to filament shorting should the filament touch the focusing cup.

(b) Multi-lense Gun (fig. 10)*

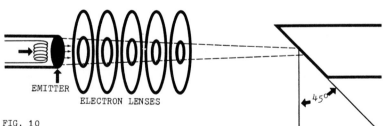

FIG. 10

The principle of the RSI microfocus x-ray tube is shown in this diagram. The arrow at the left points to the filament heater that raises the emitting surface temperature of the circular, smooth-surface cathode (second arrow) to an optimum point for electron emission. The electrons are emitted perpendicular to the smooth cathode surface and travel parallel to each other. The electron beam is focused, as shown, through a series of electron lenses to produce a circular focal spot of 0.09mm with no double-peaking or off-axis radiation. The target angle of the stationary anode (on right) is 45 degrees.

This rather sophisticated electron gun consists of a smooth, basically flat electron emitting surface and a series of lenses which allow precise focusing of the beam into a uniform circular focal spot at all mA levels. Failure of focusing -- e.g. an oversized focal spot--is not a sign of a faulty tube, but of a fault in the gun power supply. Therefore, a bad focus can be corrected easily external to the tube.

*RSI MTF-1

2. ENERGY RELATIONS

2.1 GENERAL FORMULAS

Within this category of an x-ray system, we are concerned mainly with x-ray source strength or tube load limits.

The main reason for the desire of high tube load limits is to minimize motion unsharpness. No comprehensive mathematical treatment has been made to date of imaging systems performance which includes the energy relations (via motion unsharpness) and to optimize the performance. The relation between maximum tube power and focal spot area or size is not linear. The power limits decrease by the 3/2 power with decreasing spot size on a rotating target. On a stationary target, the relation can be anything from a square law (power proportional to focal spot area) usually for very large proximity cooled source areas, to a 2/3 law for some microfocal spot anode constructions:

Rotating Anode: P proportional to $W^{3/2}$ (0.1 sec. exposure)

Stationary Anode: P proportional to $W^{2/3 \cdots 2}$, typically to W,

with P the maximum power allowed, and W the dimension of the side of the square focal spot. As an example, on a rotating anode, decreasing the size by a factor of 4 decreases load limits by a factor of 8. For a target with a target angle $\alpha = 13°$, a rotational speed of n = 10,000 rpm and a diameter of D = 100 mm, the loadability or power limit for short exposures (0.1 sec) is approximately

$$P_o = 10 \; (W/0.3)^{3/2} \; h \text{ in kW*} \tag{10}$$

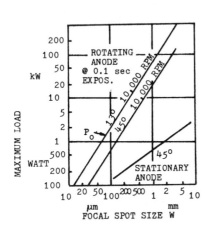

see Fig. 11. W is the width of a uniform focal spot which is projected into the central beam, h = projected length/W. For a square projected focal spot, h = 1. For focal spots with non-uniform distribution, W is the Equivalent Loadability Size W_e [1].

For other values of α, n and D, the power limit is

$$P = P_o \; \frac{\sin 13}{\sin \alpha} \; \sqrt{\frac{n}{10,000}} \; \sqrt{\frac{D}{100}} \; h, \text{in kW} \tag{11}$$

and

$$\sin 13/\sin\alpha \approx 13/\alpha \tag{12}$$

for small α ($\alpha \lesssim 20°$).

With increased exposure time, power handling capability of rotating anodes decreases, while it remains basically constant for stationary anodes.

FIG. 11
X-RAY ANODE LOADABILITY (POWER).

OTHER FACTORS: $P' = P_o \frac{\sin 13}{\sin\alpha} \frac{\sqrt{nD}}{1000}$
Rotat. Anode

2.2 EFFECT OF CHANGING RPM, DIAMETER AND TARGET ANGLE

From (10) and (11) it follows that the focal spot size for a given power limit is proportional to $n^{1/3} D^{1/3} \alpha^{-2/3}$. Table 1 summarizes the effect of changing RPM, D or α on size W or power P, as well as on anode mechanical

*Calculate : (W/0.3) times $\sqrt{W/0.3}$ on a hand calculator, W in mm.

performance. As can be seen, the effect of these changes on focal size or on power limits is surprisingly small.

TABLE 2

CHANGE	EITHER OR		FORCES ON BEARINGS	SPEED UP TIME
	SMALLER FOCAL SPOT	MORE POWER		
RPM x 2	-25%	+40%	times 4	times 4
Dia + 50%	-15%	+25%	+ 50%	times 5
Target angle -25% ($13^o \rightarrow 10^o$)	-15%	+25%	-	-

The forces on bearings are mainly unbalance and weight.

2.3 HEEL EFFECT

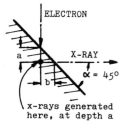

x-rays generated here, at depth a

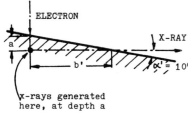

x-rays generated here, at depth a

FIG. 12
HEEL EFFECT.

This effect leads to a reduction of x-ray output with smaller target angles by a factor $H(\alpha)$ [11]. The cause is self absorption of x-rays in the upper target layer, see Fig. 12. The smaller the target angle α, the longer the path b of the x-ray beam through the target material, the more the x-rays are absorbed. The ratio in x-ray output for the following target angles: $7^o - 13^o - 45^o$ is approximately 80 - 100 - 140, for the same kV/mA factors.

2.4 DISTANCE RELATIONS

The smallest possible distance between source and recorder will maximize energy efficiency resulting in minimized exposure time, and, for rotating anodes, in increased tube power utilization which results in higher "EFFECTIVE HEAT UNIT STORAGE CAPACITY".

The x-ray intensity at the film (recorder) is

$$I = C \, H(\alpha) \, P/(SID)^2, \qquad (13)$$

with C a constant, and SID = S the source to image receptor distance: SID=S=F/tanβ, see Fig. 13. This formula holds for both rotating and stationary anodes. For a rotating anode combining (10) and (13), we get for the x-ray intensity I at the recorder, relative to the x-ray intensity I_0 at 40" SID:

$$\frac{I}{I_0} = H(\alpha) \, \frac{P}{P_0} \, \left(\frac{40}{SID}\right)^2. \qquad (14)$$

Relative to a 13° target, and a 17" field size at 40" SID:

$$\frac{I}{I_o} = H(\alpha)\,\left(\frac{W}{0.3}\right)^{3/2}\left(\frac{17}{F}\right)^{2}\left(\frac{\tan\beta}{\tan 12}\right)^{2}\left(\frac{\sin 13}{\sin\alpha}\right)\sqrt{\frac{n}{10,000}}\sqrt{\frac{D}{100}} \quad (15)$$

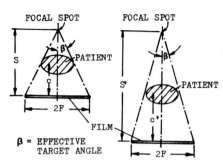

FOCAL SPOT   FOCAL SPOT

S   β   PATIENT

c

2F

S'   β   PATIENT

c'

FILM

2F

β = EFFECTIVE TARGET ANGLE

FIG. 13

DISTANCE RELATIONS.

For the special but common case, that $\beta\approx\alpha$, which means adjusting the SID such that maximum use is made of the available field coverage, the x-ray intensity is proportional to H(α) and α:

$$I \sim H(\alpha)\alpha, (\alpha \lessgtr 20°). \quad (16)$$

This result is interesting insofar as it shows that although the loadability or power limit P is proportional to $1/\alpha$ (see (11) and (12)), the x-ray intensity at the recorder is directly proportional to α, if full use can be made of the available field. For instance, if we compare a 7° target with a 16° target, we gain a factor of 3 for the x-ray intensity. For a 17" field, SID is 70" for a 7° versus 30" for a 16° target.

For a stationary target, P is approximately proportional to $1/\sqrt{\sin\alpha}$ *. For small target angles, this is about $1/\sqrt{\alpha}$, therefore:

$$I \sim \alpha^{3/2} H(\alpha) \quad (17)$$

(with a different proportionality constant than in (16)). (17) shows that in case of a stationary anode, with its inherent lower power level, it is even more beneficial to shorten SID using large target angles. If maximum field usage is made, x-ray intensity for a 16° target is 4.5 times as high than that for a 7° target.

Some of the disadvantages of the short SID - large angle system in magnification techniques and possible remedies are the following:

(1) X-ray Scatter is increased because of the smaller air gap, therefore contrast is reduced, which is particularly unwanted in mammography. However, a relatively transparent grid can be used to increase scatter rejection. The systems energy efficiency loss caused by the grid is smaller than that coming from an increased SID. The optimum is probably somewhere between the extremes of "grid-only" and "magnification-only". M. Friedrich et al[12] favor a grid-only technique over the magnification technique in mammography. They cite the impracticality of the large film format required, and the lower contrast because of a higher tube voltage used. The latter was required because with their machine the electron beam could not be focused to a small enough spot at the required mA levels at lower kV.

(2) There might be problems to fit the patient close enough to the x-ray tube.

(3) An objection heard often is that the skin entrance dose is higher for the short SID system (at same magnification). However, if we compare the integrated x-ray energy deposited in the breast, dose increase is relatively small.

*The power law for stationary targets, however, is much more dependent on target construction, focal spot size etc. See para. 2.1.

2.5 FIGURE OF MERIT

The Figure of Merit for focal spots can be defined as a number which relates loadability of the spot to its optical performance. If we request a certain focal spot "size" (RMS size B_F) for a certain procedure, we generally will be interested in a focal spot intensity distribution which allows the highest load possible, at given target angle, diameter and RPM.

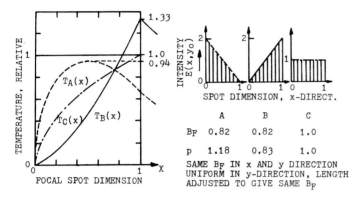

SAME B_F IN x AND y DIRECTION
UNIFORM IN y-DIRECTION, LENGTH
ADJUSTED TO GIVE SAME B_F

FIG. 14
FOCAL SPOT TEMPERATURE DISTRIBUTION FOR SAME LOAD INTO
THREE FOCAL SPOTS OF DIFFERENT INTENSITY PROFILE.

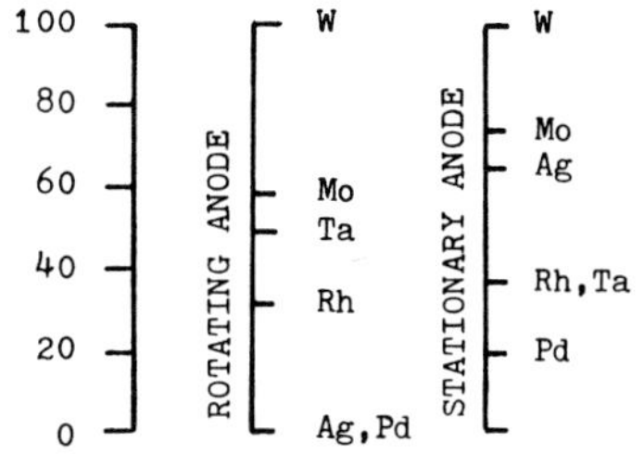

FIG. 15
RELATIVE LOAD CAPABILITY OF
VARIOUS TARGET MATERIALS

ROT.ANODE: $\sqrt{\varrho ck}\,\Delta T/(\sqrt{\varrho ck}\,\Delta T)_W$
STAT.ANODE: $k\Delta T/(k\Delta T)_W$

$\Delta T \triangleq$ TEMP. WHERE VAP.PRESS. IS
10^{-6} TORR, MINUS ANODE BASE TEMP.

In Ref. [1], various focal spots are compared on this basis. For instance, focal spot A in Fig. 14 has 40% more loadability than focal spot B. This equals the gain achievable by increasing the RPM by as much as a factor of two, see table 1. However, both spots have the same imaging performance (same B_F). It can also be shown, that on a rotating anode a cylinderical symmetric Gaussian focal spot is not necessarily the best one in the context of an optimized magnification system.

2.6 TARGET MATERIALS

The constant "10" in formula (10) for a special target contains among others, the material constants, essentially in the form [10]

$$C_R = \Delta T \sqrt{\varrho\, ck} \qquad (18)$$

for a rotating target, with ΔT the maximum permissible temperature in the focal spot, measured as the difference to the target base temperature. ϱ is the density, c the specific heat, and k the thermal conductivity of the material. For a stationary target, the power limit is proportional to

$$C_S = \Delta T\, k. \qquad (19)$$

Fig. 15 shows the relative magnitude of each of these two constants for various materials relative to tungsten. Note, that a loadability comparison can only be made here between the different materials, everything else being the same, such as target and focal spot geometries, kV/mA factors etc.

Also note, that the target base temperature of a rotating anode must be chosen sufficiently high to allow reasonably short target cooling periods (cooling takes place almost entirely by heat radiation, which increases as the 4th power of the absolute temperature). For instance, a decrease in absolute temperature by 19% cuts cooling in half. Conventional rotating targets are rated for a maximum bulk temperature of about 1200°C. The target base temperature of a liquid cooled stationary target is essentially the temperature of the cooling liquid, which is usually not higher than 150°C.

Also, total x-ray output increases with atomic number Z; the bremsstrahlung continuum intensity is roughly proportional to $Z^{0.6}$, see (14). However, if selective spectral output is desired, such as using molybdenum's K_α characteristic radiation, x-ray output obeys a different law: x-ray characteristic intensity is increasing with decreasing atomic number. The exact relationship between the image receptor response versus tube voltage and current can be very involved in this case.

The relations are different for a rotating target when the so-called "volume heating mode" become predominant[10]. However, for the low tube voltages used in mammography, this effect is so small as to be negligible.

3. BACKGROUND OR SPURIOUS PHOTONS

Both scatter and off-focus radiation belong to this systems category. As mentioned before, the means for removal of scatter usually reduce systems energy (effective source strength), and a combination of different scatter removal techniques (air gap, grid, multiple moving slit) might lead to an optimum.

Off-focus radiation cannot be removed easily, since it is generated inside the vacuum envelope of the tube. External "near shutters" are used to reduce off-focus radiation somewhat. Fig. 16 depicts the basic cause of off-focus radiation. ½% of the electrons incident on a tungsten surface generate x-rays, and 48% are back scattered, after losing some of their energy in the upper layer of the anode. These high energy back-scattered electrons move on trajectories determined by the distribution of the electrical potential (voltage) within the tube. As the electrons fly towards the cathode, they lose energy in the electrical potential field until they turn back towards the anode -- like a tennis ball, falling down and bouncing back, to a lesser height, since some energy is lost. Multiple scattering spreads the electrons further over the anode. As can be expected, the off-focus x-ray intensity distribution depends somewhat on the cathode-anode distance.

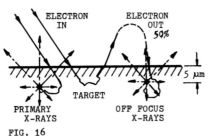

OF THOSE ELECTRONS NOT BACK SCATTERED:
1% X-RAYS - 99% HEAT

FIG. 16
OFF FOCUS X-RAY GENERATION BY BACK SCATTERED ELECTRONS.

At the beginning of the exposure (application of high voltage) many electrons fly towards the glass, charging it up. This changes the electric field distribution, which causes further electrons to return to the anode, covering its entire surface, including its back surface. Fig. 17 shows this schematically for a conventional rotary anode tube.

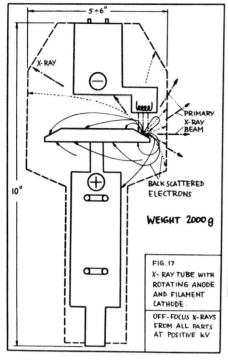

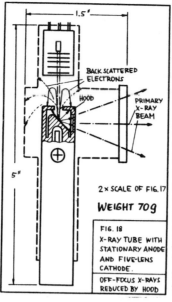

FIG.17
X-RAY TUBE WITH
ROTATING ANODE
AND FILAMENT
CATHODE.

OFF-FOCUS X-RAYS
FROM ALL PARTS
AT POSITIVE kV

WEIGHT 2000 g

WEIGHT 70 g

2 × SCALE OF FIG. 17

FIG. 18
X-RAY TUBE WITH
STATIONARY ANODE
AND FIVE-LENS
CATHODE.

OFF-FOCUS X-RAYS
REDUCED BY HOOD

Fig. 18 shows a stationary anode tube featuring a "Hood" surrounding the target surface. Inside the hood we have approximately an equipotential volume, which means a very small electrical field. Back scattered electrons therefore fly on straight lines towards the inside hood surfaces. Depending on materials and construction of the hood, only very small amounts of off-focus x-rays exit the window. R. Gould [13] reports a reduction of off-focus radiation to 1/3 with this type of tube* compared to a conventional rotating anode tube.

Can misfocused primary electrons cause off-focus radiation? The simplest mathematical model of a uniform electrical field results in an electron spread of (See Fig. 9)

$$a = 2 \sqrt{V_0/V_T} \, d + R. \tag{20}$$

eV_0 is the total of kinetic energy components perpendicular to the center line, imposed on the electrons by electric field components E_x in that direction. E_x is of any significance only near the filament. For instance, even if $V_0 = 1000V$, then with $d = 10$ mm and $V_T = 10^5 V$, a is only 2 mm. This "proximity focusing effect" prevents electrons from traveling on trajectories far away from the center line C. More accurate computer calculations confirm this. Therefore, "off-focus" radiation is usually not caused by primary "misfocused" electrons, but by back scattered electrons, as explained before.

4. X-RAY BEAM QUALITY

It seems from recent publications that monochromatic x-rays or at least a narrow spectral band would be most desirable for optimized mammographic imaging. However, much remains to be done with regard to finding the most desirable x-ray beam quality for a given mammography procedure and subject. According to Motz and Danos [15], the optimum x-ray photon energy would be in the 40-50 keV range if appropriate technologies and imaging processing would be applied, and the radiologist would be able to read "noisy" images.

A number of articles have appeared recently analyzing the effect of different target materials and external filtration on the mammographic image. [16] [17] Of particular interest has been the comparison of tungsten and molybdenum targets. [18] Also results with a rhodium target have been

* RSI Mag II system.

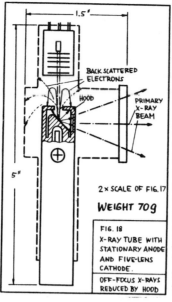

207

reported.[19]

It is generally agreed upon that a molybdenum target with it's strong K characteristic radiation at about 17.5 keV gives the highest contrast (for film mammography), but with high dose levels for thick breasts. Using target materials of somewhat higher atomic number, a trade-off between contrast and dose can possibly be made.

However, the materials to be used must meet two basic criteria: (A) they must be compatible with the high vacuum environment, and (B) they must have the required thermal stability, to assure sufficient or comparable x-ray output. Formulas (18) and (19) can be used to compare the different materials with regard to criterium (B).

For instance (Fig. 15), on a rotating anode, loadability of molybdenum is about 60% and rhodium 30% of that of tungsten. On a stationary anode, molybdenum has approximately 75%, rhodium 35%, and silver 65% of the loadability of that of tungsten. The high number for silver here follows from the superior thermal conductivity (k), which counteracts the effect of the low working temperature limits (formula (19)). Since the K_α line of silver is at 22 keV, a silver target should have a similar effect on contrast as rhodium filtration of the tungsten continuum since the K edge of rhodium is at 23.2 keV.[16]

Because of the low working temperature of silver, it cannot be used on a rotating anode, since high anode temperature levels are necessary to obtain sufficient heat radiation for anode cooling. At 400°C, heat radiation is only 10% of that at 900°C, because of the T^4 law (see paragraph 2.6).

In some instances, the low working temperature limitation can be overcome by using a composite target. An example of this for iodine contrast imaging was reported by Eisenberg et al[20], utilizing a cerium boride anode instead of the pure cerium material (see Ref. [10] for the theoretical details).

A self-filtering Anode [21] can be thought of as a transmission target with a shallow angle geometry, see Fig. 19. As with an externally filtered arrangement, with the filter being the same material as the anode material, the characteristic radiation is only minimally absorbed, since the K lines are at slightly lower photon energies than the K edge. Compared to an externally filtered x-ray beam the self-filtered anode

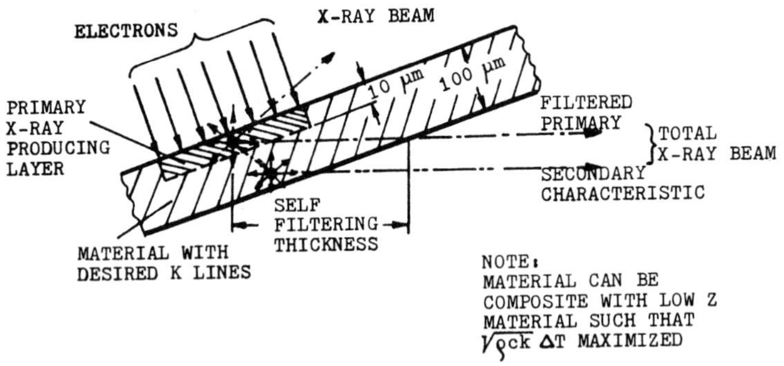

FIG. 19
SELF FILTERING ANODE.

generates an amount of characteristic radiation which is further enhanced by secondary fluoroscent x-rays, which are generated when the primary x-ray continuum above the K edge of the material is photo-electrically absorbed in the thin target layer. These secondary x-rays are then coming essentially from the focal spot area, which is the area where the primary photons are generated.

For constructional reasons, the thin target has to be supported by some kind of a low x-ray absorbing material, such as graphite.

For the case of a 20 μm thick molybdenum self-filtered anode, the "purity" of the beam, that is the characteristic radiation (plus a narrow band of continuum) as a percentage of the total output, increases from 55% to nearly 80%, as the angle decreases from 90° to 10°.

REFERENCES

(1)   M. Braun, W. Roeck, and G. Gillan, "X-ray Tube Performance Characteristics and their Effect on Radiologic Image Quality", SPIE 152, 94 (1978).
(2) K. Doi, and K. Rossmann, SPIE 47, 207 (1975).
(3) P. Sprawls, SPIE 127, 106 (1977).
(4) R.F. Wagner, Photogr. Sci. Eng. 21, 252 (1977).
(5) R.F. Wagner, K.E. Weaver, E.W. Denny, and R.G. Bostron, Med. Physics. 1, 11 (1974).
(6) NEMA Standards Publication XR5-1974. -The size derived from the star pattern image is called "Effective Size" in this publication.
(7) B.A. Arnold, H. Eisenberg, and B.E. Bjarngard, to be published in Radiology.
(8) E.A. Sickles, K. Doi, and H.G. Genant, Radiology 125, 69 (1977).
(9) B.A. Arnold, E. W. Webster, L. Kalisher, Radiology 129, 179 (1978).
(10) M. Braun, SPIE 70, 65 (1975).
(11) R.C. Placious, J. Appl. Phys. 38, 2030 (1967).
(12) M. Friedrich, and P. Weskamp, Medicamundi 23/1, 29 (1978).
(13) R. Gould, and H.K. Genant, "Comparison of Off-Focus Radiation from several Micro-Focus X-ray Tubes", AAPM 20th Ann. Meeting, 7/30-8/3 1978, San Francisco, CA.
(14) D.B. Brown, D.B. Wittry, D.F. Kyser, J. Appl. Phys. 40, 1627 (1969).
(15) J.W. Motz, and M. Danos, Med. Phys. 5, 8 (1978).
(16) M.P. Siedband, R.J. Jennings, R.J. Eastgate, and D.L. Ergun, SPIE 127, 204 (1977).
(17) G. Jotten, K. Kyser, and W.J. Oosterkamp, Medicamundi 19, 24 (1974).
(18) A.G. Haus, C.E. Metz, J.T. Chiles, and K. Rossman, Radiology 118, 705 (1976).
(19) G.A. Johnson, and F. O'Foghludha, Radiology 127, 511 (1978)
(20) H. Eisenberg, B.A. Arnold, M. Braun, and W. Holland, "A Cerium Anode X-ray Tube for Iodine Contrast Examinations", RSNA 1976, Chicago.
(21) U.S. Patent No. 3,894,239.
(22) A.G. Haus, K. Doi, J.T. Chiles, K. Rossmann, and R.A. Mintzer, Invest. Radiol. 10, 43 (1975).

FILTERS - PHOTON ENERGY CONTROL AND PATIENT EXPOSURE

R.J. Jennings and T.R. Fewell

Medical Physics Branch
Division of Electronic Products
Bureau of Radiological Health
Rockville, MD 20857

INTRODUCTION

The x-ray spectrum is one of the most important factors to be considered in any analysis of roentgenographic examinations of the breast. In this discussion, a simple theoretical model will be described which predicts the optimum x-ray energy for mammography. Comparisons of the predictions of this model with spectra currently used for screen-film mammography indicate that significant improvements can be made by using modified x-ray spectra. Examples of such spectra are presented and evaluated for use with current mammography systems on the basis of image contrast, patient exposure and dose, and tube loading. This discussion concludes with some indications of how these spectra might be used to improve the performance of mammography systems through an optimization procedure involving all of the parameters over which the system designer has control.

THEORY

A theoretical model which predicts the variation of image quality and patient exposure with x-ray photon energy can be derived by applying signal-to-noise ratio (SNR) theory to an idealized mammographic imaging task. Results of such derivations have been published by Motz and Danos (1), and by Muntz et al. (2). A simplified version of such a derivation, which neglects the effects of scatter and the influence of detector characteristics, has been found to predict optimum energies in good agreement with those predicted by Muntz. The details of the calculation have been discussed previously (3), so only the outline will be repeated here.

The mention of commercial products herein is not to be construed as either an actual or implied endorsement of such products by the Department of Health, Education and Welfare.

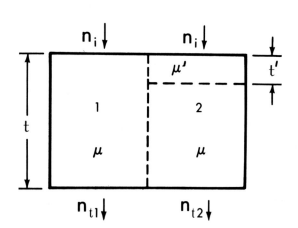

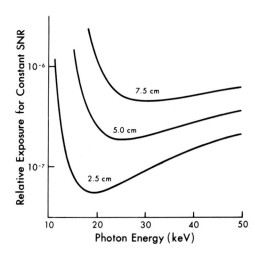

Figure 1. Simple imaging situation used to develop a theoretical model for mammography.

Figure 2. Relative exposure required for constant SNR as a function of photon energy for imaging of glandular tissue in a mixture of 50 percent adipose and 50 percent glandular tissue, for three breast thicknesses.

The imaging situation is shown schematically in Fig. 1. Photon fluence n_i is incident on a phantom consisting of a uniform region of thickness t composed of a material with linear attenution coefficient μ and another region consisting mostly of the same material, but with a small thickness t' replaced by a material with attenuation coefficient μ'. The transmitted fluences are given by n_{t1} and n_{t2}. The task is to distinguish between regions 1 and 2. The SNR is found by taking the ratio of the contrast C, given by

$$C = (\mu - \mu')\, t' = \Delta\mu t',$$

to the noise contrast C_n, for a reference area A. C_n is given by

$$C_n = (n_i A\, e^{-\mu t})^{-\frac{1}{2}}.$$

The SNR which results is given by

$$SNR = (\Delta\mu t')(n_i A e^{-\mu t})^{\frac{1}{2}}.$$

The corresponding incident photon fluence n_i is

$$n_i = (SNR)^2/\Delta\mu^2 t'^2\, e^{-\mu t}\, A.$$

For the purposes of this discussion, it is sufficient to study the relative variation of the fluence required to produce a fixed value of the SNR as a function of photon energy. The factors $(SNR)^2$, t'^2, and A are all independent of energy, and in an arbitrary system of units, each can be set equal to 1. The resulting relative fluence n_{Rel} is given by

$$n_{Rel}(E) = (\Delta\mu^2(E)\, e^{-\mu(E)t})^{-1}.$$

212

Photon fluence can be converted to the most commonly measured parameter, exposure, by multiplying n_{Rel} by the conversion factor $K(E)$ relating fluence to exposure, so that

$$X_{Rel} = K(E) \, n_{Rel} \, (E).$$

This relative exposure information can then be converted to other measures of patient risk, such as average dose, or midline dose by using, for example, the data relating exposure to dose published by the Northeast Center for Radiological Physics (4).

In Fig. 2, the relative exposure X_{Rel} has been plotted as a function of photon energy for the case of imaging glandular tissue in a breast with an average composition of 50 percent adipose tissue and 50 percent glandular tissue. This choice of materials represents the imaging of a tumor in normal tissue as well as the imaging of normal breast structure. The elemental compositions and densities of these two materials were taken from Ref. 4. Plots are shown for breast thicknesses of 2.5, 5.0 and 7.5 cm.

The plots show definite minima in the exposure required to obtain a given SNR. The energy corresponding to the minimum exposure depends on breast thickness, so that any clinical optimization must involve either varying the x-ray spectrum to match the patient or selecting a single spectrum which is a compromise. The minima fall at 19.5, 25.5, and 30.5 keV for the three thicknesses selected, showing that, for all but the thinnest breasts, the K-characteristic energies from Mo-anode tubes (17.4 and 19.6 keV) are not optimal. The strong dependence of minimum exposure or of exposure at a given energy on breast thickness shows clearly the importance of breast compression in reducing exposure.

In addition to considering the dependence of optimum energy on breast thickness, it is important to examine the dependence of optimum energy on the compositon of the object being imaged. In order to compare optimal conditions for the imaging of calcifications with those for tumor imaging, X_{Rel} was also plotted for inner bone (representing the calcification) in a 5 cm breast with the same 50 percent adipose and 50 percent glandular tissue composition used above. This is shown in Fig. 3, along with the plot for the 5 cm breast with the glandular tissue inclusion, which was reduced by a factor of 1000 to facilitate the comparison. The difference in scale simply indicates that, for any given exposure, the thickness of calcification which can just be detected is much smaller than the thickness of tumor which can just be detected. The third curve in Fig. 3 is for the case of an aluminum object in a lucite host. The optimum energy for the calcification imaging case is 25 KeV, for the tumor case 25.5 KeV, and for the phantom 24 KeV. Thus, the mammographic spectrum can be optimized simultaneously for tumor and calcification imaging, and experiments with a phantom of lucite and aluminum should give good predictions of the relative performance of different spectra in actual breast imaging, in terms of the criterion $(SNR)^2/exposure$.

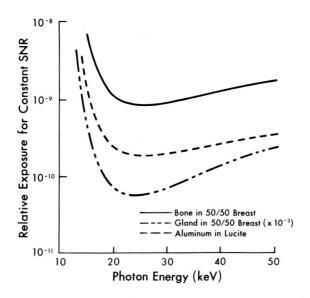

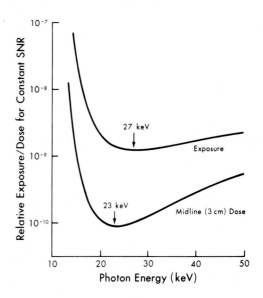

Figure 3. Relative exposure required for constant SNR as a function of photon energy for three different imaging tasks.

Figure 4. Relative exposure and relative midline dose for constant SNR compared. Imaging task is detection of bone (representing a calcification) in a 6 cm breast composed of 50 percent adipose and 50 percent glandular tissue.

Finally, spectral optimization to minimize exposure and midline dose are compared in Fig. 4. The imaging task is detection of bone, representing a calcification, in a 50 percent adipose and 50 percent glandular breast which is 6 cm thick. Midline dose was determined from the data in Ref. 4 relating midline dose to exposure and spectrum half-value layer (HVL). The optimum energies for minimizing exposure and midline dose are 27 and 23.5 keV, respectively. Although the optimum energy for dose is lower than that for exposure, it is still above the energy of the K-characteristic radiation of a Mo-anode tube.

The spectrum from a Mo-anode tube can be seen to be less than optimal for another reason. Data presented in Refs. 5 and 6 show that, even when a 0.03 mm Mo filter is used to suppress the bremsstrahlung continuum at energies above the Mo K-edge, the beam hardening effect of a moderately thick breast results in a transmitted spectrum with a significant number of photons at energies above 20 keV. These photons reduce the contrast in the image. As a result, the SNR in such an image may be lower than the SNR in an image produced with the same exposure but using only Mo K-characteristic radiation.

SPECTRA

The optimum spectrum for mammography thus has two important characteristics: (1) the mean energy is higher than 20 keV, and (2) the spectrum is distributed over a narrow range of energies. Although monoenergetic sources with these characteristics exist, they are not suitable for clinical use because of intensity limitations. Suitable spectra can be produced using a tungsten (W) anode tube with Al filtration, but, because of the very low peak tube potentials required to obtain appropriate mean energies, intensity is the limitation here as well.

However, it has been shown (3,6) that the use of filters with K-edges above 20 keV with a W-anode tube can produce suitable spectra with adequate intensity. Further experiments with these spectra are reported here, along with studies using the same filters to modify the spectrum of a Mo-anode tube.

Materials with K-edges above 20 keV which might be suitable for use as filters for screen-film mammography are ruthenium (Ru), rhodium (Rh), palladium (Pd), silver (Ag), and cadmium (Cd). Previous work (3,6) has shown that, unless other changes are made to a mammographic system to increase contrast, such as reducing scatter or using a higher contrast film, Ag and Cd filters produce image contrast which is noticeably lower than that obtained with a Mo-anode tube and Mo filter. Therefore, measurements were limited to filters of Ru, Rh, and Pd. Applications of materials with higher energy K-edges (Ag, Cd, In, Sn) in the systematic optimization of a mammographic system in which all of the relevant parameters can be manipulated will be discussed later.

Measurements of a large number of spectra were made using the equipment and techniques reported by Fewell and Shuping (7,8). Two x-ray tubes designed for mammographic imaging were used. Once was a Machlett Dynamax 69M, with a W anode and glass window. The other was a Machlett Dynamax M64, with Mo anode and glass window. Entrance spectra as well as exit spectra from phantoms of 2.5, 5.0 and 7.5 cm of lucite were measured. Data were recorded at peak tube potentials of 27.5, 30.0, 32.5 and 35.0 kVp.

Figure 5 shows the spectrum produced by the W-anode tube with a 0.051 mm Rh filter at a tube potential of 27.5 kVp. The spectrum produced by the Mo-anode tube with a 0.03 mm Mo filter at a peak tube potential of 30 kVp is shown for comparison. The W-anode spectrum has a higher mean energy and a higher HVL. Figure 6 shows the spectra which result when the spectra of Fig. 5 are attenuated by 5 cm of lucite. Note that the HVL's are closer together, and the mean energies are now nearly equal. Note also that the filter used with the W-anode tube is sufficiently thick to suppress nearly all of the radiation above its own K-edge, even after attenuation by 5 cm of lucite, while the Mo-anode tube spectrum shows a significant contribution from the photons with energies above the K-edge of the Mo filter.

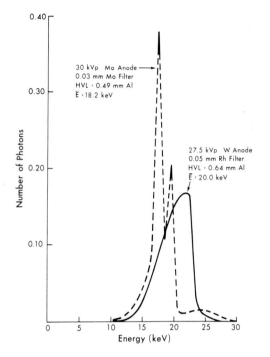

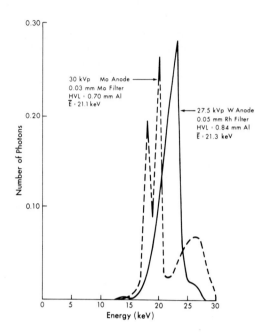

Figure 5. Solid line: spectrum from W-anode tube operated at 27.5 kVp with 0.05 mm Rh filter. Dashed line: spectrum from Mo-anode tube operated at 30 kVp with 0.03 mm Mo filter.

Figure 6. Spectra generated as described in Fig. 5 after attenuation by 5 cm lucite phantom.

It has been observed that, for very thick and/or dense breasts, a Mo-anode tube may be operated with an Al filter to produce images with satisfactory contrast, at much lower exposure and anode heat load values than are required using an Mo filter (9,10). This is due to the fact that the Mo K-characteristic x-rays are so strongly attenuated that they are no longer effective in forming the image. The use of filters with K-edges above the K-edge of Mo to attenuate the Mo K-characteristic radiation and select a narrow band of energies from the bremsstrahlung spectrum of the Mo-anode tube was studied as a possible means of refining this approach. Figure 7 shows two Mo-anode tube spectra, one produced using a 0.051 mm Pd filter, the other using a 0.03 mm Mo filter, both at 30 kVp. Figure 8 shows these spectra after being attenuated by a 5.0 cm lucite phantom. A similar approach using a thin (.025 mm) silver filter has been reported by Jotten, et al. (10).

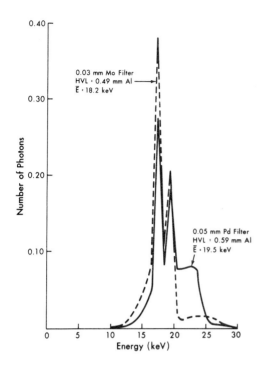

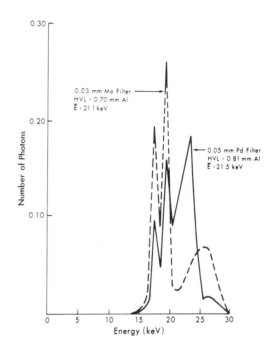

Figure 7. Spectra produced by Mo-anode tube operated at 30 kVp. Solid line: spectrum filtered with 0.05 mm Pd. Dashed line: spectrum filtered with 0.03 mm Mo.

Figure 8. Spectra generated as described in Fig. 7 after attenuation by 5.0 cm lucite phantom.

The HVL's and mean energies extracted from the measured spectra are listed in Table 1. Note that the lowest HVL shown is 0.45 mm of Al, while values of 0.3 mm are often reported for Mo-anode tubes. Since an HVL of 0.3 mm corresponds to an effective energy of about 15 KeV, the difference is assumed to be due to the added attenuation of low energy photons by the glass windows of the tubes used for the measurements, compared to the attenuation of the beryllium windows of some models of x-ray tubes used for mammography.

PHANTOM MEASUREMENTS

The spectra listed in Table 1 were also studied to determine their imaging properties. Radiographs of three phantoms were made using Kodak's Min-R screen-film combination. Each phantom consisted of a block of lucite with a 0.5 mm thick Al plate covering a portion of the area imaged, to give a measure of large area contrast. The lucite thicknesses were 2.5, 5.0, and 7.5 cm.

For each spectrum and phantom thickness, three radiographs were made, at exposure values selected so that the film densities in the lucite-only region of the image bracketed a net density of 1.0. Using the three data pairs, the phantom exposure required for a net density of 1.0 was determined. The density difference between the areas with and without the added aluminum was also measured on these films. The density difference corresponding to the exposure which produced a net density of 1.0 was used as a measure of image contrast.

Table 1. Characteristics of measured spectra

Anode	kVp	Filter	Phantom (cm of lucite)	HVL (mm Al)	E (keV)
W	27.5	None	None	0.52	19.5
W	27.5	45 mg/cm^2 Ru	None	0.61	19.6
W	27.5	45 mg/cm^2 Ru	2.5	0.72	20.5
W	27.5	45 mg/cm^2 Ru	5.0	0.78	20.9
W	27.5	.05 mm Rh	None	0.64	20.0
W	27.5	.05 mm Rh	2.5	0.76	20.8
W	27.5	.05 mm Rh	5.0	0.84	21.3
W	27.5	.05 mm Rh	7.5	0.89	21.7
W	27.5	.05 mm Pd	None	0.68	20.5
W	27.5	.05 mm Pd	5.0	0.89	21.9
Mo	27.5	None	None	0.45	18.2
Mo	27.5	.03 mm Mo	None	0.47	17.8
Mo	27.5	.05 mm Rh	None	0.55	18.9
Mo	27.5	.05 mm Rh	2.5	0.65	19.7
Mo	27.5	.05 mm Rh	5.0	0.72	20.4
Mo	27.5	.05 mm Rh	7.5	0.79	20.9
Mo	27.5	.05 mm Pd	None	0.57	19.2
Mo	27.5	.05 mm Pd	5.0	0.77	21.0
W	30.0	None	None	0.60	20.8
W	30.0	.05 mm Rh	None	0.66	20.4
W	30.0	.05 mm Rh	5.0	0.88	22.0
W	30.0	.05 mm Pd	None	0.72	21.0
W	30.0	.05 mm Pd	2.5	0.85	21.8
W	30.0	.05 mm Pd	5.0	0.94	22.4
W	30.0	.05 mm Pd	7.5	1.00	22.8
Mo	30.0	None	None	0.48	18.9
Mo	30.0	.03 mm Mo	None	0.49	18.2
Mo	30.0	.03 mm Mo	2.5	0.60	19.7
Mo	30.0	.03 mm Mo	5.0	0.70	21.1
Mo	30.0	.03 mm Mo	7.5	0.84	22.6
Mo	30.0	.05 mm Rh	None	0.56	19.0
Mo	30.0	.05 mm Rh	2.5	0.66	20.0
Mo	30.0	.05 mm Rh	5.0	0.74	20.8
Mo	30.0	.05 mm Rh	7.5	0.84	21.7
Mo	30.0	.05 mm Pd	None	0.59	19.5
Mo	30.0	.05 mm Pd	2.5	0.70	20.6
Mo	30.0	.05 mm Pd	5.0	0.81	21.5
Mo	30.0	.05 mm Pd	7.5	0.90	22.2
W	32.5	None	None	0.66	22.0
W	32.5	.05 mm Rh	None	0.70	20.9
W	32.5	.05 mm Rh	5.0	0.95	23.1
W	32.5	.05 mm Pd	None	0.74	21.4
W	32.5	.05 mm Pd	5.0	1.00	23.3
Mo	32.5	None	None	0.51	19.5
Mo	32.5	.03 mm Mo	None	0.51	18.7
Mo	32.5	.03 mm Mo	2.5	0.63	20.6
Mo	32.5	.03 mm Mo	5.0	0.77	22.6
Mo	32.5	.03 mm Mo	7.5	0.96	24.3
Mo	32.5	.05 mm Rh	None	0.58	19.3
Mo	32.5	.05 mm Rh	5.0	0.78	21.7
Mo	32.5	.05 mm Pd	None	0.60	19.7
Mo	32.5	.05 mm Pd	2.5	0.71	20.8
Mo	32.5	.05 mm Pd	5.0	0.82	21.9
Mo	32.5	.05 mm Pd	7.5	0.95	23.1
W	35.0	None	None	0.73	23.1
W	35.0	.05 mm Pd	None	0.78	22.1
W	35.0	.05 mm Pd	5.0	1.08	24.6
Mo	35.0	None	None	0.54	20.2
Mo	35.0	.03 mm Mo	None	0.53	19.4
Mo	35.0	.03 mm Mo	2.5	0.66	21.8
Mo	35.0	.03 mm Mo	5.0	0.86	24.3
Mo	35.0	.03 mm Mo	7.5	1.15	26.2
Mo	35.0	.05 mm Pd	None	0.61	20.0
Mo	35.0	.05 mm Pd	5.0	0.88	23.1

The results of the phantom imaging experiments are given in Tables 2, 3, and 4 for the 2.5, 5.0, and 7.5 cm phantoms, respectively. The tables list anode type, filter material and thickness, peak tube potential, the product of tube current and exposure time, the density difference corresponding to the areas with and withoutthe Al object, the exposure X_m required for a net density of 1.0, a figure of merit X^* which has been designated "noise-equivalent exposure," and, for the 5.0 cm phantom, the average dose corresponding to the measured exposure.

Table 2. Data for 2.5 cm lucite phantom

Anode	Filter	kVp	mAs	ΔD	X_m (mR)	X^*(mR)
W	.05 mm Rh	27.5	155	.32	130	180
W	.05 mm Pd	30	100	.29	100	170
Mo	.03 mm Mo	30	95	.38	200	200
Mo	.05 mm Rh	30	110	.34	185	230
Mo	.05 mm Pd	30	100	.32	150	210

Table 3. Data for 5.0 cm lucite phantom

Anode	Filter	kVp	mAs	ΔD	X_m (mR)	X^*(mR)	Average dose[1] (mrad)
W	.45 mg/cm^{2}Ru	27.5	1100	.26	560	700	180
W	.05 mm Rh	27.5	530	.26	440	550	150
W	.05 mm Pd	27.5	330	.22	350	610	130
Mo	.03 mm Mo	30	400	.29	1000	1000	270
Mo	.05 mm Rh	30	430	.28	720	770	220
Mo	.05 mm Pd	30	520	.27	600	700	190
Mo	.5 mm Al	35	60	.16	300	990	100

[1]Average dose was calculated using the analysis by Muntz (11), of the data in Ref. 4.

Table 4. Data for 7.5 cm lucite phantom

Anode	Filter	kVp	mAs	ΔD	X_m (R)	X^*(R)
W	.05 mm Rh	30	1340	.19	1.6	1.7
W	.05 mm Pd	30	600	.19	1.7	1.8
Mo	.03 mm Mo	30	1620	.20	5.1	5.1
Mo	.05 mm Rh	30	2400	.20	3.8	3.8
Mo	.05 mm Pd	30	1600	.19	2.6	2.9
Mo	.5 mm Al	35	200	.12	.9	2.5

Exposures were measured with a Victoreen model 555 Integrating Ratemeter using a 1DAS ionization chamber. Whenever possible, exposure times short enough to avoid reciprocity law failure were used. Where this was not possible, due to anode heat load limitations, longer exposure times were used. The data were not corrected for the reduction in film speed associated with the longer exposure times, since the measured exposures represent values which would be required under similar circumstances in clinical applications.

The concept of "noise-equivalent exposure" has been discussed previously (3). It is derived in the following way. First, it is assumed that the quantum noise in images of the same density is the same, even if they were made using different spectra. Since, according to the section on theory above, the exposure required for a given value of SNR is inversely proportional to the square of the contrast, all images can be compared on an equal SNR basis by multiplying the measured exposure by the square of the ratio of the density difference for an image produced by a reference spectrum to the measured density difference. The reference spectrum was assumed to be that produced by a Mo-anode tube with 0.03 mm Mo filter operated at 30 kVp.

The average dose which would be associated with a given exposure if it were used to image a breast having a composition of 50 percent adipose tissue and 50 percent glandular tissue was determined for the 5 cm phantom exposures from the measured exposure and the HVL of the incident spectrum using the analysis by Muntz (11) of the data in Ref. 4.

The data for the images of the 2.5 cm phantom indicate that the spectrum produced by a Mo-anode tube with a Mo-filter produces high contrast, compared to the other spectra studied, with reasonable exposures.

For a 5.0 cm phantom, however, K-edge filters with a W-anode tube can produce contrast nearly equal to the contrast obtained with a Mo-anode tube and Mo-filter, with an exposure reduction of nearly a factor of three, and a reduction in average dose of up to a factor of two. The use of Rh and Pd filters with the Mo-anode tube produces smaller but still significant exposure reductions.

Two comments should be made about these data. First, the exposure values shown for the 5 cm phantom and W-anode tube with Rh and Pd filters at 27.5 kVp and 30 kVp, respectively, are 70 percent to 75 percent higher than previously reported values (3,6). There are several possible causes for the discrepancy. The most important one is probably the difference in film sensitometric parameters caused by differences in processing conditions. Despite the differences in absolute exposure levels, the exposure reductions with W-anode tube/K-edge filtered spectra agree with previous data (3,6). The second comment to be made is that, although there is a large difference in average dose between the W-anode and Mo-anode spectra studied, the average dose corresponding to some reported values of exposure and HVL for Mo-anode spectra (e.g., 600 mR, 0.3 mm Al) is about the same (100 mrad) as shown here for the W-anode spectra.

The data for the 7.5 cm phantom show even larger advantages for K-edge filters other than Mo with both W- and Mo-anodes. The tube loading required with the W-anode tube/Pd filter combination is high but still reasonable. With the Mo-anode tube the anode heat loading is too high to permit the clinical use of the spectra studied. Note, however, the large reduction in both actual and noise-equivalent exposure. Moreover, the contrast level is much higher than that obtained using Al filtration, as in the technique proposed by Haus, et al (8). The appropriate filter, if a Mo-anode tube must be used for imaging thick breasts, would probably be Ag or Cd. These filters would reduce contrast slightly but would also decrease exposure, and would probably reduce tube loading dramatically due to the increased transmissivity of the breast at higher photon energies, and the increased x-ray production efficiency associated with operating the tube at the higher potentials which are suitable with higher K-edge energies.

CONCLUSIONS

The simple theoretical analysis of mammography presented here has shown, in agreement with Motz and Danos (1), and Muntz et al. (2), that the optimum photon energy for mammography lies above the predominant energy in the commonly used Mo-anode tube spectrum. Experimental measurements have shown that narrow-band spectra with energies appropriate for screen-film imaging of a variety of breast thicknesses and compositions can be produced using K-edge filters such as Ru, Rh and Pd with W-anode x-ray tubes. These spectra require exposure and dose levels which are significantly below those required with a Mo-anode tube and Mo filter, with anode heat loads which are less than or comparable to heat loads required with the Mo/Mo system. Aluminum filtration with W-anode tubes is not feasible for screen-film mammography since it is not possible to obtain adequate output at the very low tube operating potentials required to give satisfactory contrast. An additional advantage of the K-edge filter technique is that the W-anode tube is also well-suited for Xerox imaging of the breast, so that two x-ray systems are not required where both screen-film and Xerox modalities are employed.

Measurements using Rh and Pd filters with a Mo-anode tube instead of a W-anode tube have shown that smaller, but still significant improvements can be achieved in imaging thick and/or dense breasts, compared to results obtained with Mo or Al filtration. The experiments show that filters with K-edges at higher energies than the K-edge energy of Pd may work best.

All of the above comments are related to imaging performance using currently available x-ray systems and screen-film combinations. It is not clear, however, that these systems and image receptors cannot be improved. Magnification techniques, for instance, can be used to improve the effective MTF of a screen-film combination and reduce scatter. Muntz has discussed the optimization of mammography systems where magnification is employed (12). As he points out, x-ray tube anode head loading is one of the limits in such an optimization. The data given here and in Ref. 3 can be used to develop relationships between tube output, SNR, and dose or exposure. The optimization procedure can then be extended to include spectrum-dependent contrast effects and their influence, through focal spot and heat loading limitations, on the geometric factors involved. The computer simulation techniques for the study of x-ray spectra discussed in Ref. 3 could be used for such a study. Since substantial increases in contrast can result from the optimization techniques described in Ref. 12, the use of filters with K-edge energies higher than those of the elements studied here would be feasible. Possible choices are Ag, Cd, In, and Sn.

ACKNOWLEDGEMENTS

The authors gratefully acknowledge the capable assistance of Mark Connaughton and Earl W. Denny in performing the measurements reported here, and of Dean F. Elbert in preparing the illustrations.

REFERENCES

1. Motz, J.W. and M. Danos. Med Phys 5:8 (1978).

2. Muntz, E.P., M. Welkowsky, E. Kaegi, L. Morsell, E. Wilkinson and G. Jacobson. Radiol 127:517 (1978).

3. Jennings, R.J., R.J. Eastgate, M.P. Siedband and D.L. Ergun. To be submitted to Med Phys.

4. Hammerstein, G.R., D.W. Miller, D.R. White, M.E. Masterson, H.Q. Woodard and J.S. Laughlin. Radiol 130:485 (1979).

5. A.G. Haus, C.E. Metz, J.T. Chiles and K. Rossmann. Radiol 118:705 (1976).

6. Siedband, M.P., R.J. Jennings, R.J. Eastgate and D.L. Ergun. Proceedings of the S.P.I.E. 127:204 (1977).

7. Fewell, T.R. and R.E. Shuping. Radiol 128:211 (1978).

8. Fewell, T.R. and R.E. Shuping. Handbook of Mammographic X-Ray Spectra, HEW Publication (FDA) 79-8071, October 1978.

9. Haus, A.G., C.E. Metz, K. Doi and J. Bernstein. Radiol 124:511 (1977).

10. Jotten, G., K. Kyser and W.J. Oosterkamp. Medica Mundi 19:25 (1974).

11. Muntz, E.P. On the relative carcinogenic effect of different mammography techniques. To be published in Med. Phys.

12. Muntz, E.P. An analysis of the significance of scattered radiation in reduced dose mammography, including magnification effects, scatter suppression, focal spot and detector blurring. To be published in Med. Phys.

CHARACTERISTICS OF SCATTER

Gary T. Barnes

Department of Diagnostic Radiology
University of Alabama School of Medicine
The University of Alabama in Birmingham
Birmingham, Alabama 35233

INTRODUCTION

The contrast reducing effect of scattered radiation is a well-known phenomenon in general medical radiography, but its importance has not been appreciated in mammography until recently. It was generally believed that because of the low kVp's employed and the small volume of tissue irradiated (on most women) that the amount of scatter and its effect on contrast was small. Figure 1 compares a low scatter content image with one made under typical mammographic conditions. In both cases the test object, kVp, filtration, primary attenuation and film processing were the same. Visual comparison of the two images indicates that scatter significantly degrades mammographic contrast and information content. The objectives of this paper are to review the pertinent literature dealing with experimental determinations of the intensity of scatter in mammography, quantify the anticipated improvement in contrast or alternatively in dose reduction that can result from reducing scatter and finally compare different methods of accomplishing this reduction.

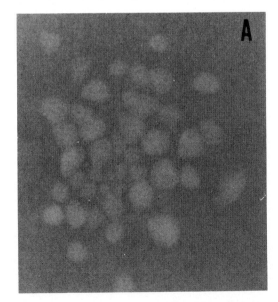 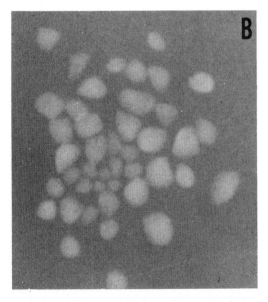

Figure 1. Comparison of Radiographs made under typical mammographic imaging conditions with (A) and without (B) the presence of scatter. 36 kVp (Mo target/filter) and a primary beam attenuation of 6 cm of Lucite was used in both cases. The images are of the simulated calcifications in a Kodak Pathe' phantom.

REVIEW OF EXPERIMENTAL RESULTS

In the late fall of 1974, Barnes et al. [1] presented a paper on an electronic mammographic system in which the application of an electronic moving slit concept to reduce scattered radiation was mentioned. Their presentation, however, did not include an analysis of the significance of scatter. The first paper to appear in the radiological literature which quantified the influence of scattered radiation on mammographic image quality was by Friedrich in 1975 [2]. His investigation revealed that the effect of scattered radiation is considerable and severely limits the visibility of small microcalcifications. For a breast thickness of 5 cm, he found the average ratio of scattered-to-primary radiation imaged(S/P) to be about 0.78. Subsequently, presentations and papers appeared by Sashin, et. al. [3,4]; Barnes and Brezovich [5-7]; Gur, Sashin and Herbert [8]; Hoeffken, Jötten and Richter [9]; Muntz [10]; Friedrich [11]; Dick and Motz [12]; Richter [13]; and Friedrich and Weskamp [14] quantifying the amount of scatter and its effect or dealing with various methods of reducing it. Other papers of interest dealing with scatter measurements in general Diagnostic Radiology whose results in light of present knowledge can be extended to the mammographic photon energy region are Stargardt and Angerstein [15] and Dick, Soares and Motz [16].

TABLE I. Quantification of Scatter in Mammography - Chronological Listing

Investigator(s)	Year	X-Ray Detector	Phantom Thickness	Scatter/Primary(S/P)
Friedrich	1975	film	5 cm	0.78
Barnes & Brezovich	1976-1978	NaI(Tl) crystal	3.6-7.1 g/cm^2	0.40-0.85
Gur, Sashin & Herbert	1977	film/screen	6 cm	0.8
Hoeffken, Jötten & Richter	1977	film	6 g/cm^2	0.79
Muntz	1977	xenon gas	3-8 g/cm^2	0.63-0.92
Dick & Motz	1978	NaI(Tl) crystal	5.5 g/cm^2	1.17

The results of the various investigators are summarized in Table 1 and indicate reasonable agreement with the exception of the slightly higher S/P ratio of Dick and Motz [12]. A subsequent investigation indicated that this result was due to additional collimator scatter arising at low photon energies [15]. Two of the more comprehensive investigations listed in Table I are tabulated in Tables II and III. In Tables I-III thickness is expressed in g/cm^2 rather than in cm. The relationship between the two is

$$\text{Thickness(g/cm}^2) \;=\; \text{Thickness(cm)} \times \text{density(g/cm}^3) \tag{1}$$

This normalizes thickness to the same mass and number of electrons (for most low atomic materials) of scattering material placed in the x-ray beam.

TABLE II. Pertinent S/P Data* of Barnes and Brezovich [6,7]

Field Size[†]	Phantom Thickness (g/cm^2)			
(cm)	3.57	4.76	5.95	7.14
4	0.32	....	....	0.54
6	0.37	....	....	0.65
10	0.39	....	....	0.80
14	0.40	0.54	0.71	0.85

*Lucite Phantom(ρ = 1.19 g/cm^3) and 32 kVp(1ϕ)
[†]Diameter of circular radiation field

TABLE III. Pertinent S/P Data* of Dick, Soares and Motz [16, 17]

Field Size[†]	Photon Energy (Monoenergetic Beam)	
(cm)	17.5 keV	32 keV
2.2	0.07	0.15
3.7	0.26	0.31
7.0	0.42	0.55
10.4	0.49	0.69
14.3	0.54	0.75

*5.53 g/cm^2 polystyrene phantom(ρ = 1.05 g/cm^3)
[†]Diameter of circular radiation field

TABLE IV. Average Energy* of Primary and Scattered Photons [6,7]

X-Ray Tube[†] Voltage(kVp)	Primary Photons(keV)	Scattered Photons(keV)
27	21.6	21.2
32	24.5	23.7
36	25.4	24.6
42	27.7	26.8

*Transmitted through a 7.14 q/cm^2(6 cm) thick Lucite phantom
[†]Tungsten target, 0.5 mm Al filtration

Barnes and Brezovich measured the average primary and scattered x-ray photon energy for x-ray tube voltages from 27 to 42 kVp(1φ) utilizing a tungsten/aluminum target/filter combination. Their results are tabulated in Table IV. Over the range of x-ray tube voltages studied the average primary x-ray energy changed by 6.1 keV and the average scattered x-ray energies were from only 2 to 3.9% less than the primary energies. This small change in the average primary photon energy along with the small scatter energy dependence (see Table III) are the reasons that they observed the relative intensity of scatter (S/P) to be independent of beam quality [6,7]. Friedrich observed a 16% increase in the S/P ratio (i.e., an 8% increase in the scatter fraction) as the x-ray tube voltage was changed from 25 to 40 kVp(3φ) [2]. He employed a molybdenum target/filter combination which would result in a greater average primary x-ray energy shift than obtained by Barnes and Brezovich and explain the difference between the two investigations. Another factor contributing to the observed difference in the beam quality dependence is in the energy dependence of x-ray detectors employed. Barnes and Brezovich used a beryllium window NaI(Tl) crystal; whereas, Friedrich used film. The absorption efficiency of the former is ~ 100% and is independent of x-ray photon energy over the mammographic region; whereas, the K-edge of silver is 25.5 keV. This strong detector energy dependence along with the slight energy degradation of scatter are also the likely reasons why investigators using film tabulated in Table I report a slightly higher S/P ratio for a given phantom thickness and field size than those employing other types of x-ray detectors.

The S/P results of Dick, Soares and Motz [16,17] and Barnes and Brezovich [6,7] are compared in Fig. 2 as a function of field size for a 5.5 g/cm² phantom thickness. The points plotted of the former investigators were linearly interpolated to an energy of 24.5 keV using Table III; while, the other investigators'points for a phantom thickness of 5.5 g/cm² were obtained from Table II in a similar manner. The results are plotted in Fig. 3 as a function of phantom thickness for a 14 cm diameter radiation field. The agreement is quite

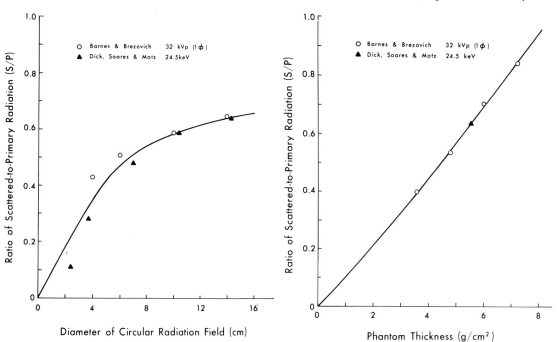

Figure 2. Effect of field size on scatter for a 5.5 g/cm² thick phantom.

Figure 3. Effect of phantom thickness on scatter for a 14 cm diameter field.

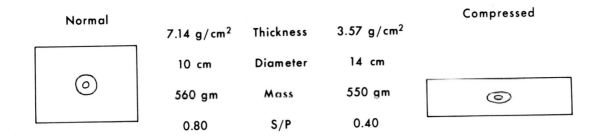

	Normal	Thickness	Compressed
	7.14 g/cm²	Thickness	3.57 g/cm²
	10 cm	Diameter	14 cm
	560 gm	Mass	550 gm
	0.80	S/P	0.40

Figure 4. Effect of compression on scatter.

good between the two studies except for smaller field sizes. Since the S/P ratio is strongly field size dependent for smaller field sizes, this lack of agreement is attributed to the increased effect of small differences in the measurement techniques employed.

Figures 2 and 3 give qualitative verification to the well known fact that in mammography, as well as in general radiography, the amount of scatter increases with field size and/or with patient thickness. The increase with thickness is supralinear, while for larger field sizes the increase is more gradual. This strong dependence on patient thickness and smaller dependence on field size is one of the reasons why compression is so advantageous in mammography. This point is illustrated in Fig. 4 using the data of Table II. That is, decreasing the breast thickness by compression reduces the amount of scatter even though the irradiated area has increased. Another more subtle advantage is that more information carrying x-rays (more primary) are employed to image a compressed breast since it is imaged over a larger area.

Typical compressed breast range in thickness from 3-7 cm with an imaged area from 80-200 cm². Exceptionally well-endowed or obese women may be larger. Taking this range of breast sizes into account and examining the data in Tables I-III, one concludes that S/P ratios in mammography range from 0.35 to 1.0.

EFFECT OF SCATTER

CONTRAST

The formation of the radiological image is illustrated in Fig. 5. Using the characteristic response of a film/screen combination to radiation exposure, one can write

$$\Delta D = \gamma \cdot \log[E + \Delta E)/E] \qquad (2)$$

or

$$\Delta D = 0.43 \cdot \gamma \cdot \ln[1 + \Delta E/E] \qquad (3)$$

where ΔD is the density difference arising from the difference in radiation exposure to two areas of the film/screen combination, γ is the slope of the film/screen combination's sensitometric curve between the two different exposure levels and E and E + ΔE are as defined in Fig. 5. Since $\ln(1 + \alpha) \simeq \alpha$ for $\alpha \ll 1$, Eqn. 3 becomes

$$\Delta D \simeq 0.43 \cdot \gamma \cdot (\Delta E/E) \qquad (4)$$

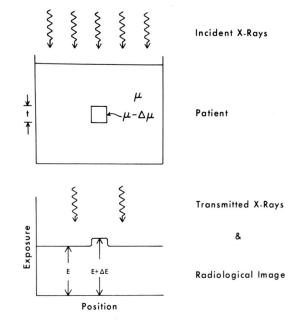

Figure 5. Schematic representation of
the formation of the radiological image.

In Eqn. 4 ΔD, γ and $\Delta E/E$ are commonly known as radiographic, film and subject contrast, respectively. Assuming that the scatter component of exposure, S, is uniform beneath the object and surrounding area,

$$E = P + S \qquad (5)$$

and

$$E + \Delta E = P + \Delta P + S \qquad (6)$$

where P and ΔP are the primary and difference in primary radiation exposure, respectively. Substituting Eqns. (5) and (6) in Eqn. 4, one obtains

$$\Delta D \simeq 0.43 \cdot \gamma \cdot (\Delta P/P)/(1 + S/P) \qquad (7)$$

The general form of Eqn. (7) in which subject contrast was separated into the primary beam subject contrast, $\Delta P/P$, and the effect of scatter on subject contrast, $(1 + S/P)^{-1}$, was first derived by Morgan [18]. $(1 + S/P)^{-1}$ has been referred to by the author as the scatter degradation factor (SDF) [5-7,19] and is the fraction of primary beam subject contrast imaged due to presence of scatter. Using this definition the subject contrast (SC) component of Eqn. 7 becomes

$$SC = C_p \cdot SDF \qquad (8)$$

where C_p has been set equal to $\Delta P/P$.

The effect of scatter on subject contrast is illustrated in Fig. 6. It is apparent that a relatively small amount of scatter significantly degrades the contrast imaged. In reviewing the experimental results of various inves-

228

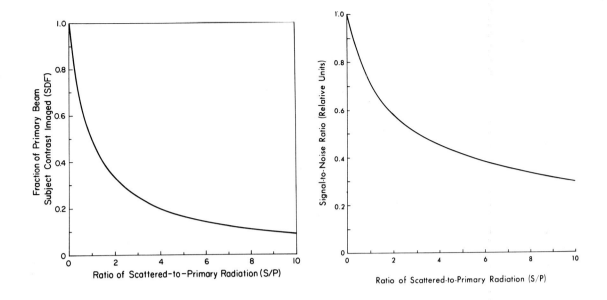

Figure 6. Plot of the fraction of possible or primary beam subject contrast
(scatter degradation factor or SDF)
versus the ratio of scattered-to-primary radiation.

Figure 7. Plot of the effect of scatter on the signal-to-noise ratio.

tigators it was concluded in the previous section that the typical imaged S/P
ratio is from 0.35 to 1.0 depending mainly on breast size. Referring to Fig.
6 this implies that only from about 75 to 50% of the primary beam subject contrast is imaged in mammography and that contrast improvements of from 35 to 100
% are possible if scatter can be eliminated.

The development in the preceding paragraphs is for the large area contrast
case of film/screen image receptors. Small object contrast is also degraded by
the imaging system transfer characteristics [20,21]. In the case of image receptors with edge enhancement such as xeroradiography or electron radiography,
γ and the image system transfer function both depend on spatial frequency [22],
and, as in the case of small objects with film/screen combinations, the resultant image contrast depends on both the image receptor transfer properties and
subject contrast spatial frequency content. It has also been pointed out by
Doi that the small angle scatter component of the SDF is spatial frequency dependent and tends to degrade object border sharpness by lowering the high
spatial frequency content of the resultant image [23]. That is, small angle
scatter arising from or absorbed by an object results in a scatter x-ray image
of greater spatial extent than that of its primary x-ray image.

SIGNAL-TO-NOISE RATIO

The noise component in the radiological image is due to the contrast fluc-
uations associated with statistical variations in the number of x-ray photons
or quantum mottle (QM) which is given by

$$QM = 1/\sqrt{N} \qquad (10)$$

where N is the average number of photons per area. For a given beam quality N is directly proportional to radiation exposure or

$$QM \simeq 1/\sqrt{E} = 1/\sqrt{(P + S)} \qquad (11)$$

The signal-to-noise (SNR) of the radiological image is

$$SNR = SC/QM \qquad (12)$$

which can be expressed using Eqns. [8] and [11] as

$$SNR \sim (C_p/\sqrt{P}) \cdot \sqrt{SDF} \qquad (13)$$

Since the SNR without scatter is proportional to $C_p/\sqrt{P}$, Eqn. (13) indicates the SNR is degraded by $\sqrt{SDF}$ when scatter is present. Expressions similar to Eqn. (13) have recently appeared in the literature [24,25].

The effect of scatter on SNR is illustrated in Fig. 7. Assuming that typical imaged S/P ratios vary from 0.35 to 1.0 in mammography, Fig. 7 (or Eqn. (13) indicates that the SNR is degraded by a factor of from 0.86 to 0.7. That is, improvements of from 16 to 41% in the SNR are possible for the same level of primary if scatter can be eliminated. This implies an increase in the perceivability of small microcalcifications and soft tissue detail since both are inherently limited by the imaged SNR [26,21, 24, 25].

SCATTER REDUCTION METHODS

TERMINOLOGY

Conventional methods of reducing scatter are grid and air gap techniques. Other methods that have been employed are dual scanning slits [27,1,28,3,4, 29,30] and multiple scanning slits [19,31]. A variety of terminology has evolved to quantify the capabilities of anti-scatter techniques with the most important terms defined in the following paragraphs.

Two basic concepts are the primary transmission (T_p) and scatter transmission (T_s) of a scatter reduction technique. These are respectively the fraction of incident primary and incident scattered radiation transmitted by the technique. The transmitted scatter/primary(S'/P') ratio is therefore related to the incident scatter/primary(S/P) ratio by

$$S'/P' = (T_s \cdot S)/(T_p \cdot P) \qquad (14)$$

Combining Eqns. (8) and (14) the subject contrast of the x-ray image emerging from an anti-scatter device (SC') is given by

$$SC' = C_p \cdot SDF' \qquad (15)$$

where

$$SDF' = 1/(1 + S'/P') \qquad (16)$$

The contrast improvement factor(K) of a scatter reduction technique is defined as the ratio of the contrast of the x-ray image transmitted by the device to that of the incident image [32,33]. That is, the ratio of Eqn. (15)

to Eqn. (8), or

$$K = SDF'/SDF \qquad (17)$$

where the C_p's have cancelled since the penetrating quality of the primary beam is assumed to be unchanged by the device.

The relative patient exposure is defined as the factor by which patient exposure has increased with an anti-scatter device to achieve the same image receptor exposure level as obtained without the device. If there is no change in geometry or beam quality, the relative patient exposure is just equal to the radiation emerging from the patient (S + P) divided by that transmitted by the device (S' + P'), which reduces to

$$\text{Rel. Patient Exposure} = K/T_p \qquad (18)$$

Taking into account inverse square law effects if a change in magnification occurs, Eqn. (18) becomes

$$\text{Rel. Patient Exposure} = M^2 \cdot K/T_p \qquad (19)$$

where M is the relative magnification.

The Bucky Factor is defined as the ratio of technique factors(mAs) with and without the device. The Bucky Factor is equal to the ratio of radiation emerging from the patient-to-that transmitted by the device divided by the fractional field of coverage(F_c) or

$$\text{Bucky Factor} = K/(T_p \cdot F_c) \qquad (20)$$

F_c is the fraction of the area of interest irradiated at any instant during an exposure and is unity for grid and air gap techniques. The Bucky Factor is the increase in tube loading required to employ the scatter reduction technique at the same kVp.

The concept of detective quantum efficiency(DQE) was adapted by Wagner to rank the relative effectiveness of scatter reduction techniques [34]. DQE is defined as

$$DQE = [SNR'/SNR_i]^2 \qquad (21)$$

where SNR' and SNR_i are the Signal-to-Noise ratios of the actual and ideal ($T_p = 1.0$, $T_s = 0$) scatter reduction methods. Utilizing Eqns. (13) and (14), Eqn. (21) reduces to

$$DQE = T_p \cdot SDF' \qquad (22)$$

It is implicit in the DQE definition that both the real and ideal scatter reduction methods are operating at the same level of primary. Employing Eqns. (13) and (22) to determine the relative primary exposure levels P_1 and P_2 for two different scatter reduction techniques to yield equal SNR's, one obtains

$$P_2/P_1 = DQE_1/DQE_2 \qquad (23)$$

Since the beam qualities are the same, patient dose will scale the same way. Assuming one device is ideal, Eqn. (23) indicates that the DQE of an actual anti-scatter device is the reduction in primary radiation and absorbed dose that could be achieved by an ideal device for the same SNR.

231

TABLE V. Characteristics of Philips Grid [13]

Physical		X-Ray*	
Grid Ratio	5:1	Primary Transmission	0.72
Lines/cm	32	Scatter Transmission	0.15
Lead Content(mg/cm^2)	55	Contrast Improv. Factor	1.55
Thickness(mm)	~ 2.5	Rel. Patient Exp.	2.15
		Bucky Factor	2.15

*Measured at 31 kVp(3ϕ) employing a molybdenum target/filter combination and a 6 g/cm^2 thick, 10 cm x 10 cm phantom with a resultant S/P = 0.79.

GRIDS

Due to their extremely small transmission of low energy x-rays conventional grids are impractical in mammography. Recently, however, Friedrich in conjunction with Philips scientists have developed and employed special mammographic grids [9,11,13,14]. The physical dimensions and x-ray data of the grid that Philips is currently marketing are listed in Table V. This remarkable grid is constructed of lead strips 16 μm wide separated by 300 μm of fibre interspacing. The height of the lead strips is 1.5 mm giving it a 5:1 grid ratio. The key to the grid's usefulness in mammography is its high primary transmission which is due in part to the carbon fibre/resin material used to encase the grid strips and give it mechanical rigidity.

AIR GAP

In medical radiography it is a well-known and often employed principle that by moving the image receptor away from the patient less scatter will be imaged. That is, due to the fact that the majority of scattered x-rays are not directed at the image receptor separating the image receptor and patient allows them to escape from being imaged. Generally, the greater the air gap and the smaller the irradiated area, the smaller the amount of scatter imaged.

References in the radiological literature dealing with the air gaps in mammography are limited and two to date have been reported [9,10]. In the study by Muntz, the scattered photon fluence values were reported in relative units and are difficult to compare [10]. The results of Hoeffken, Jötten and Richter [9] are plotted in Fig. 8 along with the higher x-ray photon energy data of Stargardt and Angerstein [15] and Dick, Soares and Motz [16]. Good agreement exists between the latter two references. The large discrepency between their results and those of Hoeffken, Jötten and Richter is due mainly to differences in measuring geometry. The latter two employed a much larger source-to-phantom distance (SPD) than the former.

The concept of virtual source has long been employed to identify the "origin" of electron beams incident on a diffusing foil [35]. Muntz has experimentally verified the validity of applying this concept in parameterizing the functional dependence of scatter on air gap [10]. The intensity of scatter, S,

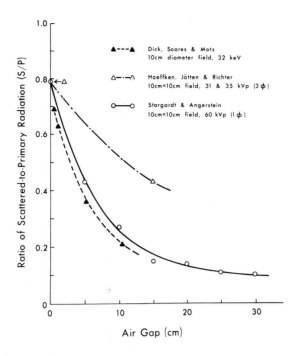

Figure 8. Effect of air gap on scatter for a 5.5 cm²/g thick phantom

is assumed to vary inversely with the square of the distance from the virtual source of scatter, or

$$S \sim 1/(\delta + d)^2 \qquad (24)$$

where d is the air gap distance and δ is the distance of the virtual source of scatter from the rear surface of the phantom or patient. Considerations of the scattering solid angle as seen by a point on the image plane and experimental results indicate that δ is a function of field size and thickness of scattering medium. It increases with increasing radiation field size and will depend to a lesser extent on the thickness of the scattering medium.

Two types of experimental geometry have been employed in measuring the S/P ratio dependence on air gap--a fixed SPD and a fixed source-to-image receptor distance (SID). In the former case the SID is equal to the source-to-phantom (rear surface) distance, D, plus the air gap distance, d, and, since the primary radiation varies inversely with the square of the distance from the source, one obtains

$$P \sim 1/(D + d)^2 \qquad (25)$$

Combining Eqns. (24) and (25) and normalizing to the rear surface of the phantom, one obtains

$$\frac{S}{P} \sim \left(\frac{\delta}{\delta + d}\right)^2 \cdot \left(\frac{D + d}{D}\right)^2 \qquad (26)$$

233

In the latter case the primary radiation at the detector does not vary. However, since scatter is directly proportional to the primary at the scatterer, it is therefore proportional to $D^2/(D-d)^2$, and one obtains

$$\frac{S}{P} \sim \left(\frac{\delta}{\delta + d}\right)^2 \cdot \left(\frac{D}{D - d}\right)^2 \tag{27}$$

An equation similar to Eqns. (26) and (27) except for the inclusion of the virtual source concept was derived by Seeman in 1938 [36].

Both Eqns. (26) and (27) indicate that at greater SPD's air gap techniques are more effective in reducing scatter(S/P). This is due to the decreased divergence of the primary beam while the divergence of scatter is basically independent of SPD. This point has previously been noted by Muntz [10].

Eqns. (26) and (27) can be applied to explain the apparent discrepancy in the results plotted in Fig. 8. Hoeffken, Jötten and Richter employed a fixed SDD of 50 cm while Stargardt and Angerstein utilized a fixed SPD of 400 cm. Substituting these values in Eqns. (26) and (27), taking the ratio for a 15 cm air gap and neglecting the virtual source terms, one would anticipate that Stargardt and Angerstein's S/P ratio would be 53% that of Hoeffken, Jötten and Richter's. The actual value is 40%. Thus, most of the discrepancy is due solely to differences in the primary beam divergence between the two investigators. The remainder is attributed to differences in measurement technique and the virtual source term in Eqns. (26) and (27) since the location of the virtual source of scatter will depend to some extent on the amount of primary beam divergence occuring in the scattering medium. It should also be noted that in the fixed SID measuring geometry the amount of primary divergence in the phantom changes with air gap. This affects the location of virtual source and limits the range of air gaps over which Eqn. (27) will be valid.

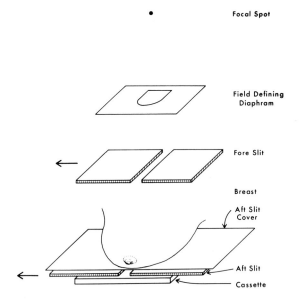

Figure 9. Principle of scanning mammographic dual slit assembly.

SCANNING SLIT TECHNIQUES

The use of a set of moving slits to reduce secondary radiation was the first scatter reduction technique suggested in the radiological literature [27] and a similar arrangement has been adapted for mammography by Gur, Sashin and Herbert [8]. Their device is illustrated in Fig. 9 and consists of a beam defining fore slit between the x-ray tube and patient and one scatter-eliminating aft slit between the patient and image receptor. The two slits move synchronously and scan the area to be x-rayed. The principle of such a device is the small radiation field defined by the fore slit produces little scatter in the area of the film irradiated by the primary beam and x-rays scattered out of the irradiated volume are not imaged because of the aft slit. However, due to the long exposure time required and increased tube loading, the employment of a single set has not proved practical for general medical radiography. In mammography, tube loading is not as limiting and with the use of compression devices to immobolize the patient long exposure times do not detract from the resultant image quality.

The physical dimensions of Gur, Sashin and Herbert's device are listed in Table VI along with its x-ray characteristics. It should be noted that a substantial improvement in contrast is obtained with the device with little or no loss of the primary x-rays emerging from the patient. Its Bucky factor is quite large due to the small percentage of the field of interest covered at any instance during the exposure (i.e., small F_c). However, it is likely that for routine work some of the contrast gained will be sacrificed by employing higher kVp's than employed conventionally to reduce patient exposure. If this is the case the Bucky factor would be less than the value listed in Table VI.

The Bucky factor problem associated with a single set of scanning slits can be reduced by employing a multiplicity of such slits. Such a device consists of an array of beam-defining fore slits that are aligned and synchronously moved with a similar array of scatter-eliminating aft slots[*]. The geometry is similar to that of a set of scanning slits with the array of fore slits and aft slots replacing the respective fore slit and aft slit depicted in Fig. 9. The employment of aft slots is essential when a multiplicity of radiation beams is used to minimize scatter contributions from neighboring beams. Such a device has been developed by Barnes et al for abdominal radiography and is referred to as the Scanning Multiple Slit Assembly or SMSA [19,31]. In such applications it is the most efficient method of reducing scatter currently available [24,31].

King, Barnes and Yester have adapted such a device for mammography [37]. Pertinent physical dimensions of their device along with its projected x-ray characteristics are listed in Table VII. The device depicted in Table VII is capable of imaging a 24 cm x 28 cm area and has an aft slot cover dimension of 46 cm. In order for a set of scanning slits to image a 28 cm long area the aft slot cover would be approximately 110 cm.

---

[*]In the literature the terms slit and slot are often used interchangeabley. In this paper a distinction is made. A slit refers to a long, narrow cut in a plate about 1.6 mm thick or less, whereas, a slot refers to a similar cut in a much thicker piece of material and a grid ratio associated with it.

TABLE VI. Characteristics of Double Slit Mammography [8]

Physical Dimensions (mm)		X-Ray*	
Focus-fore slit dist.	370	Primary Transmission	1.0
Fore slit width	5	Scatter Transmission	0.25
Focus-aft slit dist.	480	Contrast Improv. Factor	1.5
Aft slit width	6.8	Rel. Patient Exposure	1.5
		Bucky Factor[†]	22

*Calculated for S/P = 0.79
[†]10 cm field

TABLE VII. Characteristics of Mammographic SMSA [37]

Physical Dimensions (mm)		X-Ray*	
Focus-fore slit dist.	550	Primary Transmission	0.96
Fore slit width	2	Scatter Transmission	0.026
Focus-aft slot dist.	770	Contrast Improv. Factor[†]	1.75
Aft slot width/depth	3/30	Rel. Patient Exp.[†]	2.0
Aft slot interval	10.5	Bucky Factor[†]	6.4

*Projected from single fore slit and aft slot data
[†]S/P ratio of 0.79 assumed

TABLE VIII. Comparison of Grid, Air Gap*, Dual Slits and SMSA Performance Characteristics[†]

	Contrast Improvement	Rel. Patient Exposure	Bucky Factor
Grid	1.55	2.15	2.15
Air Gap*	1.25	1.6	1.25
Dual Slits	1.5	1.5	22
SMSA	1.75	2.0	6.4

*10 cm x 10 cm field and 15 cm Air Gap
[†]The initial S/P ratio was taken equal to 0.79 and an 80 cm SID was assumed in all cases

COMPARISON OF DIFFERENT METHODS

In Table VIII the contrast improvement factor, relative patient exposure and Bucky factor of the four methods of scatter reduction previously discussed are compared. The 50 cm SID Hoeffken, Jotten & Richter air gap data was corrected to an 80 cm SID using Eqn. 27 to make the comparison more valid. It would appear that for an 80 cm SID an air gap of ~ 25 cm would be required to obtain approximately the contrast improvement obtained with the grid or dual slits. The SMSA images 98% of the possible or primary beam contrast and none of the other methods approach more than 87%. The patient exposure required with the grid and air gap methods is higher than that of the dual slit or SMSA with the opposite being true for the Bucky factor.

TABLE IX. Comparison of DQE's of Different Anti-Scatter Methods

	Nothing*	Grid	Air Gap+	Dual Slits	SMSA
DQE	0.56	0.62	0.70	0.83	0.94

*The initial S/P ratio was taken equal to 0.79
+10 cm x 10 cm field, 15 cm Air Gap

The DQE's of the different anti-scatter techniques are compared in Table IX. The DQE's of the scanning slit techniques (the SMSA approaches that of an ideal anti-scatter device) are substantially better than those of the grid and air gap indicating that they reduce scatter in a more dose efficient manner. If a 25 cm rather than 15 cm air gap (80 cm SID) is compared, the resultant DQE would be ~ 0.85. Such an air gap would be more comparable to the scanning slit techniques. However, the required increase in image magnification would result in unacceptable geometrical unsharpness except for the smallest focal spots.

REDUCED SCATTER AND PATIENT EXPOSURE

GENERAL CONSIDERATIONS

It has been well documented in the general radiological literature that comparable images requiring less radiation can be obtained at higher x-ray tube voltages when less scatter is imaged [38-41, 29, 8, 31]. This is also true for mammography and can be accomplished with the image receptors currently available. An alternative method would be employing the same kVp with faster image receptors (faster film) having less contrast. Due to the limited availability of faster films this is not as easily accomplished, but since the beam quality remains the same the dose savings that could be achieved can be more readily calculated.

USE OF HIGHER KVP TECHNIQUES

The effect of kVp on mammographic contrast is illustrated in Fig. 10. It is apparent from Fig. 10 that much higher kVp techniques can be employed without scatter to achieve the same contrast. Since increasing the kVp slightly in mammography requires a substantial decrease in mAs to achieve the same radiation level at the image receptor, a net decrease in patient exposure will result.

237

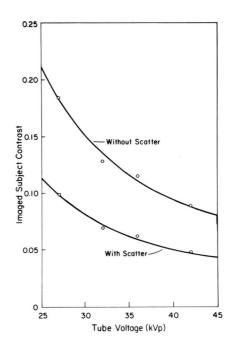

Figure 10. Effect of x-ray tube voltage and scatter on the subject contrast of a 500 μm thickness of bone and Lucite. A S/P ratio of 0.85 was assumed to obtain the plot with scatter.

Calculations similar to those depicted in Fig. 10 indicate that for S/P ratios from 0.35 to 1.0 the x-ray tube voltage can be increased from 7 to 25 kVp without scatter to achieve the same contrast for a nominal 32 kVp technique. This will increase the radiation output (mR/mAs) by a factor of from 2 to 8 [42]. Taking into account the decrease in radiation at the image receptor resulting from the removal of scatter and using the standard mammographic technique rules of thumb that increasing the kVp by 4 from 30 to 40 kVp, by 5 from 40 to 50 kVp, and by 7 from 50 - 60 kVp is equivalent to doubling the mAs, increases of from 7 to 25 kVp in x-ray tube voltage (for a nominal 32 kVp technique) would result in net entrance skin exposure reductions of from 27 to 75%. However, due to the increased penetrating quality of the x-ray beam, the decrease in the midline breast radiation absorbed dose will not be as great [43]. The above calculations are in need of experimental verification, but it is interesting to note that Gur, Sashin and Herbert have reported entrance skin exposure reductions of up to 67% with their dual slit device which transmits 25% of the scatter [8].

EMPLOYING FASTER IMAGE RECEPTORS

The effect of scatter on the SNR has been discussed in a preceeding section and it has been noted that SNR improvments of from 16 to 41% can result with the removal of scatter. The same SNR as obtained with scatter can be obtained without scatter by decreasing the number of primary photons. This increases the noise or quantum mottle, but, since the signal or contrast has increased with the elimination of scatter, the SNR can be kept the same. However, since the scattered radiation has been eliminated and the level of primary reduced, a more sensitive (and less contrasty) image receptor is required.

One obtains DQE's from 0.74 to 0.50 utilizing Eqn. (22) for S/P ratios ranging from 0.35 to 1.0. Since the DQE for a practical (or no) scatter reduction technique is the exposure reduction that could be achieved by an ideal anti-scatter device to achieve the same SNR as obtained with the practical (or no) method, the possible reduction in patient radiation absorbed dose scales the same way. The dose reduction that can be realized with current methods of reducing scatter, as indicated in Table 9, will be somewhat less than this with the exception of the SMSA.

CONCLUSIONS

Scatter significantly degrades image quality in mammography. It results in only from 50 to 75% of the primary beam or possible contrast being imaged. Signal-to-noise ratio (SNR) analysis indicates that improvements of from 16 to 41% in the SNR at current dose levels or, alternatively, dose reductions by a factor of from 1.35 to 2.0 at current SNR's are possible with its suppression. That is, in order to obtain the maximum patient information for the minimum radiation dose it is essential that scatter be eliminated.

Scatter can be reduced by air gap, special soft tissue grid, dual scanning slit or multiple scanning slit techniques. The latter two methods reduce scatter in the most dose effective manner. However, this is done at the expense of increased tube loading and mechanical complexity, and, it should be also noted that, their clinical feasibility remains to be seen.

REFERENCES

1. Barnes JO, Morris CW, Sashin D, Ricci JL, Meire H, Piasecki JO: An Electronic Mammographic System. Paper 42, 60th Scientific Assembly and Annual Meeting of the Radiological Society of North America, Chicago, Illinois, Nov. 30 - Dec. 4, 1974.

2. Friedrich M: Die Einfluss der Streustrahlung auf die Abbidldungsqualität bei der Mammographie. Forstschr Röntgenstr 123, 556-566, 1975.

3. Sashin D, Morris CW, Ricci JL, Barnes JO: An Evaluation of Low Light Level Television for Breast Cancer Detection. Proc. of the Soc Photo Optical Instru Eng, 70:384-392, 1975.

4. Sashin D, Barnes JO, Ricci JL, Gur D: Electronic Moving Slit for Scatter Reduction in Diagnostic Radiology. Pages 787-790, Proc of the 9th Midyear Topical Symposium of the Health Physics Society, Denver CO, Feb. 9-12, 1976.

5. Barnes GT, Brezovich IA: The Intensity of Scattered Radiation in Mammography. Paper 25.2, 4th International Conference on Medical Physics, Ottawa, Canada, July 25-30, 1976.

6. Barnes, GT, Brezovich IA: Contrast: Effect of Scattered Radiation in Breast Carcinoma - The Radiologist's Expanded Role, edited by WW Logan, John Wiley & Sons, New York, 1977, Pages 73-81.

7. Barnes GT, Brezovich IA: The Intensity of Scattered Radiation in Mammography. Radiology 126:243-247, 1978.

8. Gur D, Sashin D, Herbert DL: Improved Contrast in Mammography Using a

Double Slit Technique. Presented at the 25th Annual Meeting of the Association of University Radiologists, Kansas City, KS, May 1-4, 1977.

9. Hoeffken W, Jotten G, Richter D: A New Method of Reducing Radiation Exposure and Improving Image Quality in Mammography. Medicamundi 22:61-64, 1977.

10. Muntz EP: On the Significance of Scattered Radiation in Reduced Exposure Mammography. Paper 105, 63rd Scientific Assembly and Annual Meeting of the Radiological Society of North America, Chicago, IL, Nov.26-Dec.2, 1977.

11. Friedrich M: Neuere Entwicklungstendenzen der Mammographie Technik: Die Raster - Mammographie. Fortschr Röntgenstr 128:207-222, 1978.

12. Dick CE, Motz JW: New Method for the Experimental Evaluation of X-Ray Grids. Med Phys 5:133-140, 1978.

13. Richter D: Evaluation of Grid Technique in Mammography. Paper B4, 20th Annual Meeting of the Amer Assoc of Phys in Med, San Francisco, CA, July 30-Aug 3, 1978.

14. Friedrich M, Weskamp P: New Modalities in Mammographic Imaging: Comparison of Grid and Air Gap Magnification Techniques, Medicamundi 23:1-16, 1978.

15. Stargardt A, Angerstein W: Über die Streustrahlenverminderung bei der Röntgenvergrösserungstechnik. Fortschr Röntgenstr 123:364-369,1974.

16. Dick CE, Soares CG, Motz JW: X-Ray Scatter Data for Diagnostic Radiology. Phys Med Biol, in press.

17. Dick CE: Private Communication, 1978.

18. Morgan RH: An Analysis of the Physical Factors Controlling the Diagnostic Quality of Roentgenographic Images. Part III. Am J Roentgenol 55:67-89, 1946.

19. Barnes GT, Brezovich IA, Witten DM: Scanning Multiple Slit Assembly: A Practical and Effective Device to Reduce Scatter. Am J Roentgenol 129: 497-501, 1977.

20. Rossman K: Some Physical Factors Affecting Image Quality in Medical Radiography. J Photo Sci 12:279-283, 1964.

21. Wagner RF: Toward a Unified View of Radiological Imaging Systems. Part II: Noisy Images. Med Phys 4:279-296, 1977.

22. Shaw R: Some Fundamental Properties of Xeroradiographic Images. Proc. of the Soc Photo-Optical Instru Eng 70:359-363, 1975.

23. Doi K: Modulation Transfer Function of Scattered Radiation in Evaluating its Effect on Photographic Image Quality. Jap J Non-Destruct Inspect 14: 262-270, 1969.

24. Motz JW, Danos M: Image Information Content and Patient Exposure. Med Phys 5:8-22, 1978.

25. Askins BS, Wagner RF, Barnes GT: A Demonstration of the Effect of Reduced Scatter on Information Content and Patient Exposure. Paper M5, 20th Annual Meeting of the Am Assoc of Phys in Med, San Francisco, CA July 30-Aug 3, 1978.

26. Sturm RE, Morgan RH: Screen Intensification Systems and Their Limitations. Am J Roentgenol 62:617-634, 1949.

27. Pasche O: Über eine Neue Blendenvorrichtung in der Röntgentechnik, Deutsche Med Wocheuschr 29:266-267, 1903.

28. Jaffe C, Webster EW: Radiographic Contrast Improvement by Means of Slit Radiography, Radiology 116:631-635, 1975.

29. Sorenson JA, Nelson JA: Investigations of Moving Slit Radiography. Radiology 120:705-711, 1976.

30. Moore R, Korbuly D, Amplatz K: A Method of Absorbing Scattered Radiation Without Attenuation of the Primary Beam, Radiology 120:713-717, 1976.

31. Barnes GT, Brezovich IA: The Design and Performance of a Scanning Multiple Slit Assembly. Med Phys, in press.

32. Bonenkamp JG, Boldingh WH: Quality and Choice of a Potter Bucky Grid. Part K: A New Method for the Unambiguous Determination of the Quality of a Grid. Acta Radiol 51:479-489, 1959.

33. Bonenkamp JG, Boldingh WH: Quality and Choice of a Potter Bucky Grid Part II: Application of the Criterion of Quality to Various Types of Grids. Acta Radiol 52:149-167, 1959.

34. Wagner RF: Noise Equivalent Parameters in General Medical Radiography: The Present and Future Pictures. Photo Sci Eng 21:252-262, 1977.

35. Radiation Dosimetry: Electrons With Initial Energies Between 1 and 50 MeV. ICRU Report 21, Washington, D C, 1972.

36. Seeman HE: Secondary Radiation Intensity as a Function of Certain Geometrical Variables. Am J Roentgenol 39:628-633, 1938.

37. King MA, Barnes GT, Yester MV: A Mammographic Scanning Multiple Slit Assembly: Design Considerations and Preliminary Results. To be published in the Proceedings of the Conference on Reduced Dose Mammography, Buffalo, NY, Oct 4-6, 1978.

38. Trout ED, Graves DE, Slauson DB: High Kilovoltage Radiography. Radiology 52:669-683, 1949.

39. Wachsmann FK, Breuer, Bucheim E: Fundamentals and Results of Hard-Radiation Technic. Fortschr Röntgenstr 76:147-157, 1952.

40. Trout ED, Kelley JP, Cathey GA: The Use of Filters to Control Radiation Exposure to the Patient in Diagnostic Roentgenology. Am J Roentgenol 67:946-963, 1952.

41. Nemet A, Cox WF, Hills TH: The Contrast Problem in High Kilovoltage Medical Radiography, Brit J Rad 26:185-192, 1953.

42. Yester MV: Private Communication, 1978.

43. Miller DW, Hammerstein GR, White DR, Masterson ME, Laughlin JS: Radiation Absorbed Dose in Mammography. Paper E5, 19th Annual Meeting of the Am Assoc of Phys in Med, Cincinnati, OH, July 31-Aug 4, 1977.

A MAMMOGRAPHIC SCANNING MULTIPLE SLIT ASSEMBLY:

DESIGN CONSIDERATIONS AND PRELIMINARY RESULTS

Michael A. King, Gary T. Barnes,
and Michael V. Yester

Department of Diagnostic Radiology
University of Alabama School of Medicine
University of Alabama in Birmingham
Birmingham, Alabama 35233

INTRODUCTION

The fact that scattered x-rays reduce contrast is a well known phenomenon in medical radiography. In mammography, it has been estimated that the presence of scattered radiation results in only from 54 - 71% of the primary beam or possible contrast being imaged [1]. The application of conventional grid and air gap techniques have not proved to be practical in mammography--the former because of the poor primary transmission of conventional grids at mammographic kVp's and the latter because of the increase in the geometrical unsharpness with the use of air gap techniques on conventional units. The use of a single fore slit coupled with a single aft slit [2-8], multiple fore and aft slits [5,6], and multiple fore slits and aft slots [3,7] have been suggested as techniques for improving radiographic image quality by reducing scatter with little or no loss of primary. The latter type of device, referred to as a scanning multiple slit assembly or SMSA, has been built for use in abdominal radiography and found to be a practical and efficient method of reducing scatter [9,10].

At the University of Alabama in Birmingham (UAB), a prototype mammographic SMSA has been designed and adapted to a commercial unit (GE MMX-2). In this paper, the important design features and a preliminary evaluation of the performance of the device are reported. The principal of the mammographic SMSA is illustrated in Fig. 1. The collimating or fore slits define a plurality of long, narrow beams of radiation which are aligned and synchronously moved during an exposure with an array of scatter eliminating aft slots. Such a device is effective because little scatter results from the small volume of tissue irradiated with each long, narrow beam of radiation, and because the deep aft slots clean-up scatter from neighboring beams. It can virtually eliminate scatter in mammography with little or no loss of the primary x-rays emerging from the breast.

The disadvantages of an SMSA are an increase in mechanical complexity and tube loading. The latter is due to the reduction of scatter and the fact that only part of the x-ray beam is used. Also, in the prototype device another disadvantage is a slight increase in geometrical unsharpness due to the increased image magnification imposed by the aft slots. This increased magnification, however, can actually be advantageous for small focal spot tubes as will be shown later.

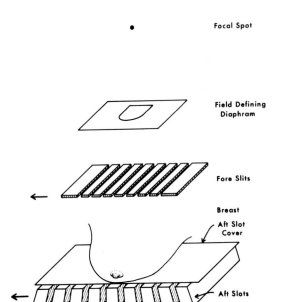

Focal Spot

Field Defining Diaphram

Fore Slits

Breast

Aft Slot Cover

Aft Slots

Cassette

Figure 1. Principle of SMSA.

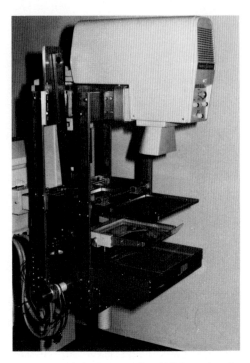

Figure 2. Mammographic SMSA, showing fore slits, compression device, linkage arm and aft slot cover and face plate.

DESIGN OF SMSA

DESCRIPTION OF UNIT

The mammographic SMSA is shown in Fig. 2. It is capable of imaging a 23 × 25 cm area and consists of 31 beam-defining fore slits and scatter eliminating aft slots. The fore slits and the bottom of the aft slots are located at distances of 55 and 80 cm, respectively, from the focal spot. The aft slot width, spacing between slots and slot depth are 3 mm, 7.5 mm and 3 cm, respectively. That is, a 10.5 mm slit interval and a 10:1 aft slot grid ratio. The focal spot-to-film distance (FFD) is 81 cm with the aft slot cover positioned approximately 4.5 cm above the film. The length of the aft slot cover is 46 cm. The unit was designed so the aft slots come to within 1/8 inch from the front of the device to maximize the amount of breast tissue imaged.

The aft slots are constructed of two slit plates 3 cm apart. The size and spacing of the slits in each plate is determined by the projection of the fore slits onto each of the respective planes. Each slit plate has 1.4 cm high by 3 mm wide anti-scatter vanes located centrally in the space between slits that constitute the aft slot septa. These anti-scatter vanes eliminate any possibility of scatter penetrating the aft slot septa. The fore slit plate and both of the aft slot slit plates are mechanically connected by a linkage arm which pivots in the plane of the x-ray tube focal spot and maintains alignment of all plates during a scan. Thus, during a scan the lower aft slot slit plate moves slightly faster than the upper and eliminates grid cutoff. During

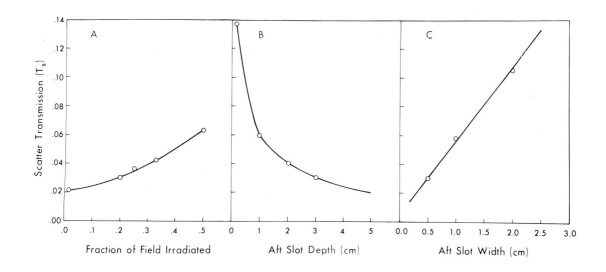

Figure 3. Plot of SMSA scatter transmission vs: A. field coverage for 5 mm wide and 3 cm deep aft slots; B. aft slot depth for 5 mm wide aft slots and 20% field coverage; C. aft slot width for 3 cm deep aft slots and 20% coverage.

an exposure the assembly scans through 7 slit intervals (i.e., a distance of 7.35 cm in the plane of the lower aft slot slit plate). The fact that the unit scans through 7 slit intervals reduces the clinical effect of radiation start/stop overlap banding and imperfections in slit fabrication.

SCATTER AND PRIMARY TRANSMISSION CONSIDERATIONS

Scatter/primary ratios and the distribution of scatter in the plane of the image receptor were measured as a function of slit width and slot depth for a single long, narrow beam geometry and can be used to calculate the antici- pated performance of a SMSA for certain design configurations [7]. Such calculations give good agreement with actual performance [10]. The scatter transmission (ratio of scatter obtained with the SMSA to that obtained without) for variations in slot spacing, slot depth, and slit width are plotted in Fig. 3. The data upon which these calculations are based were obtained at 80 kVp (1ϕ) and a systematic error is introduced extending them to mammographic kVp's. However, the trends they represent should be valid and they allow one to obtain an indication of the device's performance.

Figure 3A indicates that a reduction in the scatter transmission occurs when the field of coverage (fraction of the area of interest irradiated at any instant during an exposure) is reduced. The mammographic SMSA was designed to have a 29% field of coverage. Decreasing the field of coverage further results in increased tube loading and little gain in scatter reduction. With industri- al film, mammographic units were operated at near maximum output. The advent of low dose film/screen combinations have substantially reduced the loading and have made possible the use of a SMSA with its fractional field of coverage to reduce scatter in mammography.

In Fig. 3B, it can be seen that an increase in scatter reduction can be realized for a given slit width and field of coverage by utilizing deeper aft slots. However, the scatter transmission of the current design is sufficiently low that aft slots deeper than 3 cm are not warranted. Also, the geometrical unsharpness that would have resulted from deeper slots would have decreased the clinical usefulness of the prototype device. This latter point will be subsequently discussed in more detail.

The scatter transmission can also be decreased by decreasing the fore slit width and distance between slits (i.e., slit interval) for a given slot depth and field of coverage as can be seen in Fig. 3C. However, this gain is eventually limited by the loss of primary radiation due to the geometrical unsharpness of the fore slits at the level of the aft slots. This was an important consideration for the GE MMX unit, which has nominal 1.0 and 2.0 mm focal spots whose effective sizes are somewhat larger, and limited the distance between the fore slits and aft slots. This is conceptually illustrated in Fig. 4A. In Fig. 4B the aft slot primary transmission is plotted as a function of aft slot width for ghe geometry previously mentioned and an effective focal spot size of 1.4 mm. The calculations plotted in Fig. 4B are for aft slots that are geometrical projections of the fore slits. The fore slit and aft slot width selected for the SMSA were 2.1 and 3.0 mm, respectively which resulted in a calculated primary transmission of better than 96%.

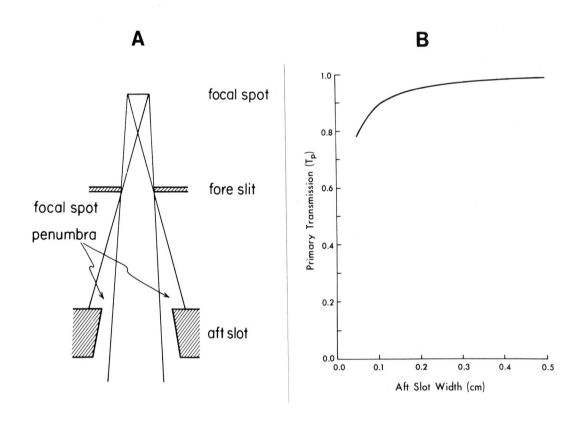

Figure 4: Loss of primary due to unsharpness of fore slits at aft slots. A Geometry of focal spot, fore slit, and aft slot. B. Plot of primary transmission vs aft slot width for 1.4 mm effective focal spot and 1.46 magnification of fore slit at aft slot.

GEOMETRY AND IMAGE QUALITY CONSIDERATIONS

As mentioned above a problem with the prototype mammographic SMSA is the increased magnification and associated geometrical unsharpness occurring because the object-to-film distance imposed by the aft slots. However, when small focal spots are employed this increased magnification can result in improved image quality [11-13]. The reasons are twofold: 1.) a decrease in the relative unsharpness of the object and 2.) a decrease in the effective noise. The former advantage is due to the fact that for small focal spots the slight amount of geometrical unsharpness occurring with magnification is more that compensated for with the decrease in the relative screen unsharpness [13]. The decrease in effective noise results from the fact that more x-ray photons are used to image a magnified object thereby decreasing the quantum and radiographic mottle associated with the object's imaged area. This point has been thoroughly discussed and demonstrated by Doi [11].

The total relative unsharpness, U_r, is plotted in Fig. 5 as a function of image magnification for various focal spot sizes. Appendix A contains a derivation of the expression that was used to calculate the results plotted in Fig. 5. A screen unsharpness of 0.15 mm was assumed, which is typical of mammographic screens [14]. On a conventional GE MMX unit (65 cm FFD) object magnifications vary from 1.0 to 1.1 for a 6 cm thick breast. For the SMSA the FFD was increased to 81 cm (i.e., 1.06 to 1.15 object magnifications) so that the resultant U_r's were somewhat comparable to those of a conventional unit for 1.0 to 2.0 mm focal spots. Fig. 5 also illustrates that significant improvement in U_r can be realized by using a smaller focal spot in conjunction with from 1.2 to 1.3 object magnifications.

The most efficacious criteria for optimizing an imaging system geometry is to maximize the (signal-to-noise ratio)^2 per unit absorbed dose to the breast (SNR^2/rad). The derivation of an approximate expression for the SNR^2/rad in the case of no scattered radiation (the SMSA) is given in Appendix B. Results calculated for different focal spots using this expression are plotted in Fig. 6 for two different object sizes. The plots have been normalized to unity at a magnification of 1.0 for each object size. This masks the fact that the larger object, because of its larger area and differential attenuation, has an inherently larger SNR and SNR^2/rad. The larger relative increase in the SNR^2/rad of the smaller object is a subtle advantage of direct geometrical magnification with small focal spots. It can be seen from Fig. 6 that the most dose effective SMSA geometry would be to employ a small focal spot in conjunction with a certain amount of magnification. A small focal spot would also allow one to decrease the already small loss of primary radiation due to fore slit penumbra and to position the fore slits closer to the x-ray tube target.

PRELIMINARY RESULTS AND DISCUSSION

The projected scatter transmission for an SMSA having 3 mm wide and 3 cm deep aft slots with a 20% field of coverage is ~ 0.020 (See Fig. 3C). Interpolating to a 29% field of coverage using Fig. 3A, one obtains a projected scatter transmission of ~ 0.026. For a 6 cm thick and 14 cm diameter Lucite phantom (S/P = 0.85) this results in a S/P ratio of 0.026 assuming a primary transmission of 0.86 (i.e., an aft slot primary transmission of 0.96 and an aft slot cover transmission of 0.90). Preliminary measurements give a S/P ratio of 0.06 ± 0.02 (39 kVp, Mo target/filter combination) for the same phantom [15] and are in reasonably good agreement with the projected value. Assuming a S/P ratio ranging from 0.40 to 0.85, such a device would result in contrast improvements of from 1.36 to 1.75 [1].

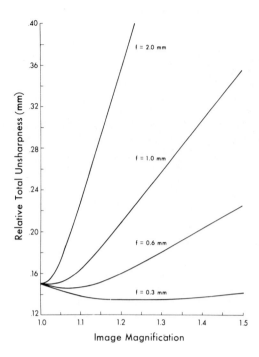

Figure 5. Plot of relative total unsharpness vs. magnification for representative focal spot sizes.

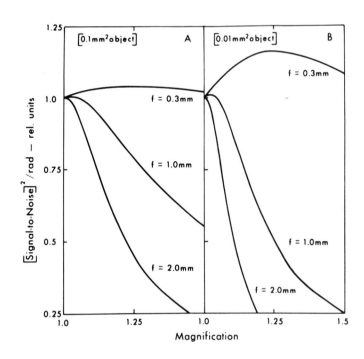

Figure 6. Plot of (signal-to-noise ratio)^2 per rad vs. magnification for representative focal spot sizes. A. 0.10 mm^2 object. B. 0.01 mm^2 object.

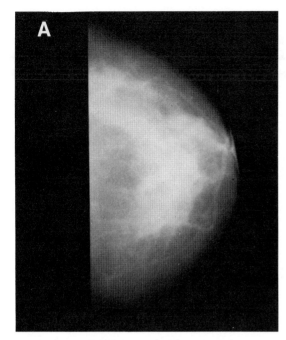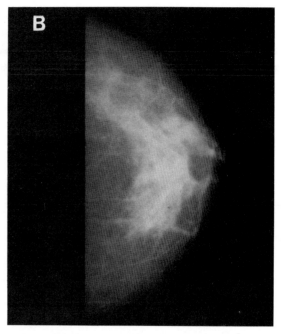

Figure 7: Comparison mammograms of a 66 year old woman with a compressed breast thickness of 5 cm illustrating the contrast improvement achieved through use of the SMSA. A. Conventional film. B. SMSA film. Both were made at 32 kVp and 200 mA utilizing a molybdenum target/filter combination (0.27 mm of Al HVL). The conventional film's exposure time and skin dose values are 1/4 sec and 420 mrad; while, the respective SMSA values are 2 1/4 sec and 730 mrad.

Figure 7 compares conventional (non adapted GE MMX-2) and SMSA mammograms. Both films were obtained employing a Kodak min-R film/screen combination at the same kVp and filtration. The improvement in contrast obtained with the SMSA is readily apparent and results in increased clarity of soft tissue detail. The longer exposure time required for the SMSA film is due primarily to the fractional field of coverage and larger FFD. Other factors requiring increased primary to maintain a proper exposure level at the image receptor are the decrease in scatter, primary losses due to the unsharpness of the fore slits at the aft slots, attenuation by the aft slot cover and decreased film speed arising from reciprocity failure. The latter factors are also the reasons for the resultant increase in skin dose with the SMSA.

Preliminary experimental results indicate that an SMSA can virtually eliminate scatter in mammography. Patient comparison films verify this qualitatively and indicate that such a device is clinically practical. At the same beam quality as employed conventionally an SMSA results in increased radiation dose. However, this improved image quality can be compromised to reduce patient dose either by employing a faster image receptor or a more penetrating beam [1]. That is, compared to conventional techniques an SMSA can either be employed to obtain improved images at comparable dose levels or to obtain comparable images at reduced dose.

The current device is a prototype adapted to a conventional unit, and, as such, its design options were limited. Improvements in performance can be realized by using a smaller focal spot and optimizing the system geometry as discussed in the preceding section. Incorporating these improvements would make it the most dose effective method of reducing scatter in mammography currently available.

APPENDIX A: RELATIVE UNSHARPNESS

If we neglect motion and film unsharpness, the total unsharpness, U_t, can be expressed as

$$U_t = (U_g^2 + U_s^2)^{\frac{1}{2}} \tag{A1}$$

where U_g is the geometrical unsharpness associated with the finite size of the focal spot and U_s is the screen unsharpness. The concept of unsharpness as employed in Eqn. (A1) is defined as

$$U^2 = [\iint MTF^2(f_x, f_y) \cdot df_x \cdot df_y]^{-1} \tag{A2}$$

where $MTF(f_x, f_y)$ is the associated component or system modulation transfer function and f_x and f_y denote the spatial frequencies associated with the x and y dimensions. Eqn. (A1) is an approximation, but has been shown to be strictly valid for Gaussian MTF's [16].

Eqn. (A1) refers to the unsharpness in the image plane and in comparing the unsharpness of images at different magnifications it is more pertinent to determine the unsharpness in the object plane or relative unsharpness, U_r. The unsharpness in the object plane is simply the unsharpness in the image plane divided by the object magnification factor, M, or

$$U_r = U_t/M \tag{A3}$$

Using Eqn. (A1) and setting U_g equal to $f \cdot (M - 1)$, where f is the effective focal spot size, Eqn. (A3) becomes

$$U_r = [f^2 \cdot (M - 1)^2 + U_s^2]^{\frac{1}{2}}/M \tag{A4}$$

It is interesting to note that Eqn. (A4) has minimum at a magnification of

$$M_{min} = (f^2 + U_s^2)/f^2 \tag{A5}$$

APPENDIX B: (Signal-to-Noise Ratio)^2/rad

Our derivation of an expression for the $[SNR]^2$/rad as function of object magnification is based on the approximate SNR formulation of Wagner [16] and is similar in certain respects to that of Muntz [17] except for our neglect of scatter (the SMSA case) and our assumption that the image receptor is always exposed to the same number of photons. Following Wagner [16] the signal contrast, C_s, is given by

$$C_s = C_0 \cdot A_0 \cdot M^2/A_i \tag{B1}$$

where C_0 is the inherent subject contrast of the object due to differential attenuation, A_0 is the area of the object and A_i is the imaged area of the object taking into account the blurring effects of the focal spot and screen. Equation (B1) indicates that the imaged signal contrast is equal to the inherent subject contrast times the ratio of projected object area-to-blurred object area. The latter is given by

$$A_i = (A_o \cdot M^2 + U_t^2) \tag{B2}$$

which is an exact expression for objects with a Gaussian attenuation profile and a Gaussian imaging system MTF [16]. It is an approximation for real objects and imaging systems. The noise contrast, C_n, or contrast fluctuations associated with quantum mottle and the imaged object area is given by

$$C_n = (N \cdot A_i)^{-\frac{1}{2}} \tag{B3}$$

where N is the effective number of x-ray quanta per unit area detected by the image receptor.

The SNR is given by the ratio of signal contrast-to-noise contrast or

$$SNR = C_s/C_n \tag{B4}$$

Substituting Eqns. (B1) and (B3) into Eqn. (B4), one obtains

$$SNR = C_o \cdot A_o \cdot M^2 \cdot [N/(A_o \cdot M^2 + U_t^2)]^{\frac{1}{2}} \tag{B5}$$

For a fixed FFD system in the absence of scattered radiation, the radiation absorbed dose in rads to the object for a given number of x-ray quanta at the image receptor simply scales as M^2. Using this fact and Eqn. (B5), the relative SNR^2/rad as a function of magnification is given by

$$SNR^2/\text{rad} \sim M^2/(A_o \cdot M^2 + U_t^2) \tag{B6}$$

Substituting in Eqn. (A1), the above expression becomes

$$SNR^2/\text{rad} \sim M^2/(A_o \cdot M^2 + f^2 \cdot (M - 1)^2 + U_s^2) \tag{B7}$$

It is interesting to note that the SNR^2/rad will have a maximum independent of object size at the magnification given by Eqn. (A5) where the relative unsharpness has a minimum.

REFERENCES

1. Barnes GT, Brezovich IA: Contrast - the Effect of Scattered Radiation In Breast Carcinoma: The Radiologist's Expanded Role, edited by WW Logan, John Wiley & Sons, New York, 1977, pp 73-81.

2. Pasche O: Über eine neue Blendenvorrichtung in der Röntgentechnik. Deutsche Med Wochenschr 29:266-267, 1908.

3. Jaffe C, Webster EW: Radiographic Contrast Improvement by Means of Slit Radiography. Radiology 116:631-635, 1975.

4. Sashin D, Barnes JO, Ricci JL, Gur D: Electronic Moving Slit for Scatter Reduction in Diagnostic Radiology. In Proc of the Ninth Midyear Topical Symposium of the Health Physics Society, Denver, CO, Feb 9-12, 1976, pp 787-790.

5. Sorenson JA, Nelson JA: Investigations of Moving Slit Radiography. Radiology 120:705-711, 1976.

6. Moore R, Korbuly D, Ampaltz K: A Method to Absorb Scattered Radiation Without Attenuation of the Primary Beam. Radiology 120:713-717, 1976.

7. Barnes GT, Cleare HM, Brezovich IA: Reduction of Scatter in Diagnostic Radiology by Means of a Scanning Multiple Slit Assembly. Radiology 120: 691-694, 1976.

8. Gur D, Sashin D, Herbert DL: Improved Contrast in Mammography Using a Double Slit Technique. Presented at the 25th Annual Meeting of the Association of University Radiologists, Kansas Cit KS, May 1-4, 1977.

9. Barnes GT, Brezovich IA, Witten DM: Scanning Multiple Slit Assembly: A Practical and Efficient Device to Reduce Scatter. Am J Roentgenol 129:497-501, 1977.

10. Barnes GT, Brezovich IA: The Design and Performance of a Scanning Multiple Slit Assembly. Med Phys, (in press).

11. Doi K: Advantages of Magnification Radiography. In Breast Carcinoma: The Radiologist's Expanded Role, edited by WW Logan, John Wiley & Sons, New York, 1977, pp 83-92.

12. Haus AG: Effect of Geometric Unsharpness in Mammography and Breast Xeroradiography. In Breast Carcinoma: The Radiologist's Expanded Role, edited by WW Logan, John Wiley & Sons, New York, 1977, pp 93-108.

13. Sprawls P: Focal Spots in Mammography. In Breast Carcinoma: The Radiologist's Expanded Role, edited by WW Logan, John Wiley & Sons, New York, 1977, pp 117-120.

14. Wagner RF: Physical Factors that Affect Mammographic Images. In Breast Carcinoma: The Radiologist's Expanded Role, edited by WW Logan, John Wiley & Sons, New York, 1977, pp 61-71.

15. Yester MY, Barnes GT, King MA: Experimental Measurements of the Scatter Reduction and Contrast Improvement Obtained in Mammography with a Scanning Multiple Slit Assembly. Paper 277, 64th Scientific Assembly and Annual Meeting of the Radiological Society of North America, Chicago, IL, Nov 25- Dec 1, 1978.

16. Wagner RF: Toward a Unified View of Radiological Imaging Systems Part II: Noisy Images. Med Phy 4:279-296, 1977.

17. Muntz PE: On the Significance of Scattered Radiation in Reduced Exposure Mammography. Paper 105, 63rd Scientific Assembly and Annual Meeting of the Radiological Society of North America, Chicago, IL, Nov 26 - Dec 2, 1977.

EVALUATION OF GRID-TECHNIQUE IN MAMMOGRAPHY

Gerhard Jost

Philips-Mueller Medical Systems Division, 2000 Hamburg, Germany

This paper is the result of our applied studies and theoretical considerations which started 2 1/2 years ago due to publications of A. Haus[1] (long
distance technique) and M. Friedrich[2] (influence of scatter).

As the visualization of slight density differences is of decisive significance in mammography the aim of this paper is to discuss additional measures
which improve the quality of the primary x-ray image. Such optimization has to
take various conflicting requirements into account. On one hand, to reduce the
radiation exposure in mammography, and on the other hand, to achieve this aim
without reducing image quality.

Although there might be an additional change in the future, the x-ray
spectrum will not be considered here. In other words, we are assuming a spectrum emitted by a molybdenum anode with an additinal molybdenum filter.

With the availability of film-screen combinations, attention began to be
paid to ways of improving the radiographic contrast. The x-ray beam exiting the
object consists of primary radiation and depending on the thickness of the
object, 30 to 50% scattered radiation (Fig. 1).

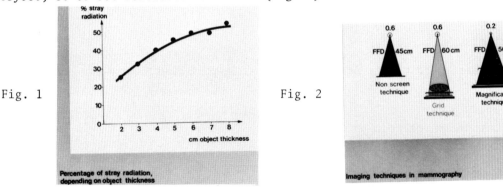

Fig. 1   Fig. 2

The use of methods for suppressing scattered radiation could not be considered
when non-screen films were used, owing to the required increase in radiation
exposure. Nowadays, however, film-screen combinations offer two possibilities:
the grid technique and the magnification technique (Fig. 2). We have tested
both of these techniques in clinical practice, using experimental equipment.

For magnification technique a focal spot size of less than 0.3 mm is required. The suppression of scattered radiation in the magnification technique
by the airgap effect is relatively poor. With a 5 cm thick object and a magnification factor of 1.6, for example, the reduction will be from 45% to about 30%
(Fig. 3).

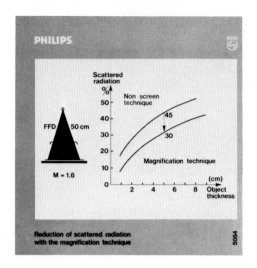

fig. 3

An advantage however, is that magnification increases the size of object details with respect to the granularity of the imaging system. On the basis of
practical experience and the theoretical considerations, the magnification
technique has the following limitations in mammography.

1. Magnification requires a larger film size than the standard 18 x 24 cm
   A format of at least 24 x 30 cm is required for survey exposures, with
   the associated problems of filing and higher cost. (18 cm x 24 cm) x
   1.6^2 = (28.8 cm x 38.4 cm).

2. The larger area to be studied may increase the time and effort required
   for diagnosis.

3. Patient and film positioning are more complicated and it is more difficult to obtain adequate visualization of details adjacent to the thorax.

4. A higher skin dose is unavoidable, in view of the reduced focus-skin
   distance.

5. Reduced loadability of the microfocal spot, which limits the choice of
   recording systems.

6. The reduction of local density gradients, which gives a subjective
   impression of reduced contrast.

An improved reduction in scattered radiation can be obtained with the GRID
technique. Taking a 5 cm thick object, as in our previous example, this gives
a reduction in scatter from 45 to 15% (Fig. 4). A prerequisite for this technique is the use of a special soft-radiation grid. It should give adequate
suppression of scattered radiation, but without an excessively high grid factor.
This is realized at a grid ratio about 5, small lead content and low absorption
of the interspace and cover materials. The grid technique still permits a
greater focus-film distance than the non-screen technique, thus reducing the
effect of geometrical unsharpness due to the focal spot.

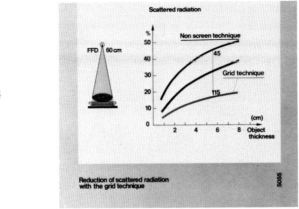

fig. 4

One tool for the explanation of the image quality is the modulation transfer function (MTF). The MTF is the result of measurements and mathematical
calculations. It gives an indication of how details of an object are trans-
fered to the image, taking into consideration the focal spot size, the FFD, the
FOD and the resolving power of the image carrier. A comparison of the modulation transfer functions for the magnification and grid techniques may lead to
the conclusion that, for an object of average thickness, the two techniques
give comparable results (fig. 5). However, this is only true of MTF calculations which do not take the effect of scattered radiation into account.
Such a comparison does not, of course, reflect the real situation.

A true comparison of the modulation transfer functions must take into
account the improvement in image quality by suppression of scattered radiation.
The mathematical step in calculation of the MTF is multiplication of the ordinate by a factor equivalent to the proportion of primary radiation at the detector. The real difference between the MTF curves of the two systems now becomes
clear (fig. 6).

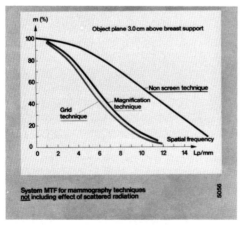

fig. 5

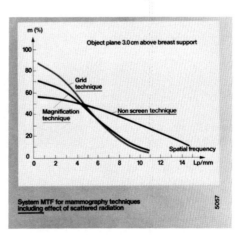

fig. 6

The increased contrast of the grid technique for details in the spatial frequency range up to five (5) line-pairs per millimeter, which is the most important range for mammography, is also confirmed by practical results. Five line-
pairs per mm means a detectability of 100 micron details. Due to the improved
contrast sensitivity the grid technique yields more information in low contrast
high scatter areas, for instance in dense glandular tissues, which have been

until now the most difficult cases for diagnosis.

Comparison between microdensitometer measurements made with the non-screen technique, and the grid technique clearly show the increased contrast of the latter (fig. 7):

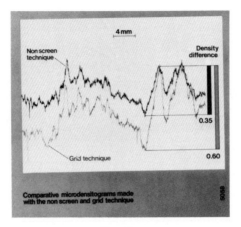

fig 7

the difference in blackening caused by the structure of the object increases from 0.35 with the non-screen technique to 0.60 with the grid technique which means that small details with grid technique are more detectable. Copies of mammograms may show the differences, although it is difficult to judge on a copy, especially because the average blackening in non-screen film has to be higher than in film-screen combination (fig. 8, fig. 9).

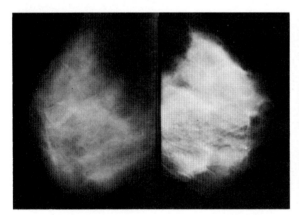
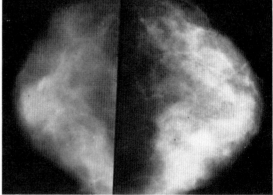

| Industrial film non-grid | Screen film grid | Industrial film non-grid | Screen-film grid |

fig 8   fig 9

The results obtained with the grid technique can be summarized as follows:

- With the increased focal-film distance of 60 cm the nominal 0.6 mm focal spot presents no serious limitation due to geometrical unsharpness.

- The increased loadability of the 0.6 mm focus does not limit the user's choice of imaging systems. In other words, he can apply both the grid technique with film-screen combinations and, as before, xeroradiography or non-screen film.

- With a proper selection of film-screen combination an image quality even superior to that of non-screen film can be obtained with less radiation exposure.

- Although the special soft-radiation grid and the object holder increase the radiation exposure by a factor of 2, a sensitive film-screen combination results in 4 to 5 times less radiation exposure as compared to non-screen film.

It would also be possible to use the higher contrast (obtained by reduction of scattered radiation) to increase the tube voltage, and thus to reduce the radiation exposure even more. The increase in high voltage, for instance, from 31 kV to 35 kV, reduces the entrance exposure by a factor of 1.5.

The use of the grid should, for the sake of patient dose, be used, when the compressed thickness is more than 3 cm, because then the amount of scatter reaches a considerable level. According to statistics of Dr. Bjurstam, who investigated the distribution of compressed breast thickness, the grid can be applicable to 93% of the patients because only 7% are below the level of 3 cm (fig. 10).

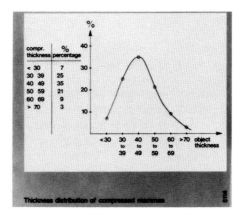

fig. 10

As a result of clinical studies, we stopped further activities with the magnification technique, and a mammography unit was developed for the grid technique permitting the use of several recording systems (fig. 11, fig. 12).

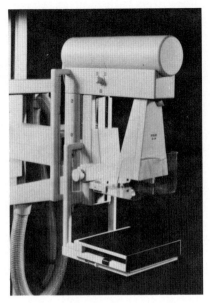

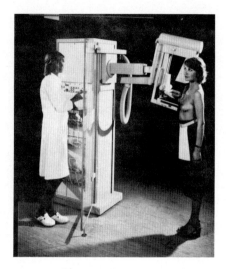

fig. 11   fig. 12

The film-focus distance is fixed to 60 cm.

The grid mechanism is easily removed, allowing one to work with or without a grid according to the clinical requirements. With the recent results achieved, we feel that there is no longer a need for non-screen films.

Because the inherent problems of dust between the film and screen and artifacts on the film still remains, the film manufacturers should develop a closed film loading system, to remedy this situation.

REFERENCES

1. Friedrich, M., Weskamp, P.: New modalities in mammographic imaging: Comparison of grid and air gap magnification techniques. Medicamundi 23:1-16, 1978.

2. Haus, A.G.: The effect of geometric unsharpness in mammography and xeroradiography. In, Breast Carcinoma: The Radiologist's Expanded Role, W.W. Logan, editor, J. Wiley and Sons, New York, 1977, pp 93-108.

MAMMOGRAPHY WITH MAGNIFICATION AND GRIDS:
DETAIL VISIBILITY AND DOSE MEASUREMENTS

Leonard Stanton, M.S.

Department of Radiation Therapy and Nuclear Medicine
Hahnemann Medical College and Hospital
Philadelphia, Pa. 19102

Wende W. Logan, M.D.

Consultant, Roswell Park Memorial Institute
1351 Mt. Hope Ave, Rochester, N.Y. 14620

At present the Xerox 125 system demonstrates finer anatomic details than screen film combinations. However, this is at the cost of twice as great exposure to the breast glandular parenchyma, even with high kVp/filtration technique (1). Apparently a "low dose" Xerox system is not in prospect. Consequently it is important to improve screen film images while retaining low patient exposure. Fortunately both scatter reduction and direct magnification can improve these images.

Barnes' work indicates that 50% greater mammographic image contrast should result from total scatter removal (2). Friedrich's study using the Philips mammography grid supports this view (3). Sickles (4) and Haus (5) reported substantial image improvement from use of direct magnification. However, fast image receptors were not used in all these image evaluations. As a result, patient exposure was at least double that of conventional "low dose" screen technique. Therefore these studies did not address the important question: Can one significantly improve screen film images, while retaining "low dose" patient exposure?

The present paper present preliminary results of a study designed to answer this question. Both direct magnification and grid images were compared with those obtained using conventional molybdenum target tube technique. In addition:

1. A very fast film was used to achieve "low dose" operation.

2. Visibility of calcific and soft tissue detail was measured using a quantitative breast phantom.

3. Average glandular parenchymal exposures were compared for various techniques, using a novel dosimetry breast model and procedure.

MATERIALS AND METHODS

We used two mammography machines: a Philips Mammo Diagnost, operated both with and without the new Philips mammography grid, and an RSI magnification unit*. Figure 1 gives exposure details. A single Kodak Min-R screen was used throughout, with a Picker vacuum bag system to assure good screen/film contact. In addition to the Min-R screen, a new fast experimental film, designed by Eastman Kodak, was also used (which, in this paper we shall refer to as "X" film). This was of single emulsion, orthochromatic design and 2.5 times faster than Min-R film. It also has more contrast. Development was carried out in a well-stabilized Kodak X-omat processor during a single seven-hour period. mAs values were chosen to yield as close to 1.3 total film density as practicable.

Visibility measurements were made with a breast phantom containing simulated calcifications and water-like fibrils in fat, of graded sizes**. In evaluating images, one is interested in both the ultimate resolution during clinical search, and the ease with which objects are seen. The former affects the possibility; the latter the probability of detection in routine clinical search.

There is great ambiguity in "dose to the breast" as reported in the literature. Thus, excellent investigators still report "skin exposure" (4,5) and "absorbed dose at 3 cm depth" (7). One of us (L.S.) has discussed elsewhere a more biologically relevant approach to radiation carcinogenesis risk (6). Since we compare below values of "mean exposure to the glandular parenchyma of a 5 cm compressed breast", a brief description is in order of the proposed model and computation procedure.

1. Biologic Model. The glandular epithelium and its stroma are taken as tissues at greatest risk. In the "average" 5 cm compressed breast, they are assumed to constitute a central water-like 2.5 cm thickness, between two adipose tissue sections (Figure 2A). The average rather than maximum dose to this central volume is computed. The result is believed to be a reasonable index of the mammography carcinogenesis hazard in a large middle to older age (35 to 65) female population.

2. Computation. There are four steps. First, the skin exposure per examination is determined from air measurements and backscatter factors. Second, the exposure at depth vs that to the skin is estimated from Hammerstein's curves (7), for a uniform composition breast. This relationship is then converted to that appropriate for the model (Figure 2B), the average ratio determined, and the mean exposure computed for the central portion. Finally, the average absorbed dose can be obtained using appropriate roentgen to rad conversion factors.

*Radiologic Sciences Inc., Santa Clara, California

**See paper by one of us (L.S.) in discussion on breast phantoms, and reference (I). Companion paper (W.W. Logan) presents clinical comparisons of conventional with grid and magnification technique.

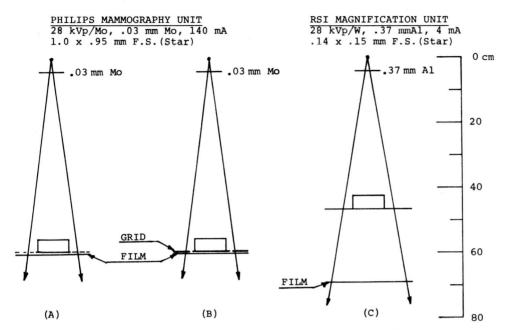

PHILIPS MAMMOGRAPHY UNIT
28 kVp/Mo, .03 mm Mo, 140 mA
1.0 x .95 mm F.S.(Star)

RSI MAGNIFICATION UNIT
28 kVp/W, .37 mmAl, 4 mA
.14 x .15 mm F.S.(Star)

.03 mm Mo

.03 mm Mo

.37 mm Al

0 cm

20

40

60

80

GRID

FILM

FILM

(A)

(B)

(C)

Figure 1.   Exposure geometry and technical factors.

(A)   Conventional screen film technique
(B)   Philips mammography grid -- Min-R and fast films
(C)   Magnification mammography -- Min-R and fast films.

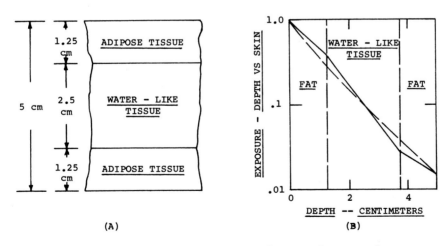

1.25 cm   ADIPOSE TISSUE

5 cm   2.5 cm   WATER - LIKE TISSUE

1.25 cm   ADIPOSE TISSUE

(A)

(B)

Figure 2.   Dosimetry model and procedure.

(A)   Compressed breast model. Vulnerable water-like central
        portion assumed, between layers of adipose tissue.
(B)   Computational procedure.
        Dashed curve -- measured in phantom of BR12 mix.
        Solid curve --- corrected for model distribution.

261

As noted above, we seek estimates of the smallest size objects visible as well as the ease with which they are seen. We now compare results for the three techniques, in tables I and II.

Table I. Smallest Visible Test Object Diameters -- mm

	Simulated Calcifications		Simulated Fibrils in Fat	
Technique	Min-R	X^+	Min-R	X^+
Conventional*	.176	.205	.425	.460
With grid	.158	.165	.410	.432
Magnification - RSI#	.159	.167	.375	.406

$^+$Experimental fast film. Both films used with a single
       Min-R screen.
*Philips 28 kVp/Mo, .03 mm Mo; 60 cm TFD.
#Radiologic Sciences, Inc., Santa Clara, Calif.

Table II. Entrance and Average Exposure
To Breast Glandular Parenchyma

Breast Thickness	Technique	Entrance Exposure -- R*		Mean Glandular Exposure -- R	
		Min-R	X^{**}	Min-R	X^{**}
5 cm	Conventional	1.31	0.44	0.181	0.061
5 cm	With grid	2.52	0.92	0.349	0.127
5 cm	Magnification	3.69	0.96	0.537	0.140
4 cm	Conventional	0.67	0.22	0.128	0.043
4 cm	With grid	1.29	0.47	0.247	0.090
4 cm	Magnification	1.80	0.47	0.355	0.093

*Including backscatter.
**Experimental fast single emulsion film.

CONVENTIONAL TECHNIQUE. Contrast is generally low, necessitating very careful detail search, unlike Xerox images. The experimental fast film exhibits poorer resolution than the Min-R film when both are used with a Min-R screen, requiring 16% larger calcific and 8% larger fibrillar objects for detection. This is evidently due to greater quantum mottle.

GRID TECHNIQUE. Contrast improvement is significant, yielding greater ease of visualization for all object sizes. In addition, calcific resolution is improved (10 and 6% smaller objects seen with the Min-R screen and fast film, respectively). However, much less improvement is noted with soft tissue fibrils (4% and 0).

MAGNIFICATION. Visibility is improved because the x-ray image is enlarged relative to the receptor; this reduces the effect of receptor blur and noise*. In addition, some contrast increase is achieved with the larger air gap we used (22.5 cm). As with grid technique, detail search is greatly facilitated for all size objects. The minimum object size for calcific details is also decreased from that of conventional technique (8.5 and 6%). Moreover, unlike grid technique, smaller soft tissue fibrils are seen (7 and 4%).

Dosage estimates for the several techniques are given in Table II. In general about 30% lower exposure is delivered with the preferred grid and magnification techniques (underlined)** Possible errors arise from uncertainties in the experimental film sensitivity, development, and the application of the Hammerstein curves to another machine; we therefore estimate errors of the order of ± 20% in the stated exposure figures. However, the data does prove low dose operation is achieved for the grid and magnification techniques using fast film.

CONCLUSIONS

1. The possibility has been demonstrated of significant image improvement in screen film mammography without increase in relevant patient dose. Improvement in both detail resolution and ease of visualization are observed.

2. Greater improvement is noted in visibility of calcific than soft tissue details. However, the latter appear to be seen better in magnification than in grid images.

3. Further work is in progress to improve the accuracy of both visibility and dosage determinations.

*This is accomplished by effectively scaling down the signal frequencies by the magnification factor, thus reducing the required recording system frequency band width.
**Data underlined for preferred combinations in Tables I and II.

REFERENCES

1. Stanton L, Villafana T, Day JL, et al: A breast phantom method for evaluating mammography technique. Invest. Radiol. 13:291-297, 1978.

2. Barnes GT and Bresovich IA: The intensity of scattered radiation in mammography. Radiology 126:243-247, 1978.

3. Friedrich M and Weskamp P: New modalities in mammographic imaging: Comparison of grid and magnification techniques. Medicamundi 23:1, 1978.

4. Sickles EA, Doi K and Genant HK: Magnification film mammography: Image quality and clinical studies. Radiology 125:69-76, 1977.

5. Haus AG, Paulus DD, Dodd GD, et al: Evaluation of magnification mammography. Proceedings of SPIE International Symposium on Medical Imaging, August 28, 1978 (In press).

6. Stanton L, Villafana T, Day JL, et al: A study of mammographic exposure and detail visibility, using three systems: Xerox 125, Min-R and Xonics. 125, Min-R and Xonics. Radiology, in press.

7. Hammerstein GR, Miller DW, White DR, et al: Radiation absorbed dose in mammography. Radiology (in press).

GRID VERSUS MAGNIFICATION USE IN CLINICAL MAMMOGRAPHY

Wende W. Logan, M.D.
Consultant, Roswell Park Memorial Institute
1351 Mt. Hope Avenue, Rochester, New York 14620

Leonard Stanton, M.S.
Department of Radiation Therapy and Nuclear Medicine
Hahnemann Medical College and Hospital
Philadelphia, Pa., 19102

Preliminary breast phantom image evaluations (see Stanton's chapter on grids and magnification) have indicated that the use of faster screen-film combinations with the use of a grid, or in magnification, can result in improved images without an increase in average breast glandular dose.

GRID

The Philips grid for mammography[1] (see Jost's and Barnes' chapters), has been evaluated clinically for the past six months, in Rochester, New York (see figures 1-5).

Mammograms obtained with the grid have demonstrated a dramatic improvement over mammograms obtained without the grid use. A double-blind study is now underway, using the Philips Diagnost-M unit, comparing mammograms obtained without the grid, utilizing the Kodak Min-R screen-Min-R film combination, to mammograms performed with the grid, utilizing an experimental single-coated film*, designed for automatic processing, used with the Min-R screen. This experimental film is 2.5 times faster than Min-R film, and has more contrast. The average glandular dose** utilizing the latter combination (with grid), is about 20% less than that of the former combination (without grid). Yet, the resultant images are far superior with the faster film, because of the scatter removal. The most dramatic improvement occurs in breasts which are least compressible (i.e. 5 cm or more compressed thickness). In dense dysplastic breasts, the elimination of scatter has also resulted in improved contrast, enabling improved calcification and small tumor detection. However, even with the 60 cm focal spot-film distance, the large focal spot size (star measurement of 1.2 mm) creates some difficulties, in that geometric unsharpness is a problem in patients with larger, less compressible breasts, particularly since pressure to utilize faster screen-film systems with less detector system resolution is being continually applied to radiologists in the United States.

MAGNIFICATION

Magnification has been performed in Rochester for the past three years, utilizing the RSI Microfocus mammography unit, which has a measured 150 micron tungsten target.[2] Aerial image resolution is thus excellent for both contact

---

*The experimental film was provided by the Research Laboratories of the Eastman Kodak Company.

**All average glandular doses referred to in this paper have been determined without assuming an adipose-skin shield, since its average thickness is not yet known.

and magnification mammograms.

Because of the spectral distribution of the tungsten target, however, lack of contrast is a problem with this unit (effective contrast can usually be obtained if the patient's breast can be compressed to 4 cm or less, but increasing scatter in thicker breasts can interfere significantly in terms of calcification detection, when screen-film combinations are used (this is not a problem in xeromammography use with this unit). For this reason, Kodak NMB film (single emulsion, more contrast than Min-R film, and 20% faster) is routinely utilized with the Min-R screen, instead of Min-R film.

For the past 8 months, contact mammograms obtained with the Min-R screen-NMB film combination have been compared with 1.3 magnification mammograms utilizing the Min-R screen in combination with the Eastman Kodak experimental film (described earlier in this chapter . The film has slightly more contrast than NMB film, and is 2 times faster). Both studies have been obtained at a 45 cm focal spot-breast base distance. The NMB film-Min-R screen combination has been placed just beneath the breast. The experimental film-Min-R screen combination has been placed 10 cm below the breast (10 cm air gap). The average glandular x-ray dose has been equal with both methods, but the image quality is improved on the magnified view (in terms of calcification detection, contrast, and clarity of tissue outline - see figures 6,7). Therefore, a routine microfocus mammogram in my office now consists of a 1.3 magnification craniocaudad view with the Min-R screen-experimental film combination, and an oblique (see chapter on proper screen-film technique) 1.5 magnification view (10 cm air gap) with the Min-R screen-NMB film combination (see figure 8). The average glandular x-ray dose is 300 millirads for the two view study. The RSI unit compression device (see chapter on screen-film techniques) enables a maximum amount of posterior breast tissue to be visualized on the film. Small breasted women (even those with dense dysplastic tissue) are therefore optimally evaluated with the RSI unit, because the smaller target size results in more scatter reduction with the 10 cm air gap.[3]

A major advantage of the RSI unit is the option to perform magnification spot views of suspicious areas visualized on the routine mammogram, or to perform spot views of palpable densities on patients who have "normal" mammograms (see figure 9). Routine magnification mammograms cannot be performed on large breasted women, however (approximately 10-15% of women examined) since the magnified images cannot be projected to within a 8" x 10" film. Furthermore, the increased scatter obtained with the large target size of a large breast (coupled with the often concommitant poor compressibility of large breasted women), can create serious problems, because of the decreased contrast (see Barnes' chapter).

DISCUSSION

It has become increasingly apparent that magnification and/or grid utilization enable mammogram image improvement without an increase in average glandular dose. The advantages and disadvantages of the state of the art of these methods have been discussed (see table I for summary). Geometric unsharpness is the only major problem encountered with the Philips unit. Diminished contrast is the major problem encountered with the RSI unit. These major disadvantages of each unit would be overcome if a grid were to be utilized with a small (measured 300 micron or less)[3] tungsten target focal spot unit, thus combining optimum aerial resolution with improved radiographic contrast. Contact mammograms could be performed with the grid, on large breasted women. The grid could be removed for mammograms on small breasted women, and/ or spot magnification views. The use of the grid would allow the use of the

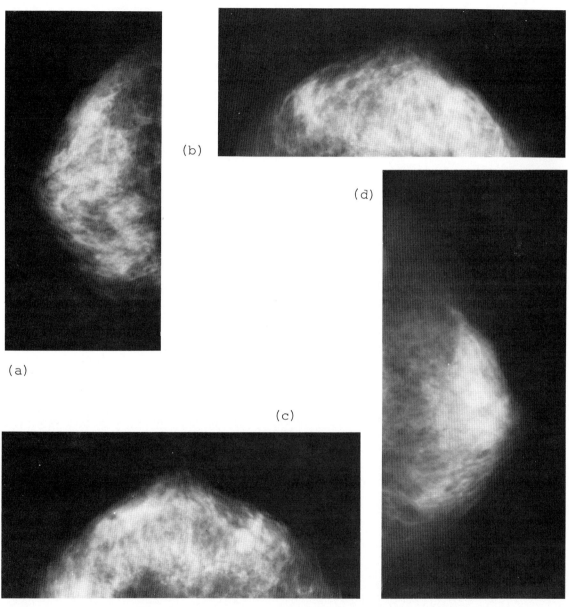

Figure 1: This patients' mammogram, performed on the Philips unit, shows the
value of the grid in delineating outlines of breast tissue. (A) is
an oblique view of the right breast (Kodak experimental film - Min-
R screen) with the grid, at 100 mR av. gl. dose. (B) is a C-C view
(Min-R screen-film) of the same breast, with grid, at 250 mR. (C)
is a C-C view (Kodak experimental film - Min-R screen) of the left
breast at 100 mR av. gl. dose. (D) is an oblique view (Min R
screen-film) of the same breast <u>without</u> grid, at 100 mR av. gl.
dose. Breast compression was 4 cm.

harder beam necessary to penetrate breasts with dysplastic tissue (the major type of problem encountered in diagnostic mammography), because the grid would absorb the scatter which now interferes with calcification and tumor detection in these same patients. The use of the tungsten target harder beam would also result in diminished breast entrance x-ray exposure, and diminished average glandular dose.

SUMMARY

The advantages and disadvantages of small focal spots, and grids, for mammography have been discussed. An ideal mammographic unit consisting of a small tungsten focal spot and a grid, should allow excellent mammography to be performed on all breast sizes and tissue consistencies.

TABLE I

	Magnification (RSI Unit)	Grid (Philips Unit)
Advantages	- Excellent aerial resolution - Magnification spot views can elucidate suspicious areas	- Excellent contrast (better visualization of tissue of poorly compressible and dysplastic breasts)
Disadvantages	- Cannot routinely magnify largest breasts - Less contrast (as breast thickness and size increase)	- Geometric unsharpness - Can't visualize posterior 5 mm of breast - ↑ av. gl. dose (Moly target)

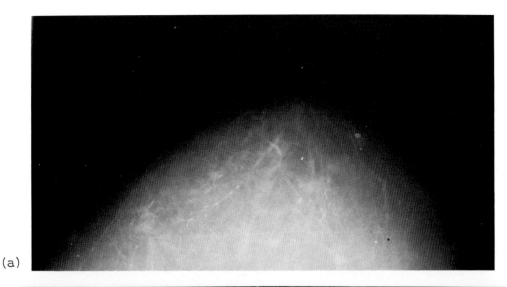

(a)

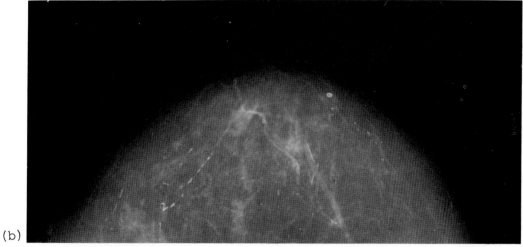

(b)

Figure 2: Philips unit, same breast - (A) was performed without grid,
(Min-R screen-film) at 150 mR av. gl. dose. (B) was performed
with the grid (Agfa Gevaert MR 30 single emulsion mammographic
film, with the Min-R screen) at 120 mR av. gl. dose (the film is
2.5 times faster than Min-R film). Breast compression was 6 cm.
Note that the improvement in contrast, with grid use, is more
dramatic, with increased breast thickness.

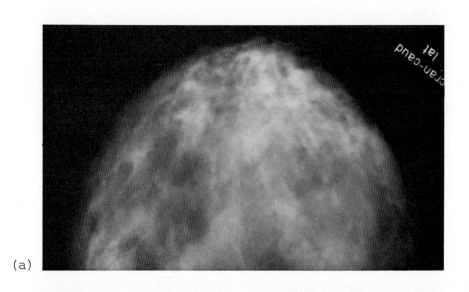

(a)

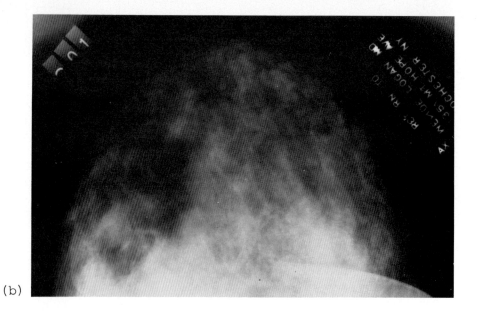

(b)

270

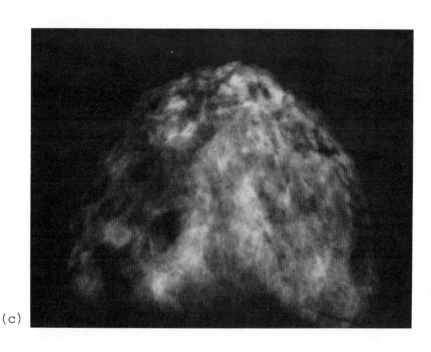

(c)

Figure 3: (A) was performed with the Philips unit, using Kodak industrial
AA film (hand processed), without the grid, at 2000 mR av. gl.
dose. (B) was performed one year later, with a GE Mammex unit,
using the Min-R screen-film combination, without the grid, at 200
mR av. gl. dose. (C) was performed on the Philips unit, with the
grid, utilizing Kodak experimental film with the Min-R screen, at
150 mR av. gl. dose. The breast compression was 4 cm. Numerous
small punctate calcifications denoting sclerosing adenosis, were
seen throughout the breast, on (C), not able to be identified on
(A) and (B) mammograms performed without the grid.

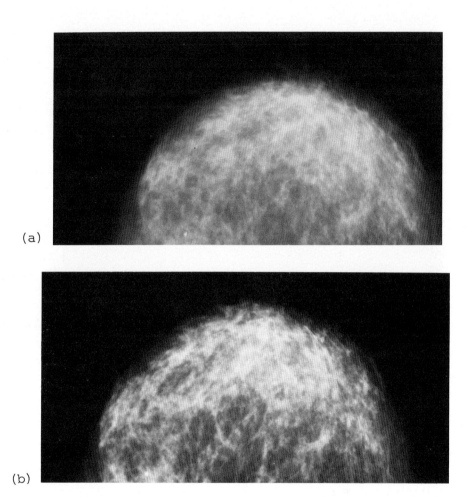

(a)

(b)

Figure 4:   Philips unit, same breast. (A) was performed (Min-R screen-film
            combination) without the grid, at 150 mR av. gl. dose. (B) was
            performed using Kodak experimental film with the Min-R screen, at
            120 mR av. gl. dose. Breast compression was 4.5 cm. Contrast is
            significantly improved.

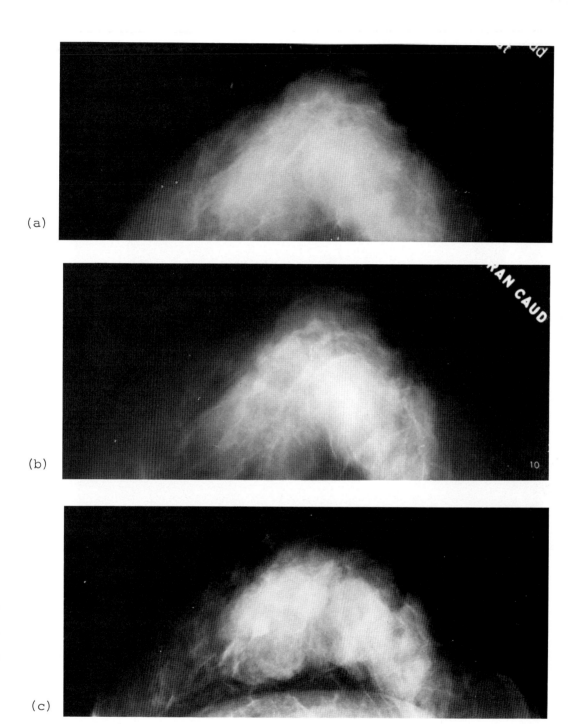

Figure 5: The Philips unit, same breast, over a 3 year period - (A) was performed using hand-processed AA industrial film (no grid), at 2000
mR av. gl. dose. (B) was performed utilizing the Min-R screen-film
combination (no grid), at 150 mR av. gl. dose. (C) was performed
using Kodak experimental film with the Min-R screen (with grid),
at 150 mR av. gl. dose. Breast compression was 5 cm.

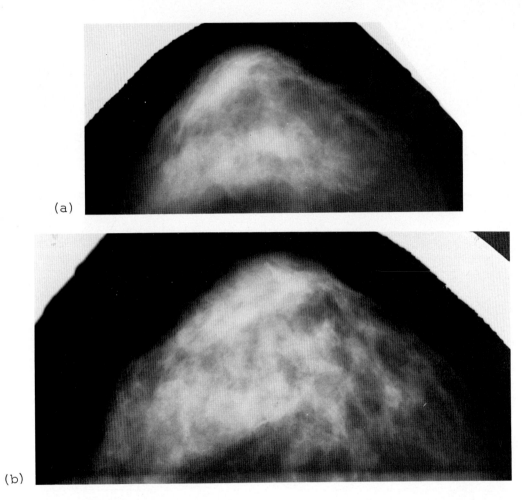

(a)

(b)

Figure 6:   RSI microfocus unit - contact vs. 1.3 magnification at the same
             dose. (A) is a contact C-C view of the left breast, using Kodak
             NMB film - Min-R screen, with a focal spot to breast base distance
             of 35 cm, at 100 mR av. gl. dose. (B)(same breast)was performed
             with experimental Kodak film with the Min-R screen, placed 10 cm
             beneath the breast (10 cm air gap, 35 cm focal spot to breast base
             distance - 1.3 x mag.), at 100 mR av. gl. dose. Note the improved
             contrast between soft tissues and surrounding fatty density, as
             well as increased detail of the outline of the glandular tissue,
             at no more increased average glandular dose to the patient's breast.

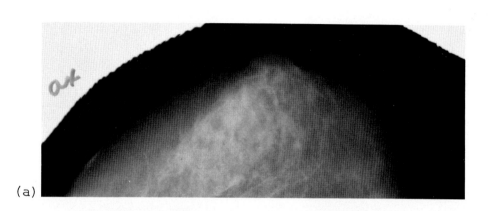

(a)

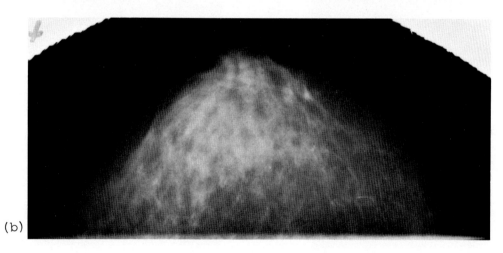

(b)

Figure 7:   RSI unit - same breast. (A) is a contact mammogram performed with
the Kodak NMB - Min-R screen, at a focal spot to film distance of
35 cm, at 100 mR av. gl. dose. (B) is performed with the Kodak
experimental film (2 times faster and slightly more contrasty than
NMB film), with the Min-R screen, placed 10 cm beneath the same
breast as (A) (10 cm air gap, 35 cm focal spot to breast base distance - 1.3 mag.). Again, note the increased contrast and delineation of the outline of the glandular tissue.

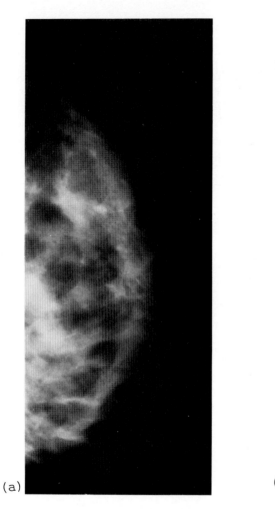
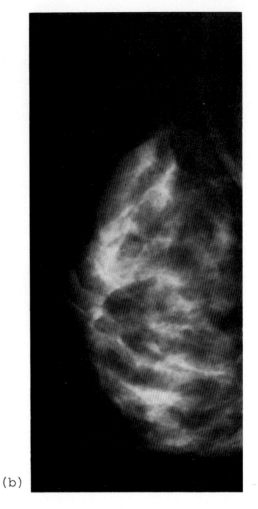

(a)

(b)

Figure 8: (A) is a lateral view performed utilizing AA Kodak industrial film, with the Philips unit (no grid), at 2000 mR av. gl. dose. (B) is an RSI 1.5 mag. 60° oblique view (same breast), on the RSI unit (25 cm focal spot to breast base distance, 10 cm air gap), at 150 mR av. gl. dose. Breast compression is 4 cm. The images have been reversed for easy comparison. Although the av. gl. dose is much less in (B), note the increased contrast and clarity of tissue outline, due to scatter removal, and excellent aerial resolution of the small focal spot.

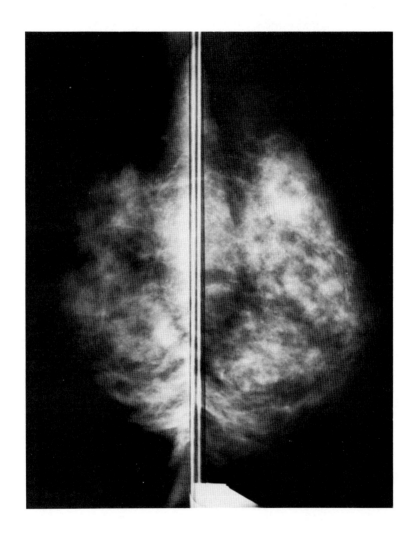

Fig. 9(a)

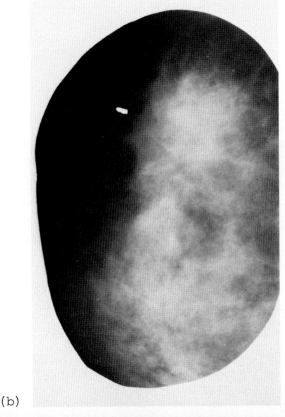

(b)

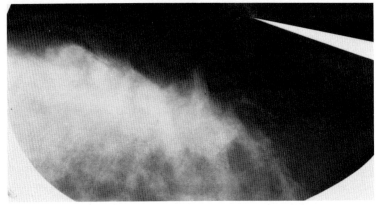

(c)

Figure 9:   The value of a tangential coned down magnification view - (A) re-
            veals left and right lateral mammograms performed with the RSI
            microfocus unit, on a patient with a palpable right breast upper
            outer quadrant 10:30 density. (B) is a coned down magnified spot
            view performed with the same unit. Carcinoma cannot be identified
            on this view. (C) reveals a tangential coned down magnified view
            of the palpable density. Fine lines can now be seen radiating from
            the border of a 1.5 cm diameter carcinoma. Without the tangential
            positioning of the density, enabling its outline to emerge from
            overlapped dense glandular tissue, the necessary surgery would
            have been delayed (this patient's mass had been felt to represent
            fibrocystic disease only, per surgical evaluation for four months
            prior to the mammogram). Surgery had not been contemplated prior
            to the mammogram results.

278

REFERENCES

1. Friedrich, M. and Weskamp, P.: New modalities in mammographic imaging:
    Comparison of grid and magnification techniques. Medicamundi 23:1, 1978.

2. Logan, W.W.: Overview of the radiologist's role in breast cancer detection.
    In, Breast Carcinoma: The Radiologist's Expanded Role, W.W. Logan, editor,
    Wiley and Sons, New York, 1977, pp 344-352.

3. Muntz, E.P., Logan, W.W.: Focal spot size and scatter suppression in
    magnification mammography. Amer. J. Roentgenol. 1979 (in press).

CONTRAST ENHANCEMENT OF LOW DOSE MAMMOGRAMS

by

B. M. Galkin*, G. Shaber*, M. Lassen*, S. Feig*, W. Logan**,
R. Nerlinger*, R. O. Gorson*

*Department of Radiology   **Rochester, New York
Thomas Jefferson University
Philadelphia, Pennsylvania

INTRODUCTION:

In spite of technical improvements in x-ray equipment, exposure techniques, and film-screen systems mammograms are often of limited value because of poor radiographic contrast. This results mainly from the small differential absorption of the x-ray beam in various parts of the breast i.e. poor subject contrast.

Since little can be done to significantly increase subject contrast recent efforts to improve the radiographic image have been directed at improving film contrast and a number of techniques have been proposed:
   a)   minimizing x-ray scatter to the film by the use of grids, moving slits, or an air gap [1-6]
   b)   electronic enhancement of the image using special equipment such as "Log Etronics" [7,8]

None of these seems to be in widespread clinical use at present -- probably because they either increase the radiation dose to the patient, are cumbersome to use, increase the liklihood of patient motion, require special costly equipment which is generally not available, or result in only limited contrast improvement.

One means to increase mammographic image contrast seems not yet to have been fully explored -- that is, the use of photographic techniques. It has long been known that image contrast can be enhanced photographically. In theory the process is simple, requiring only that the original be copied on a film which has an average gradient (gamma) > 1.0. The copy film then acts as a contrast amplifier. The problem has been that the photographic methods are time consuming, require specialized equipment and photographic emulsions that need special handling. As a result photographic contrast enhancement has not been a practical solution to the problem affecting mammograms.

Fortunately there are now several types of readily available <u>radiographic</u> films which are both rapid-processable and have an average gradient $>$ 1.0. Moreover, the degree of contrast enhancement can be controlled by a judicious selection of film and exposure technique. For example, it has recently been shown that the gradient of Kodak's rapid-process mammography film can be increased to values $>$ 3.0 by merely exposing it to visible light (from intensifying screens) instead of to x or gamma rays as intended by the manufacturer. [9-12]

In another report Kodak's rapid-process duplicating film (XD) which exhibits an increase in gamma when exposed to white or pink light, was used to improve the contrast of mammograms. Contrast enhancement of 1.8x over the original was achieved and the visibility of the tiny calcifications was maintained. [13]

Recently a photographic method for increasing the contrast of high energy teletherapy localization radiographs was described. [14] As part of this process contact prints of the original were obtained with Kodak's XTL and XV film exposed to white light. The prints showed 2-3x more contrast than the original. This prompted the application of the same contact printing process to mammograms and in the same and subsequent reports [14,15] it was shown that 1) the contrast of mammograms could be significantly increased 2) even greater contrast could be obtained by repeating the process 3) the visibility of the tiny breast calcifications was maintained 4) overexposed and underexposed mammograms could be salvaged and 5) all the above could be achieved with no additional radiation dose to the patient.

The mathematical basis for the contact printing contrast enhancement process has been described in a recent report in which XTL and XV film were used to increase the contrast of high energy radiotherapy films. [16]

Contact printing with Kodak's X-omatic Subtraction film (XS) has also been used as a means to salvage mammograms that would otherwise have to be repeated and to extract additional information from normally exposed mammograms. [17]

We have recently applied the contact printing contrast enhancement technique to mammograms obtained with various low-dose imaging systems -- Kodak's Min-R, DuPont's Lo-Dose and Xonics' XERG. [18] The details of the process are given below along with clinical examples.

CONTRAST ENHANCEMENT TECHNIQUE:

The basic idea is to make a contact print of the original mammogram using a printing film which has the desired average gradient (gamma). The higher the gradient the more contrast in the print. Table I shows the difference in densities that can be obtained with different copying films. A density difference of 0.10 appears in the contact print as a density difference of as much as 0.36 - depending on the type of film and light spectrum used for the exposure.

Table I

Original	Type of Film $\longrightarrow$	Difference in Optical Density			
		Contact Print of Original*			
		XS	XD	XV	XTL
.10		.11	.21	.27	.36

*All prints made on Kodak film exposed to white light and processed in a 90-second processor with standard chemistry.

The XS, XV, and XTL copies are "negatives" of the original, that is, the densities are reversed.

MATERIALS NEEDED:

Film: Kodak's XTL Rapid-Process Therapy Localization
                                 XM   Rapid-Process Mammography
                                 XV   Rapid-Process Verification

                 Notes: XTL and XM are the same emulsion with different names. XTL comes in larger sizes than XM.
                        XTL has more contrast than XV (see Table I above)
                        XTL is about twice as fast as XV when exposed to white light (see below under Copying Unit)

Copying Unit: The usual radiographic copying unit -- the type used to obtain subtraction radiographs. We have used the Delta-X but others are equally useful.

                 "White" light means light from the incandescent bulb used for subtraction.

Film Processor: The usual automatic rapid-processor with regular chemistry.

METHOD:

1) Obtain a mammogram using the usual technique -- low kVp, low filtration, low-dose screen-film combination. Process the film in the automatic processor.

2a) Place the mammogram on the glass (plastic) plate of the copying unit and overlay it with a sheet of copying film.

 b) Close the cover to ensure good film-to-film contact. THIS IS IMPORTANT. Poor contact will increase image unsharpness.

 c) Set the exposure switch to the shortest time possible and make an exposure with XTL film. Develop the film in the automatic processor. If the copy is too dark proceed as in 2c) below for underexposed mammograms or use XV film. If the XV copy is still too dark a neutral density filter must be used as explained below.

3) View the enhanced radiograph side-by-side with the original mammogram. The enhanced image is intended to reveal supplemental information and has been found to be most valuable in retrospective viewing of the original.

Variations

For Overexposed Mammograms

2c) Extend the exposure time to around 5 seconds. It is easy to find the correct time by making exposures of the same duration on both XTL and XV film. The XTL film is about twice as fast as the XV.

For Underexposed Mammograms

2c) The light intensity from the copying unit may be too great for even the shortest exposure possible. In this instance, cover the glass (plastic) plate of the copying unit with a neutral density filter before the mammogram is put down. A neutral density filter can be made by taping together several sheets of 14" x 17" cleared radiographic film. Use 14" x 17" film to cover the whole glass plate.

Note: If two mammograms are of approximately the same density they can be copied on a single 14" x 17" film.

RESULTS:

Clinical Examples of Low-Dose Mammograms

Mammograms with normal density and contrast

Often a mammogram has a good range of densities and good contrast except for a few areas Figs. 1(a) and 2(a). The contrast enhanced copy can improve the image in such areas enabling the radiologist to extract additional information Figs. 1(b) and 2(b). Note that the densities are reversed from the original. Sometimes the skin line is less visible on the copy depending on the degree of enhancement. However, this is not a problem because it can usually be seen on the original. The enhanced copy is meant to reveal supplemental information -- e.g. an area of calcifications in Fig. 2(b) (see also below under Calcifications).

Overexposed Mammograms

Mammograms with densities much greater than 2.5 are of little value even if viewed with a bright light Fig. 3(a). Photographic methods to salvage overexposed radiographs have been reported previously but the films used were not completely compatable with rapid-processing. [19-21] It is possible to salvage these mammograms by contact printing with Kodak's XS film. [17] Now by using XTL or XV film the overexposed image can be contrast-enhanced as well as salvaged Fig. 3(b).

Underexposed Mammograms

It has long been felt that there is little useful information in underexposed mammograms, as for example Fig. 4(a). However, this is not necessarily true. An autoradiographic method to intensify the image in underexposed radiographs has recently been reported. [22-25] Another more practical way to make the information visible is by contact printing with a high gamma film Fig. 4(b). Another example is shown in Figs. 5(a) and (b).

Calcifications

Fig. 6(a) is a mammogram taken with the Xonics' XERG system. There is a small cluster of calcifications located at the arrow. Fig. 6(b) is a contrast enhanced contact print of Fig. 6(a). Note the calcifications appear as black specks instead of white. There is a small loss in resolution which, theoretically, should adversly affect their visibility. However the increased contrast seems to offset this loss and they appear even more visible.

Since radiologists often use a low power magnifier to look at the images of small breast calcifications a comparison of magnified views of Figs. 6(a) and (b) is shown in Figs. 7(a) and (b). The calcific areas have been enlarged 2x. Many more calcifications are visible in the enlarged contrast enhanced copy than in the enlarged original. The same is true in the enlarged images of Fig. 2 shown in Figs. 7(c) and (d).

CONCLUSIONS:

This report describes a relatively simple way to enhance the contrast of mammograms. The technique is rapid and inexpensive and requires no special equipment other than a film copying unit and an automatic film processor which are usually available in radiology departments and radiologists' private offices.

The enhancement process does not appear to adversly affect the visibility of tiny calcifications - in fact, it often seems to make them more discernible.

Overexposed and underexposed mammograms can often be salvaged.

The enhancement process involves <u>no additional radiation dose to the patient.</u>

Because of the above we feel that further investigations in this area are warranted. A number of questions remain to be answered. For example:

1)   What is the best film and light spectrum to use?

2)   Can the copying unit itself be improved? Should there be built-in light filters? If so, what colors? Should there be a built-in timer permitting shorter exposures?

3)   One of the vexing problems of mammography still remaining is the risk-benefit ratio for younger women with dense breasts. The availability of a method to easily improve radiographic contrast suggests that it might be possible to tolerate original mammograms with less contrast thus permitting the use of higher energy photons and lower patient dose. [26] To what extent is this possible?

     If higher energy photons can be used would there be a need for special x-ray units designed exclusively for mammography?

Much remains to be done to objectively evaluate photographic contrast enhancement of mammograms. We hope this report stimulates others to join in investigating the many facets of the problem.

ACKNOWLEDGEMENTS:

We would like to thank Carolyn Parry, M. D. and Harold Isard, M. D. for the use of some of the mammograms and Ellen Merritt and Gail Vogel for valued technical assistance.

Supported in part by NIH Grant No. CA-11602.

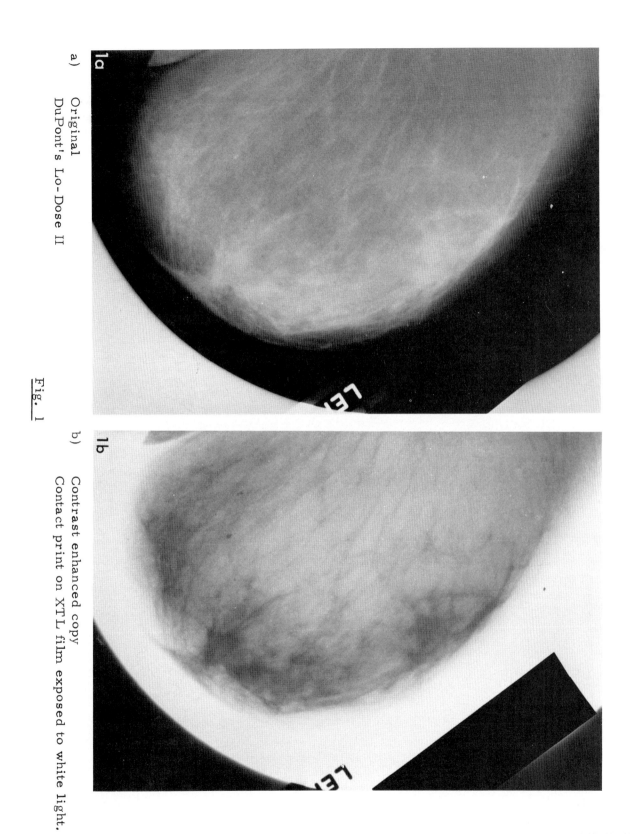

a) Original
DuPont's Lo-Dose II

b) Contrast enhanced copy
Contact print on XTL film exposed to white light.

Fig. 1

287

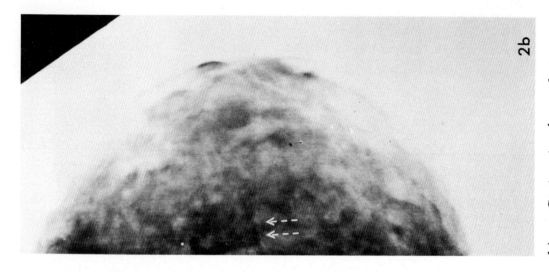

b) Contrast enhanced copy
    Contact print on XTL film exposed to white light.

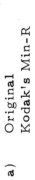

2b

Fig. 2

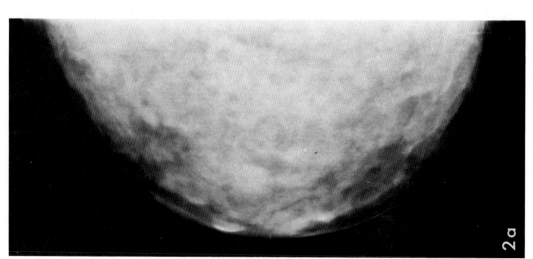

2a

a) Original
    Kodak's Min-R

288

a)   Overexposed original

Fig. 3

b)   Contrast enhanced copy
      Contact print on XV film exposed to white light.

289

b) Contrast enhanced copy
   Contact print on XTL film exposed to white light.

Fig. 4

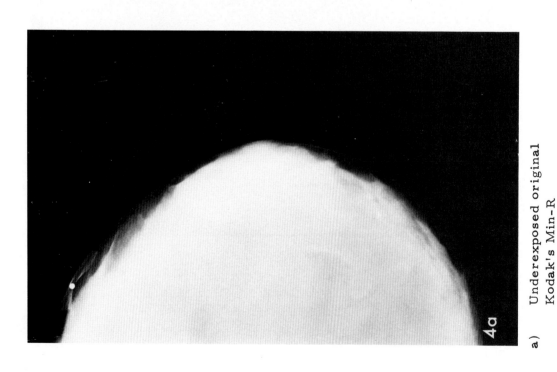

a) Underexposed original
   Kodak's Min-R

290

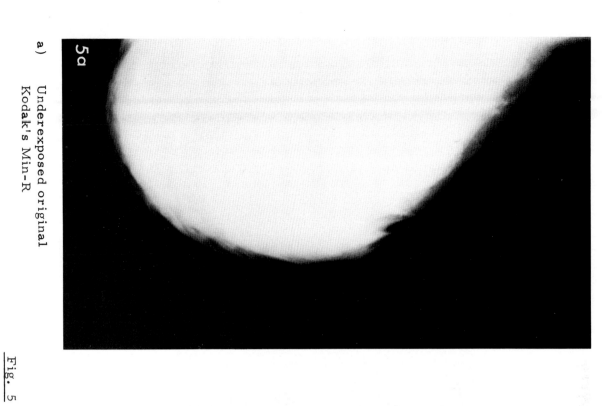

5a

a) Underexposed original
Kodak's Min-R

Fig. 5

5b

b) Contrast enhanced copy
Contact print on XTL film exposed to white light.

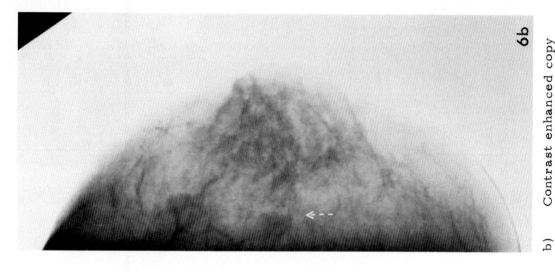

a) Original
    Xonics' XERG

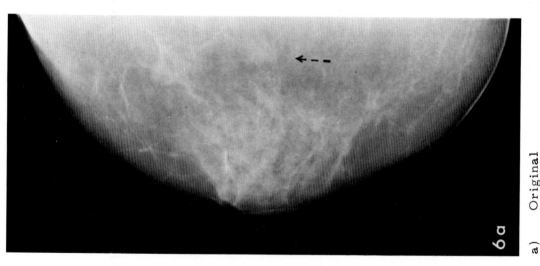

b) Contrast enhanced copy
    Contact print on XTL film exposed to white light.

Fig. 6

292

a)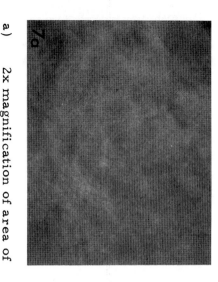

2x magnification of area of calcifications in Fig. 6(a)

b)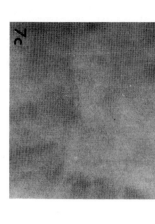

2x magnification of area of calcifications in Fig. 6(b) Note that many more calcifications are visible.

c)

2x magnification of area of calcifications in Fig. 2(a)

d)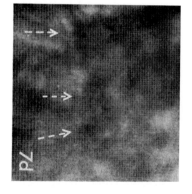

2x magnification of area of calcifications in Fig. 2(b) Again many more calcifications are visible.

Fig. 7

BIBLIOGRAPHY

1. Richter, D., Evaluation of Grid Technique in Mammography. Presented at the 20th Annual Meeting of the American Association of Physicists in Medicine, San Francisco, California, 30 July - 3 August 1978.

2. Jaffe, C., Webster, E., Radiographic Contrast Improvement by Means of Slit Radiography. Radiology 116: 631-635, September 1975.

3. Moore, R., Korbuly, D., Amplatz, K., A Method to Absorb Scattered Radiation Without Attenuation of the Primary Beam. Radiology 120: 713-717, September 1976.

4. Barnes, G., Cleare, H., Brezovich, I., Reduction of Scatter in Diagnostic Radiology by Means of a Scanning Multiple Slit Assembly. Radiology 120: 691-694, September 1976.

5. Sorenson, J., Nelson, J., Investigations of Moving Slit Radiography. Radiology 120: 705-711, September 1976.

6. Sickles, E., Doi, K., Genant H., Magnification Film Mammography: Image Quality and Clinical Studies. Radiology 125 (1): 69-76, October 1977.

7. Marmarsht in SIa, Ostrovskaia, I., Lipkovich, V., Method of Electronic Enhancement (Logetroning) of Breast Radiographs. Vestn. Roentgenol. Radiol. (2) 77-82, March-April 1975.

8. Laconi, A., Sasso, F., Polizzi, A., Reproduction and Magnification of Radiograms with Log Etron. Minerva Med. 63 (78): 4245-55, November 1972.

9. Galkin, B., Suntharalingam, N., Mansfield, C., Cobalt-60 Teletherapy Localization and Verification Radiographs Using Rapid Process Films and Intensifying Screens. American Association of Physicists in Medicine Quarterly Bulletin 6: 97, 1972. Scientific Exhibit, Annual Meeting of American Association of Physicists in Medicine, Philadelphia, Pennsylvania 1972.

10. Galkin, B., Suntharalingam, N., Mansfield, C., Greenhawt, M.H., Quality Control in the Delivery of External Beam Radiation Therapy. Digest of Third International Conference on Medical Physics, Including Medical Engineering, Goteborg, Sweden, p. 38.7, 1972.

11. Galkin, B., Wu, R., Suntharalingam, N., Methods for Improving Contrast in Therapy Localization Radiographs Obtained with ^{60}Co, 4 MV and 45 MV Photons. Scientific Exhibit, 61st Scientific Assembly, RSNA, Chicago, Illinois, 30 November - 5 December 1975.

12. Galkin, B., Wu, R., Suntharalingam, N., Improved Techniques for Obtaining Teletherapy Portal Radiographs with High Energy Photons. Radiology 127: 828-830, 1978.

13. Dronkers, D. and van der Zwaag, H., Photographic Contrast Enhancement in Mammography. Radiol. Clin. Biol. 43(6): 521-8, 1974.

14. Galkin, B., Strubler, K., Suntharalingam, N., Contrast Enhancement of High Energy Localization Radiographs. Presented at the Annual Meeting of the American Society of Therapeutic Radiologists, Denver, Colorado, November 2-5, 1977.

15. Galkin, B., Strubler, K., Feig, S., Dobelbower, R., Technique for Contrast Enhancement of Teletherapy Localization Radiographs and Mammographs. Presented as a Scientific Exhibit and written report, 20th Annual Meeting of American Association of Physicists in Medicine, San Francisco, California, 30 July - 4 August 1978.

16. Reinstein, L. and Orton, C., Contrast Enhancement of High Energy Radiotherapy Films. Oral Presentation and Scientific Exhibit at 20th Annual Meeting of the American Association of Physicists in Medicine, San Francisco, California, 30 July - 4 August 1978.

17. Orloff, T., Contrast Enhancement of Mammograms. Medical Radiography and Photography 54 (2): 38, 1978.

18. Galkin, B., Shaber, G., Lassen, M., Feig, S., Logan, W., Nerlinger, R., Gorson, R., Contrast Enhancement of Low Dose Mammograms. Scientific Exhibit Presented at 64th Scientific Assembly and Annual Meeting, Radiological Society of North America, Chicago, Illinois, 25 November - 1 December 1978.

19. Mittelstaedt, G., Method of Density Differentiation in Radiography. U. S. Patent Office Serial No. 113,582, 18 February 1964.

20. Chait, A. and Hale, J., Positive Prints of Dense Roentgenograms. Radiology 101: 331-334, November 1971.

21. Hale, J. and Chait, A., Positive Prints of Dense Roentgenograms. American Association of Physicists in Medicine Quarterly Bulletin 6: 97, 1972.

22. Askins, B., Photographic Image Intensification by Autoradiography. Appl. Optics 15: 2860-2865, November 1976.

23. Askins, B., Autoradiographic Image Intensification: Applications in Medical Radiography. Science 199: 684-686, 10 February 1978.

24. Rao, G.U.V. and Askins, B., Potential Reduction of X-ray Exposure Through Autoradiographic Intensification of Underexposed Radiographs. Presented at the 19th Annual Meeting of the American Association of Physicists in Medicine, Cincinnati, Ohio, 31 July - 4 August 1977.

25. Askins, B., Wagner, R., and Barnes, G., A Demonstration of the Effect of Reduced Scatter on Information Content and Patient Exposure. Presented at 20th Annual Meeting of the American Association of Physicists in Medicine, San Francisco, California, 30 July - 4 August 1978.

26. Orton, C. Private communication.

TECHNICAL CONSIDERATIONS PANEL

Roger Schneider, Moderator

Attendee: I have a question for Dr. Wagner. I'd like to know which x-ray energies and which type of filtration he used for his comparison of Min-R and the XERG system.

Wagner: The spectrum used for the Min-R study was 30 kVp, .002" paladium filter, 5 cm. of lucite, with the Min-R cassette. The average energy that reaches the casette is 22.4 kEv. The XERG samples were prepared with a spectrum that had an average energy of about 1 kEv less. There is a slight discrepancy there but I don't think it's a serious difference for the comparison.

Dr. Rao: This afternoon we have been introduced to 3 types of elimination of scatter: (1) the scanning slit beam, (2) the dual moving slits, and finally, (3) the Philips grid. I would like to know from either or the gentlemen, Dr. Barnes or Dr. Jost, how the contrast improvement factor compares with each of them, and also, if the some degree of contrast improvement can be expected if you use a xeromammography image system rather than film-screen?

Jost: I think it wouldn't be a fair comparison to do this with the xeromammography system. The MTF is different in both systems.

Barnes: As far as comparisons are concerned, in the grid technique, based on some Philips data, was of contrast improvement of about 55%. The dual scanning slit also obtained about a 50% improvement in contrast. One can also gain that type of improvement in contrast with air gap techniques, especially with a large air gap (30 cm. or more). The improvement in contrast with the scanning multiple slot assembly (you're imaging 98% of the possible contrast) is a contrast improvement of 1.75 in the scatter to primary ratio that I assumed. One point I was trying to make, that Phil Muntz made some time ago at the RSNA, was that in order for the air gap to be effective, you have to get far away from the focal spot with the target.

Rao: Gary, in your curve showing the effect of scatter to primary radiation as a function of air gap, you pointed out that the closer you get to the focal spot, the higher the scatter to primary ratio. You use as an explanation, the divergence of the field, and I was wondering whether the absolute intensity of the scatter being greater closer to the focal spot might be an alternative explanation.

Barnes: The particular point that you raised was published by Seeman in 1938. The difference is due to the beam divergence. The assumption is that the scatter diverges the same in both cases, and the difference is in the divergence of the primary. That is, the further away you get from the focal spot, the more parallel are the primary rays. The closer you get to the focal spot, the more rapidly do they diverge.

Attendee: Right now I'm using xeromammography but thinking of going to film-screen mammography, and there hasn't been a discussion of film processing.

How would the processing affect the film mammography as far as contrast is concerned? I'm thinking of putting film through a 90 second processor. Would it be better to modify the processor?

Masterson: We did a study of various film-screen combinations that are out now, with various chemistry types and developer temperatures, and found factors of 4 difference in exposure levels required, and very different responses based on the type of film-screen combination that was being used, so I think that might be of interest to the questioner.

Logan: It's probably best to check with the manufacturer of the film-screen system that you are using, for the optimum processing and temperature factors.

Muntz: I would like to ask Bob Jennings exactly why he used mid-line dose instead of average dose. Many people we heard today have said "average is a good adea, but I'll use mid-line anyway, because everybody else uses it". It seems to me we ought to really get away from using mid-plane dose, and use average dose. I've yet to hear an argument which would say that mid-plane should be better; in fact, there can be as much as a factor of 3 difference between mid-plane and average dose, particularly for the softer beams. I think that we ought to be fairly clear on that.

Jennings: First of all, I concur. I would have liked to have been able to quote average dose but I didn't feel I could make the extension from the Northeast CRP data to the kind of spectra I have, because I don't know what the depth dose or exposure as a function of depth distributions really look like. I have a feeling that these spectra harden in a different way; that is, with a molybdenum spectrum, you have a bimodal distribution, part of which goes away very rapidly, and part of which goes away less rapidly. I am not sure how that averaging process works out, so I'm looking into that.

Muntz: Average dose correlates quite well with half value layers for most of the measurements of the Northeast Center, so you can do this (see Muntz chapter on Dose). You can get within 10% accuracy, I'm sure, which is all we are talking about. I'll reverse the argument: you are using mid-plane measurements which have the same problem, in that the beam hardening rate varies with depth, so I think you can use the average as accurately as the mid-plane from the Northeast data. One should be no better or worse than the other.

Attendee: Dr. Jost, the grid films that I have seen were very impressive. Is this grid a stationary grid, a movable grid, an available grid?

Jost: It is a moving grid, not an oscillating grid. It moves in one direction only. It's available within a few months. We have about twenty prototypes now and we will have it available for sale and delivery starting the first three months of the new year. The grid mechanism can be adapted to previous Philips units, so it is not necessary to buy a new unit.

Barnes: Can you buy the grid separately?

Jost: Yes

Rao: Mel Siedband had raised a question about the normalization of the MTF in xeromammography. I would like to comment on that. It's very difficult to do when there is no response at zero frequency, but a more fundamental question is, how do we quantitate the resolution of xeroradiography? As Gary Barnes pointed out, we are even having difficulty understanding how scatter affects quality in xeroradiography. When we try to apply concepts like MTF, the problem becomes even more complicated because it is essentially a nonlinear system. If you try to determine the MTF, using any particular method, that particular curve will not help you to predict the response due to any other object configuration, especially complex anatomical objects such as microcalcifications or ductal patterns. So the entire concept of the MTF itself, does not, at least to my understanding, seem to have much value when you come to nonlinear systems, such as XERG, or xeroradiography.

Wagner: For the XERG system, things are not as bad as you may think. We worried about taking the MTF out of noise. The MTF was measured at large contrasts, and noise is very low contrast, so you have to wonder, is this a linear system? Phil Muntz published a paper at the Columbia meetings sponsored by the BRH in 1974, indicating that if the toner particles fall along the field lines, in fact, the system is linear. They probably don't do quite that, but it's not enough to get upset about. At the experimental level, for the XERG system, the large area contrast is quite linear, and in fact, the peak to peak contrast in an edge trace is also quite linear for short swings, so that in the limits of going to small signals, it is very reasonable to hang on to our linear hopes and dreams. For large signals, I am as intimidated as perhaps you or anyone else. It's just a very insurmountable problem for me. We have to read these plates with some other technique. Obviously, the big hangup in here is the eye. If it weren't for eyes, we'd have had this problem solved a long time ago.

Siedband: I think one thing to keep in mind about MTF'S is what they are used for. It's really not just a neat little map, but an extremely valuable tool in designing a system in order to get a reasonable match between focal spot sizes, since we know we do not want to make the focal spot too big, and lose resolution, or too small, and get patient blur. What we could do would be to just try to find some noise equivalent aperture in a narrow region, and not worry about normalizing the end tip to zero, at all. In other words, maybe we should try to find what the noise and aperture is, of any of these systems, such as the films, XERG, and the Xerox-like systems, and not worry about the normalization. On that basis, I'm questioning whether you can talk about these things peaking at two, three, or four times some reference level. I don't think that question can be answered that quickly here.

Wagner: CT is the eminently archetypical answer to this, I think. CT is a high pass filter and we just completed a study with that. We think that an Otto Schade approach to the effect of aperture works fantastically. The low pass filter part is part of the Otto Schade aperture theory analysis, and the high pass filter part is just a ramp, right? You can throw away the DC and do that separately. It is really very straightforward to model that as a simple extension of the Schade analysis. I like the engineering approach, too.

Egan: Bob Wagner said, if I quote him correctly, "If you don't see noise, you can reduce dose." What I would like to know, is, if we see noise, can we reduce the dose?

Wagner: I've seen some films in the last few days that have convinced me that we're no where near the ultimate sensitivity of mammography as a diagnostic tool, so if you can see the noise, maybe you should increase the dose. However, Motz and others have shown that we can go one or two orders of magnitude lower, in dose, than what people are using now, without losing information. That's really frightening; it really means that if we really had picture processing schemes to maximally extract the information in the films, we should be able to extract more than we get with the human eye. I know we're really infatuated with our eyes, because it's the greatest instrument that we know of, but it's nowhere near ultimate, as far as extracting information from films.

Barnes: I think there is a difference when you have a lot of anatomical structure in there. A simple object with a uniform background, and the clinical situation are just two different things. I'm not convinced.

Wagner: I basically agree with you.

Fatouros: I would like to make a final comment on the MTF of the xeroradio-graphic process. It is very legitimate to apply in xeromammography because if you observe very carefully, there are no white gaps; there are no density deletions. Instead, what you get is a continuous density profile across the edges, so that it is very legitimate to apply, therefore. A second comment is, that from the point of your theory, the modulation transfer function approaches a finite value at zero frequency because of the existence of a bias potential, and the existence of a grounding plate in the developing chamber. If you try to expose the plate without the presence of a bias potential, then, in that case, MTF goes to zero, but in the present situation, MTF does not go to zero, so there is no theoretical problem. There is absolutely no problem with applying MTF in xeromammography. I will discuss that in detail on Friday.

Muntz: I think I'd like to point out that if you do a calculation relevant to the Min-R system, and take all the degrading elements out, but leave the mammogram as it stands, with all its complexities, then it's possible to get a factor of about 10 improvement (maybe not a factor of 100, because we don't know quite how much information you need to filter through all the anatomic complexities).

Wagner: That's why I made that comment this morning, that there is not room for euphoria, now that the state of things in mammography in the country are near optimum.

WISCONSIN MAMMOGRAPHIC PHANTOMS

by

Larry A. DeWerd, John F. Wochos and John R. Cameron
Department of Radiology
University of Wisconsin
Madison, Wisconsin   53706

INTRODUCTION

Phantoms play an important role in the evaluation of imaging systems. They evaluate the entire imaging system and can detect faults in the generator, focal spot, receptor, and image processor. It is probably impossible to obtain unanimous agreement on an ideal phantom for any radiological imaging system; however, we suggest the following general requirements:

(1)   The phantom should be made of a material which closely simulates the x-ray attenuation characteristics of the body section of interest.

(2)   The phantom should contain a variety of test objects that simulate clinically important structures.

(3)   The sizes of the test objects should be quantitatively determined and should have a range of sizes from objects which are too small to be imaged by even the best systems to objects which will be visible on a poor system.

(4)   The location of the test objects in the phantom should preferably be randomizable so that the viewer will not know where to look for a given test object. This will avoid the phenomena of "if I hadn't believed it with my own mind, I never would have seen it."

(5)   The phantom should avoid high contrast objects which can be clearly seen by a very poor system. These objects give a false impression of imaging quality to a naive observer.

(6)   The phantom should be readily available and should be standardized such that one laboratory can intercompare its results with other laboratories.

(7)   The phantom should be usable on all common imaging systems.

Our group has developed three mammographic phantoms which we feel meet many of these criteria. This paper describes the characteristics of these three phantoms.*

CONSTRUCTION AND CHARACTERISTICS OF THE PHANTOM

All three of the phantoms include test objects of various sizes which are imbedded in a special wax to give contrast and resolution similar to that of clinically important structures in the mammogram. The first phantom which we developed is called the Wisconsin Mammographic Phantom (The Random Phantom).

*These phantoms are available commercially from Radiation Measurements, Inc. (RMI), Middleton, WI 53562

Many of the features of this phantom are modifications of the Stanton Phantom[1] which is not commercially available. The Random Phantom is of uniform thickness and does not simulate the clinical situation of varying breast thicknesses. To evaluate this aspect of mammography we developed the Mammograph Latitude Phantom (MLP). The MLP is wedge shaped with test objects in its base. Since the imaging system may change abruptly during use and the change not be detected until the phantoms are used at some later time, we felt it desirable to have a small mammography phantom which could be included with every mammography image. For this purpose, we developed the Individual Mammography Phantom (IMP). In the following paragraphs we describe in detail each of these phantoms.

The Random Phantom is made up of a 5 cm thick lucite base with a built in tray that holds sixteen color-coded wax blocks (Fig. 1). A 3 mm thick lucite cover keeps the wax blocks in position. The thickness of the entire phantom gives an attenuation similar to that of an average breast for the effective energies commonly encountered in mammography. The rounded half cylinder on the front of the base is designed to give a "halo" similar to that seen on a good xeromammogram. The wax blocks are made of a special dental wax which is dimensionally stable when solidifying. Five of the wax blocks contain test objects consisting of a few Al_2O_3 specks to simulate calcifications. Speck sizes range from 0.20 mm to 0.74 mm diameter. Six of the wax blocks contain a 1.5 cm long nylon fiber ranging in size from 0.40 mm to 1.56 mm diameter. The fibers are designed to simulate fibril and ductal structures in the breast. Four of the wax blocks contain spherical caps of Bakelite ranging from 0.5 mm to 4 mm in thickness. The spherical Bakelite caps simulate tumor like masses. The tapered edges of the spherical caps do not cause an abrupt change in contrast and no edge enhancement appears on the xeroradiographic image. One of the wax blocks contains no test objects. A unique feature of this phantom is the users ability to rearrange the test objects so that the viewer will not know where to scrutinize the image for the smaller objects. The color coding of the wax blocks permits easy determination of their contents.

The Mammographic Latitude Phantom allows a quick and simple test of the recording latitude of the mammographic system. It consists of a 9 cm wide lucite wedge ranging from about 0.7 to 10 cm in thickness. The bottom part contains a wax block with various sizes of low contrast nylon fibers and medium contrast Al_2O_3 granules (Fig. 2). The test objects extend in rows from the thin to the thick edge of the wedge. There are seven parallel fibers with diameters ranging from 0.22 mm to 1.15 mm. Interspaced between the fibers are six parallel rows of granules—each row contains only one size granule. The granule sizes range from 0.16 mm to 0.74 mm diameter. Because lucite simulates the linear attenuation coefficient of the breast for the normal range of mammographic energies, the phantom can be used for evaluating both film-screen and xeromammography systems.

The Individual Mammography Phantom consists of a small wax strip (1 cm x 6 cm x 0.8 cm) mounted on a 3 mm thick aluminum base (Fig. 3). The wax strip contains alternating rows of low contrast fibers and medium contrast specks which run across the width of the phantom. The five fibers range from 0.4 mm to 1.15 mm diameter; the five rows of granules range from 0.20 mm to 0.74 mm diameter. The aluminum base has space for placing xeroradiographic markers if they are used. The IMP is intended to be used with every mammographic image. It is placed in the x-ray beam so as not to interfere with the breast image. The sizes of the smallest fibers and granules visible on the resulting image are a measure of the resolution of that image. When repeat x-rays are taken at a later time, comparison of the IMP image on the mammogram is useful for a comparison of the overall resolution of the images.

EVALUATION OF THE PHANTOMS

Laboratory evaluations have been done of the Random Phantom and of the Mammography Latitude Phantom. All three phantoms are being used clinically in a number of medical centers. Clinical evaluation of these phantoms will be the subject of a later paper.

In evaluating the Random Phantom it is important to realize that when different observers are searching for objects at the threshold of visibility there is a considerable variability in the results. Because of the difficulty in viewing the small test objects, laboratory studies on the phantom showed viewer-to-viewer variability, similar to the viewer variability one would find in detecting subtle features in a roentgenogram. The error bars shown on the data points in Figure 4 represent the standard deviation of three observers. The data shown in Figure 4 represent measurements using film-screen (Lo-Dose/2) system. The graph shows the better detectability of test objects for low kVp. The detectability is comparable to that for xeroradiography.

Figure 5 shows the number of test objects in xeroradiographs of the Random Phantom correctly identified by three observers as a function of focal spot size. Note that there is an incremental jump of one test object identified at a focal spot size of ∿2.7 mm. We anticipate that if a finer gradation of test objects were used that this abrupt change would be less noticeable. An additional useful feature of this phantom is the qualitative appearance of the visible test objects. For example, all observers could arrange the radiographs in order of decreasing focal spot size. This is most easily done by observing the larger size specks. There is clinical usefulness of both qualitative and quantitative analysis of this and other phantoms in a quality assurance program.

Figure 6 shows the effect of decreased visibility of the test objects as the kVp increases in xeroradiography. In this study, the mAs was varied so that the exit exposure of the phantom was approximately constant for all images. The same type of incremental jump in visibility is noted in this graph. As indicated in Fig. 6, the detectability of small objects is better at lower kVps for a flat phantom with constant exit exposure. This is expected since the subject contrast is increasing as the x-ray energy decreases. In the clinical situation, the variable thicknesses of the breast causes the thinner portion of the breast to be overexposed and the chest region to be underexposed.

The Mammography Latitude Phantom is designed to evaluate the effect of the variability of thickness across the breast. The MLP is radiographed with the thick portion of the wedge in the location of the chest wall. The radiographic image of the wedge shows various lengths of fibrals and granules
It is desirable to have a quantitative expression for the measurements done with the Latitude Phantom. It seems logical that smaller test objects should not be compared on an equal footing with larger test objects which are naturally easier to see over a greater distance. We define a parameter, S_i, for the specks which is equal to the visible length of a row of specks divided by the diameter of the specks. A similar parameter, F_i, for fibers is defined as the visible length of the fiber divided by the diameter of the fiber. The latitude number, $L\,N$, is defined by the following equation:

$$L\,N = \frac{\sum F_i}{\sum F_{imax}} + \frac{\sum S_i}{\sum S_{imax}}$$

Where F_{imax} and S_{imax} are the latitude values one would have for an imaging system with perfect latitude, i.e., the entire length of the fibers or specks is visible. If the latitude were perfect, LN would be 2.0.

Our results on latitude measurements of film-screen systems and xeroradiographic systems show that screen-film radiography has a smaller latitude number than does xeroradiography. In measurements on six mammography units in three breast screening centers using the xeroradiographic technique the latitude number averages 1.01 + 0.24.   These measurements were made using exposures suitable for the average breast.

When the Latitude Phantom is used by technologists it is convenient to use a simpler method of calculating the latitude number. For this purpose the rows of fibrils and specks are given integral values 1, 2, 3, . . . where the largest object has the lowest number. The latitude number is arrived at by multiplying this number times the visible lengths of the given test object and summing the results. Using this technique, a perfect score would be 287 and typical values for a good xeroradiographic system are about 200.

We also define a skew number as a measure of the displacement of the visible specks or fibers toward the thin or thick portion of the phantom. For a given test object, the skew number is obtained as shown in Figure 2a. That is, the length of the visible portion from the midline towards the thicker edge is subtracted from the length of the visible portion from the midline toward the thinner edge. If the test objects are more easily seen in the thicker portion of the phantom, this will result in negative skew number. Conversely, if they are more visible in the thinner portion of the phantom this results in a positive skew number. A skew number of 0 indicates equal imaging on each side. If we assume that this is an optimum condition, a negative number indicates an overexposure and a positive number indicates an underexposure. The results are obviously dependent on both the contrast (determined primarily by the kVp) and the millampere-seconds (mAs).

For the six x-ray machines discussed above, the average skew number for the xeroradiographic images was 1.7 + 5.9 with a range from -10 to +10. We suggest that a skew number outside of these values would be an indication of a poor technique, while a latitude number around 1 or 2 indicates a good technique.   This phantom can be used to find approximate techniques which then can be adjusted by the radiologist to his or her taste. The Mammography Latitude Phantom is thus a useful quality assurance check on the mammography imaging system.

Over 50 medical centers have purchased the Individual Mammography Phantom. The IMP is useful for both film-screen and xeromammography. An example of its usefulness was demonstrated at a center using film-screen mammography where the processor was becoming defective over a period of time. The chief technician was able to demonstrate that there was a problem by noting that fewer test objects were visible on the images of the IMP over a period of time. This led to the evaluation of the film processor and the location of the problem. This example also indicates that the IMP serves as a useful test of the entire radiographic system. We feel that the IMP can be a useful tool for the initial screening of mammograms by the technician or radiologist. Often times, the viewer will not be certain whether that technique was adequate and the IMP can give an additional, objective analysis for the viewer.

CONCLUSIONS

We feel that the three phantoms described have the following advantages:

(1) The phantoms give an adequate simulation of the breast attenuation.

(2) The phantoms are sensitive to technique change in the mammographic energy region.

(3) The phantoms are useful for both film-screen and xeroradiographic systems.

(4) The phantoms give a quantitative measure of the overall imaging properties of the mammographic systems.

(5) Although the phantoms are basically quantitative they can also be used in a qualitative manner.

(6) They are relatively low in cost.

As a service to the radiologic community doing mammography the University of Wisconsin Medical Physics Laboratories provides low cost rental of the Random Phantom and the Latitude Phantom. This service is referred to as the Mammography Image Evaluation Service (MIES). A related service is our Radiation Monitoring by Mail (RM[2]) in which the on patient exposure can be measured using TLD crystals.

REFERENCES

1. L. Stanton, Proc. Summer School on Physics of Diagnostic Radiology, D. John Wright (ed.), USDHEW pub. No. (FDA) 74-8006, p. 148 (1973).

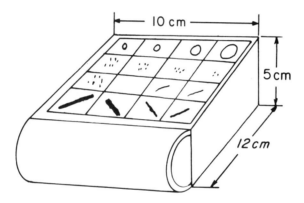

Figure 1   Schematic of the Wisconsin Mammography Phantom (The Random Phantom) showing test objects

MAMMOGRAPHY LATITUDE PHANTOM

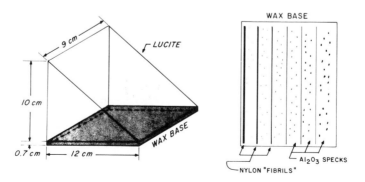

Figure 2   Schematic of the Mammographic Latitude Phantom showing wedge and rows of test objects

305

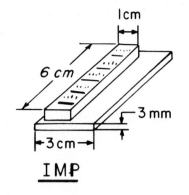

Figure 3   A schematic of the Individual
Mammographic Phantom

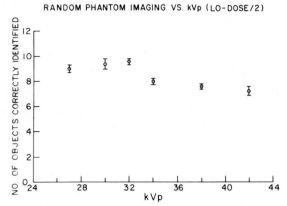

Figure 4   Results of the detectability
of test objects in the Random Phantom
as a function of kVp for a film-screen
system

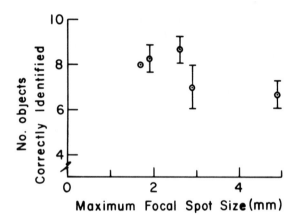

Figure 5   Detectability results of 3 observers of
xeroradiographic images of the Random
Phantom as a function of focal spot size.
The FSD was 75 cm.   The error bars indicate
one standard deviation

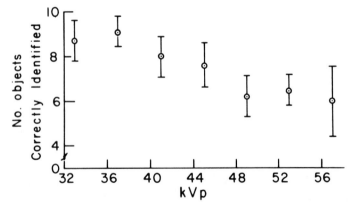

Figure 6   Detectability results of 3 observers of xeroradiographic images of the Random Phantom as a function
of kVp.   The mAs was varied to keep a constant exit
exposure

MAMMOGRAPHY PHANTOM DEVELOPMENT AT THE
NORTHEAST CENTER FOR RADIOLOGICAL PHYSICS
Daniel W. Miller, Ph.D. and Mary Ellen Masterson, M.S.
Memorial Hospital
1275 York Avenue
New York, New York 10021

The NECRP has been active in the development of mammography image evaluation methods for several years. Our goal is to develop a phantom system for testing overall imaging performance which has maximum relevance to clinical needs.

A. DESIGN CONSIDERATIONS

The following design characteristics should be considered.

1. Tissue Equivalency

Phantom materials should have the same x-ray interaction properties as the tissues being simulated. This is essential for dosimetry phantoms. For imaging phantoms absolute tissue equivalency of both object and surrounding medium may be unnecessary. However, subject contrast of phantom structures must match that of corresponding real structures over the mammography energy range.

2. Size and Shape of Internal Structures

The configuration of internal structures depends on 1) the size and shape of corresponding breast structures and 2) the system for quantifying image performance with respect to that structure. For example different systems may require a statement of the smallest observable size of a sequence of objects, resolvability of bar patterns, or analytical treatment of optical density data obtained from a single object.

3. External Size and Shape

The provision of a realistic skin contour should be considered. This is essential for providing a realistic skin line halo for Xeroradiographs. Simulation of overall thickness and density variation from chest wall to nipple is needed for testing imagability at the limits of the required latitude range.

4. Sensitivity

Indices of imaging performance derived from the phantom should be at least as sensitive to changes in radiographic parameters (eg. kVp) as observations by radiologists of clinical image response to a similar change.

5. Quantitation

Phantom systems should yield observer independent, numerical indices or imaging performance which relate directly to clinical experience. In addition, the quantitative system should have sufficient comprehensiveness and versatility to accomodate individual preferences of different radiologists.

6. Preservation

In order to make long term comparisons, phantoms should not be biologically, or otherwise degradable with time.

B. MEMORIAL-BARTS PHANTOM

A tissue equivalent mammography phantom has been developed by the Northeast Center for Radiological Physics, Dr. D.R. White of St. Bartholomew's Hospital and Ruth Snyder of the Department of Radiology of Memorial Hospital. This is the first generation of a series of systems we intend to study which will consist of two components:

1) A qualitative section for evaluation by radiologists and
2) A quantitative section from which numerical indices of image quality are derived from microdensitometric scans.

Radiologists' assessment of the qualitative portion are used to guide the development and evaluate the effectiveness of the quantitative system. The qualitative section of the M-B phantom consists of a preserved mastectomy specimen embedded in a block of tissue equivalent plastic. The specimen is approximately 4cm thick and has an area of about 10cm^2. The "D" shaped base block which contains both the specimen and the quantitative test strip is equivalent to 50% fat/50% water in its radiation interaction properties.

Several interchangeable quantitative test strips have been produced. Each of these inserts contains a number of quasi tissue equivalent structures arranged in a linear pattern so that a single microdensitometric trace passes through all of the objects. The most commonly used insert contains the following items:

1) Three blocks of water equivalent material having 5mm x 5mm cross sections and thickness of 2,4 and 6mm.
2) A 1mm diameter water equivalent cylinder, 5mm in length.
3) Three square-cut elemental silicon filaments 5mm long with thicknesses of 0.1,0.2 and 0.3mm.

The sensitivity of the quantitative system is very high for radiographic parameters affecting contrast. For example, a change in tube voltage from 28 kVp to 32 kVp with compensation by mAs to keep optical density constant produces a significant change in the computed contrast indices for both soft tissue and calcific objects. Limitations associated with our microdensitometer's analogue output have prevented quantitation beyond simple indicators of noise and contrast. However, these indices have generally agreed well with radiologists' assessment of images of the tissue portion of the phantom.

The embedded tissue specimen has shown some degradation in the three years since the phantom was constructed. However, this deterioration has not reached the point of interfering with the usefulness of the qualitative section.

USE OF A BREAST PHANTOM TO EVALUATE DETAIL VISIBILITY OF MAMMOGRAPHIC IMAGES

Leonard Stanton

Department of Radiation Therapy and Nuclear Medicine
Hahnemann Medical College and Hospital
Philadelphia, PA 19102

Image quality has been traditionally described by physical measurements. However, it is also vital to evaluate the end product: the visibility of diagnostically important items such as small calcifications and soft tissue details. Various approaches have been used to study detail visibility of mammographic images. This paper first discusses these approaches, to explain why our breast phantom was developed. The phantom and its use are then briefly described, and visibility measurements reported for three imaging systems: Xerox 125, Min-R and XERG.

WHY THE BREAST PHANTOM?

Mammographic details of interest may be extremely small by usual standards: soft tissue structures 0.8 mm and smaller, and calcifications from 0.25 down to 0.1 mm in size. Consequently subject contrast is minimal at usual beam energies, necessitating very low energy x-ray beams unless the Xerox 125 system is used. Mammographic systems must therefore produce images of very high contrast and resolution -- with low artefact and noise levels as well. The choice among systems is further complicated by many variables: x-ray tube target material and focal spot size; filter materials; image receptors; and dedicated vs multi-purpose machines. The result is that the selection of "the best" system and techniques is an extraordinarily difficult task.

Early investigators relied on clinical images to evaluate technique, usually experimenting with selected cooperative patients. Aside from cumulative dosage considerations, such comparisons are of limited value because it is hard to position a breast reproducibly, as well as for other reasons. To avoid such problems breast specimens have been used: directly after surgery, as by Millis (1); preserved, as by Friedrich (2); and sealed in a plastic block, as by Egan (3) and Snyder (4). Millis quantified visibility by measuring radiographic yield of calcifications, which were confirmed microscopically. The others' results were essentially qualitative. Snyder provided silicon and "soft tissue" rods to permit contrast measurements by microdensitometry, but made no attempt to measure detail visibility directly. Hence results of these scans are essentially similar to more conventional physical measurements.

Commercial breast phantoms have been designed to provide simple but rugged and permanent gauges of routine image quality. They generally use non-anatomic test objects sealed in plastic, such as wire mesh, steel wool, step wedges, etc. The Wisconsin units more closely resemble our basic design. They provide test objects of graded sizes, simulating calcific and soft tissue fibrillar breast details. These units are intended to provide a commercially available modified version of our design, with additional features of their own.

THE PHANTOM AND ITS USE

Our phantom differs from others in three basic ways. First, the test objects are designed to closely match the contrast of water-like soft tissue in fat* as well as breast calcifications. In addition, they are carefully shaped, oriented, and positioned to assure reproducibility and uniqueness of indicated visible size. Second, the assembly design permits varying both thickness and equivalent composition of the phantom, to evaluate the effect of breast characteristics on detail visibility. There are options of 4.7, 5.9 and 7.2 cm total thickness, and compositions of 25/75, 50/50 and 75/25% water/fat equivalent by volume. Figure 1 shows the phantom unit with the test objects in the usual position -- 3.6 cm from the exit surface. Details of the object assembly are given in Figure 2; other design and construction details are in Reference (5).

Third, we have developed a special methodology for determining visible object size, to assure reproducible and clinically relevant results. Three steps are involved: careful study of the fibril and speck images, noting the contrast and image degradation with decreasing object size; selection of sizes seen unambiguously; and final interpolation to $\pm$ 1/4 of an object size interval (5). Tests on a large series of Xerox 125 and Min-R images yielded reproducible readings among four observers, with standard deviations less than .006 and .025 mm for calcific and fibrillar test objects, respectively. These results characterize the reading uncertainty for a single roentgenogram using our method. There are somewhat greater uncertainties in repeat exposures using a given technique, with all three receptors, due to system noise. Data averaging was therefore used in deriving the curves shown below.

Thus far we have dealt with the phantom design and image study methodology. In addition, one must carry out exposures in such a way as to assure the best possible image quality for each technique studied. In this study, geometric blur was carefully controlled: MTF of the x-ray images at the receptor exceeded 10% at 9.5 cycles/mm in all cases (5). Also, since each receptor has a preferred exposure range for maximum contrast, exposures were also controlled. Min-R films were exposed to yield as close to 1.3 total density as practicable, with low fog levels; XERG films about 1.0. Extensive electrostatic voltmeter measurements were performed on Xerox 125 plates, to determine residual voltage after various single exposures. The resulting curves indicate maximum receptor contrast results with 70% voltage discharge from 1600 V initial, in good agreement with Zeman (6).

An important incidental finding is considerable variability in the sensitivity of Xerox 125 plates. In three experiments, standard deviations in plate roentgen exposure required for 70% discharge were as follows:

1. Six older plates, 32 tests .... = 15.5%

2. A single new plate, 10 tests .... = 10%

3. A single older plate, 10 tests .... = 15%

Although this result does not affect clinical use significantly, it is of great importance to those seeking to establish "the" breast dose per exposure using the Xerox 125 mammography system.

---

*For brevity "fat" and "adipose tissue" are used interchangeably in this paper.

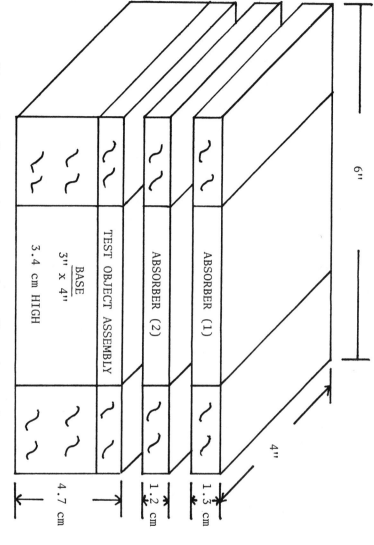

Figure 1: Breast phantom -- three dimensional view.

At the bottom is the 4.7 cm thick phantom, consisting of its base and the common test object assembly. Two absorbers (1) and (2) are shown displaced above the test object assembly; these can be added to yield a total thickness of 5.9 or 7.2 cm. The labelled central parts simulate the center of the compressed breast; the lateral shaded polyethylene blocks, adipose tissue at the sides. Three different sets of base and absorber blocks are provided, to simulate central breast densities equivalent to 25/75, 50/50 and 72/25% water/fat equivalent by volume.

311

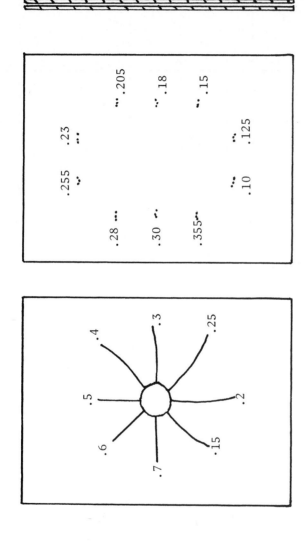

Figure 2: Common test object assembly -- sizes in millimeters.

Fibrils: Eight cylindrical acrylic rods are arranged radially about a thin plastic disc, and then immersed in a suitable oil sealed in a flat plexiglas box.

Specks: Ten groups of three each (Al) are taped to a thin acrylic plate, in air. Specks in each group have the same diameter, and lengths slightly greater than the diameter. Their axes are all parallel to each other and to the plate.

Assembly section: Speck plate is at left. Specks are adjacent to the box containing the acrylic rods, which are shown as black sloping lines.

312

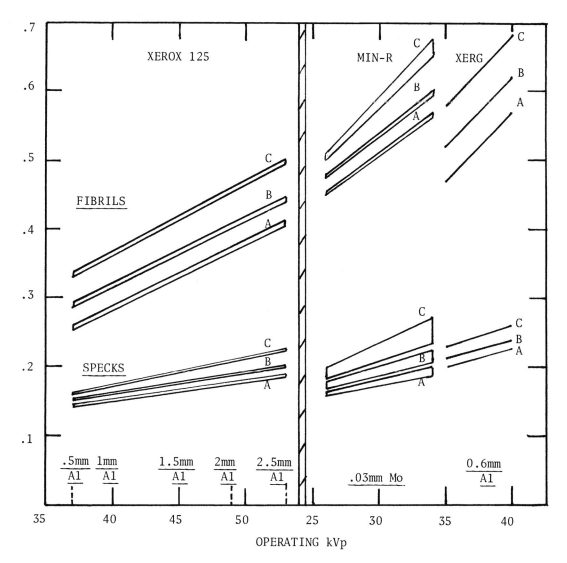

Figure 3: Visible object size vs beam energy

The upper curves are for fibrillar, the lower for speck objects. From left to right are Xerox 125, Min-R and XERG curves. Bands rather than line curves are shown for Xerox 125 and Min-R. These encompass the range of visible sizes for a great change in breast composition: 25/75 to 75/25% water/fat by volume equivalent. A, B and C refer to 4.7, 5.9 and 7.2 cm thicknesses, respectively. XERG data is for 50/50% composition only.

RESULTS AND DISCUSSION

Visible object size is plotted vs beam energy in Figure 3, for all three image receptors*. Fibrillar and speck object data are given for three phantom thicknesses: 4.7, 5.9 and 7.2 cm, labelled A, B and C, respectively. Xerox 125 and Min-R data are shown by bands rather than single line curves, for each thickness. These bands encompass the range of visible sizes for a great change in breast composition: 25/75 to 75/25% water/fat by volume equivalent. XERG data is shown for 50/50% water/fat only, as the unit is still being evaluated.

Detail resolution is consistently best for the Xerox 125 images; those of Min-R and XERG are reasonably similar to each other. This superiority results from the extreme edge enhancement of the Xerox development process; there are accompanying limitations of the system (5).

The data of Figure 3 indicate a very slight dependence of detail visibility on breast composition, of the same order as measurement uncertainties noted above. This at first appears to be in conflict with clinical experience. However, the explanation lies in the fact that the phantom subject contrast is unaltered by the composition change. In the actual breast, however, soft tissue contrast tends to be reduced in the denser breast, because this density results from greater water-like content in centrally located structures (glandular and fibrous content, fluid accumulation, cysts, etc). There is thus a significant likelihood of loss of contrast against adipose tissue. What our curves show is that where such subject contrast is preserved, mere increase in breast density in itself should not reduce detail visibility. Of courese, there is often also an increased breast structure noise in the dense breast, as well as a shift beyond the range of the receptor response; as a result, even calcifications may not be demonstrated as well in the dense breast in practice.

Increasing breast thickness seriously degrades all images. This results from increased beam scatter, and hardening, which reduce image contrast. The great importance of breast compression technique is thus confirmed by direct measurement of detail visibility.

ACKNOWLEDGEMENTS

Several colleagues have contributed to our mammography studies, which span more than a decade. These include David A. Lightfoot, M.A., John L. Day, Ph.D. and Richard Tobin of our Department, as well as Theodore Villafana, Ph.D., Department of Radiology, Temple University Medical Center. The project has received much departmental support, and I am especially grateful to Luther W. Brady, M.D., Professor and Chairman, for his outstanding encouragement and support over the years.

REFERENCES

1. Millis, R.S., Davis, R. and Stacey, A.J.: The significance of calcifications in the breast: a radiological and pathologic study. Br. J. Radiol. 49:12, 1976.

2. Friedrich, M. and Weskamp, P.: New modalities in mammographic imaging: comparison of grid and magnification techniques. Medicamundi 23:1, 1978.

3. Egan, R.L. and Fenn, J.D.: Phantoms for evaluating mammography technqiues and roentgenographic detail. Am. J. Roentgenol. 102:936, 1968.

4. Snyder, R.E., Masterson, M.E., Miller, D.W., et al: Image quality control and radiation exposure in mammography. In, Breast Carcinoma: The Radiologists Expanded Role, ed. Logan, W.W., John Wiley publisher, New York, 1977.

5. Stanton, L., Villafana, T., Day, J.L., et al.: A breast phantom method for evaluating mammography technique. Invest. Radiol. 13:291, 1978.

6. Zeman, G., Rao, G.U.V. and Osterman, F.A.: Evaluation of xeroradiographic image quality. Radiology 119:689, 1976.

---

*See Reference (5) for machine and exposure details

PHANTOMS FOR STANDARDIZED QUALITY AND RADIATION EXPOSURE IN MAMMOGRAPHY

Robert L. Egan, M.D.
Chief, Mammography Section
and
Professor of Radiology

Perry Sprawls, Ph.D.
Professor and Director
Division of Physics and Engineering
Department of Radiology

Patricia A. O'Brien, R.T.
Chief Mammography Technologist

Emory University
Atlanta, Georgia

Phantoms for evaluation of mammographic techniques have special prerequisites to: 1) evaluate object sizes of 0.05 mm as compared with 1.0 or 2.0 mm in general radiography; 2) demonstrate the low subject contrast range of adipose and fibroglandular breast tissues as opposed to the wide range of contrast of air and bone; 3) remain constant over long periods of time; and 4) simulate breast radiography.

Alteration of a single component factor producing a radiograph may be evaluated under laboratory conditions but the complexity of the interrelationship of the many factors producing the clinical radiograph and the relative contribution of each factor under varied conditions cannot be readily measured. The often-used methods of modulation transfer analysis and visual inspection of non-mammary objects such as wire mesh or aluminum rods result in significantly different results.[1,2] The estimate, and that is often misleading, of physical factors as film-screen speed, focal spot size, geometric unsharpness, density and contrast contributed very little to the evaluation of the radiographic quality, or resolution of the breast structures on the mammogram. The retinal response, the subjectivity and the psychic response of the radiologist to these strange shadows further complicated image analysis.

With such breast phantoms our results were inadequate and inappropriate for application to the well established mammographic technique that had been devised empirically through use of mastectomy specimens and the intact breast. Thus, it became necessary to devise suitable phantoms utilizing breast tis-

315

sues for evaluation of the individual factors producing mammograms and assessment of radiographic detail.[3] Two thicknesses of breast tissue were embedded in plastic to prevent liquefaction or any possible change. Fine irregular flecks of Al_2O_3 particles (Z number of 11 as compared with 7 for soft tissues and 14 for breast calcifications) were sprinkled within a 1 cm circle formed by a 0.25 mm steel wire. The evaluation of the quality of the resultant radiograph, mounted in a 35 mm slide holder and magnified 60 x by projection, required only the ability to see and count the flecks. Due to the toner robbing characteristics of xeroradiography, it became necessary to search further for an all-purpose breast phantom applicable to both film and Xerox receptors.

MATERIALS AND METHODS

Five commercially available phantoms for mammography and three Emory University produced phantoms were investigated. Receptors were Xerox, Eastman Kodak M, AA and Min-R and DuPont Lo-Dose. M and AA emulsions were hand processed while Min-R and Lo-Dose were processed in the Kodak RP X-omat Processor. Hundreds of exposures were required to obtain the same radiographic densities on the various receptors using the different mammographic units. Evaluations were only carried out on optically similar density studies. X-ray tube anodes included molybdenum, tungsten and mixed molybdenum and tungsten, with combinations of beryllium window, conventional glass and ground glass windows. Equipment included conventional, conventional units modified for mammography and units designed specifically for mammography. Radiation exposure at the surface of the phantoms (R) was measured simultaneously by TLD and a direct reading chamber with appropriate correction. After selection of the most useful phantom, numerous x-ray units in the Southeast and 7 nationally known mammography laboratories in the United States were evaluated under actual operating conditions.

Various materials were used to construct phantoms from non-mammary structures that would simulate the intact breast during radiography in the 20-50 peak kilovoltage range. It was found that finely and coarsely crushed sheets of plastic suspended in paraffin poured into a 6 cm thick container constructed from thin sheets of plastic simulated readily the breast tissue phantom.

RESULTS

The acceptability of the phantoms varied widely with the different receptors. Some phantoms proved excellent for film and poor for xeroradiography or vice versa, Table 1. The relative density of the phantoms can be judged by the surface dose needed to produce optimal studies with M film or the Xerox receptor. Further evaluation included the usefulness for all receptors, the radiographic quality produced on each receptor and the degree of simulation of breast radiography. The Emory-8 phantom, by no means the ideal, was chosen for these reasons and for its relative radiographic density being that of a more glandular medium to large sized breast.

Phantom Emory-8 was then radiographed on representative x-ray units used for mammography using 4 receptors under as similar conditions as possible to produce optimal studies. The surface dose varied widely in many instances both for receptor and x-ray unit, Table 2. The kVp, the target-film distance and filtration were kept close to that which had been recommended by the manufacturer or that found to be optimal under production of clinical mammography.

Use of Emory-8 phantom revealed wide variation in surface exposure and subjectively evaluated radiographic quality simulating clinical mammography at 6 mammography laboratories, Table 3. Again no attempt was made to alter conditions of mammography, but the phantom did give a good insight into the dose-quality relationships.

The phantom constructed entirely of non-mammary materials proved almost as useful as the more expensive and difficult to produce mammary tissue phantoms.

DISCUSSION

A distinct advantage of a tissue phantom in addition to its constancy is that the final product is a summation of all the known, and unknown, contributing factors and their interrelations to forming that study. Thus, taken into account simultaneously are blur, mottle, contrast, geometric unsharpness, etc. Obviously a great disadvantage is the subjectivity in judgment and personal preferences of each observer particularly when high definition may be underestimated in comparison with high contrast studies. All of the phantoms listed were useful in special situations. One of the most difficult problems is producing a single phantom that does justice to both xeroradiography and film receptors. The construction of the Emory-8 phantom being dense tends to favor xeroradiography while the thinner Emory-69 phantom favors the finest grain film emulsion.

The kVp-phantom thickness relationship is apparent. In Table 2, the Emory-8 phantom on M film at 22 kVp produces exceptional detail with only slightly greater exposure than that of xeroradiography at 48 kVp. The thin homogeneous Xerox phantom cannot be used with film yet it is quite acceptable for xeroradiography. The dense, homogeneous 3M phantom is 2 times the density of a medium to large breast and is too dense even with the higher kVp of xeroradiography.

The bias of building a phantom to your own desires and rebuilding numerous times to meet your own preferences must be considered in our choice of Emory-8 phantom.

We did not have the opportunity to use the precisely fabricated White-Memorial phantom[4] but have seen a number of studies made with it. These compare roughly with the Emory-TH phantom which we consider too thick for appraisal of the average clinical mammographic techniques. The surface exposures of these two phantoms are also comparable.

We produced eight paraffin-plastic phantoms that simulate breast tissues which have proved as useful in most situations as Emory-8 phantom. This is a distinct advantage as they can be rather cheaply produced and obviate the necessity of obtaining large quantities of breast tissue.

The several Dupont Lo-dose systems were evaluated. As there was very little difference in the film-speed and no vast difference in quality when compared with Min-R, the study was simply limited to the 4 representative receptors. One added parameter to a study even with these limited variables adds thousands of exposures.

Although M film is being used less and less in clinical mammography it still serves as the best yardstick for laboratory studies. Even with modification of conventional x-ray equipment, M film can be used with 22 kVp with moderately low exposures to the skin (with a much less relative midline dose) and produce the unanimously agreed far superior resolution.[5] Our previous reports of 2 r skin exposure for an average breast with M film and conventional x-ray equipment have consistently been lower exposures than when a molybdenum anode or beryllium window has been substituted in that conventional x-ray unit.

The RSI system was included in the investigation but there were so many added variables (particularly as we mounted and used the tube) that it is in a class by itself and creates confusion when compared with the less variable mammography units. In magnification radiography with this system, increased skin exposure is produced by the inverse square law (about 5 fold increase as the target skin distance is reduced from 17.5 inches to 7.5 inches), the closeness of the skin to the target and the lack of collimation.

CONCLUSIONS

There is a wide assortment of mammography phantoms available that can be used to standardize mammograms both in radiographic quality and exposure to the skin. Some are better suited for evaluating certain systems. There is no all-purpose or ideal phantom for all applications but we have produced ones that are quite acceptable.

Use of such phantoms indicate a wide range of skin exposure and quality of mammograms. Intercomparison of x-ray units, technical factors and receptors allow a more objective selection of mammographic units and technical factors.

There is a wide range in skin exposure and quality of mammograms produced in various mammography laboratories.

Although sophisticated and expensive breast phantoms may aid in evaluation of minute differences in the laboratory, a good estimate of clinical mammography can be obtained with an inexpensive phantom containing simulated breast structures.

TABLE 1. Subjective evaluation and selection of plastic embedded mammography phantoms, rated 1 to 8 with 1 most desirable and relative density based on surface dose at relatively low and high kvp to produce optimal images.

Phantom	Description	Advantage	Disadvantage	Rating - Receptor Quality					Exposure Tube-side Surface (R)	
				M	AA	Lo-Dose	Min-R	XRO	M	XRO
Kodak	coarse and fine wire grids calcific flecks (chalk) step wedges plastic tubing steel wool	many sized and density structures	mainly homogeneous plastic non-breast structures	6	4	3	3	2	3.42	1.63
3M	five wires dense block two capsules	shaped as breast	very dense amphorous plastic, dense structures, bone chips in capsules move (all non-breast)	7	7	6	6	8	5.49	2.98
Stanton	varying sized calcific particles	calcification simulated	amphorous plastic limited breast structure	5	5	4	4	3	2.42	1.32
Wisconsin	2 dozen color-coded blocks containing calcific flecks, nylon fibrils, drops or blank	blocks interchangeable, unknown phantom variable upper plastic thickness	2.5 cm of solid, dense homogeneous plastic base; breast not simulated	4	6	5	5	4	3.66	1.73
Emory-69	Al_2O_3 on actual breast tissue, breast structures finite area outlined for counting	calcification well simulated, not adaptable simple construction, actual breast structure	too thin, not adaptable readily to XRO	3	2	1	1	6	1.33	4E
Emory-TH	As EM-69 with other objects added	as EM 69, infinite scatter at this KVP	too thick and too much plastic poor for XRO	2	3	6	7	5	4.99	1.3E
Emory-8	As EM-69 with a plastic ring added to count XRO image Al_2O_3 flecks, can have 0.5 or 2.5 cm O-F-D; slightly denser than average breast	as EM-69 readily adaptable to XRO	nearest to breast but still not an intact breast	1	1	2	2	1	2.63	1.3E
Xerox	Aluminum rods; nylon fibrils, line pairs	readily constructed	too thin, not applicable to film	8	8	8	8	7	-	-

See Table 2 for x-ray factors.

TABLE 2. Salient characteristics of x-ray units for mammography with surface exposures for optimal images of Emory-8 phantom.

Unit	Anode	Tube window	Filter mm	FSS	Range kvp	Range ma	Range TFD	Exposure factors mas	Exposure factors kvp	Exposure factors TFD	Receptor	Surface exposure tube-side (R)
Conventional GE	W-Mo	gr. glass	.5 Al	1-2 mm	50	300	to 40"	1200	22	75	M	2.63
								600	26	"	AA	1.50
								90	26	"	Min-R	0.20
								180	48	"	XRO	1.38
Conventional GE	W	Be	1.2 Al	1-2 mm	50	300	to 40"	875	22	75	M	5.04
								312	22	"	AA	2.66
								50	26	"	Min-R	0.38
								60	48	"	XRO	0.93
Modified Conventional Profex-ray	Mo	Be	.5 Al	1-2 mm	50	300	to 40"	1200	33	75	M	3.45
								460	33	"	AA	1.94
								45	30	"	Min-R	0.104
								210	41	86	XRO	1.52
Senograph CGR	Mo	Be	.03 Mo	0.6 mm	22-40	40	to 18"	1200	25	45	M	17.6
								400	25	"	AA	5.87
								90	25	"	Min-R	1.58
Diagnost M Phillips	Mo	Be	----	0.6 mm	25-50	200	to 20"	1600	25	56	M	17.66
								640	25	"	AA	5.77
								64	25	"	Min-R	0.66
Mammomat Siemens	Mo	Be	.03 Mo	0.6 mm	28-49	300	18"	1000	28	46	M	21.258
								320	28	"	AA	11.86
								40	28	"	Min-R	1.56
MMX - 2 GE	70% Mo 30% W	Be	.03 Mo	1-2 mm	26-60	200-S 400-L	25"	2000	25	62.5	M	20.59 (S-FSS)
								2000	25	"	M	20.13 (L-FSS)
								600	25	"	AA	6.2 (S-FSS)
								600	25	"	AA	6.1 (L-FSS)
								80	25	"	Min-R	0.86 (S-FSS)
								80	25	"	Min-R	0.82 (L-FSS)
								300	43	"	XRO	1.09 (S-FSS)
								320	41	"	XRO	0.98 (L-FSS)

TABLE 3. Application of phantoms to evaluate exposure to the skin, receptors and radiographic quality at six national known mammography centers. Emory – 8 phantom.

Center	Receptor	Anode	Window	FSS mm	Filtration mm	kvp	mas	TFD cm	Exposure at skin in R	Quality*
A	Min-R	W	glass	0.7	0.7 AL	25	250	83	0.31	8.2
	M	W	"	0.7	(inherent)	25	3000	83	4.20	8.3
	AA	W	"	0.7	"	25	1000	83	1.38	8.6
	XRO	W	"	0.7	1.7 Al add.	48	312	83	0.81	12.3
B	Min-R	Mo	Be	0.5	0.5 Mo	28	32	56	0.55	9.3
	M	Mo	Be	0.5	0.5 Mo	28	1280	56	19.25	17.4
	AA	Mo	Be	0.5	0.5 Mo	28	400	56	7.29	13.6
	XRO	Mo	Be	0.5	0.5 Mo	50	128	56	1.14	12.0
C	Min-R	W	glass	0.6	0.5 Al+1.0 Al	28	180	43	0.28	8.3
	M	W	"	0.6	1.0 Al	28	1200	43	1.35	11.7
	AA	W	"	0.6	1.0 Al	28	400	43	0.453	8.3
	XRO	W	"	0.6	1.0 Al	48	25	46	0.44	11.3
D	Min-R	Mo	Be	0.6	0.04 Pb	28	64	45	1.56	11.7
	M	Mo	Be	0.6	0.04 Pb	28	1600	45	21.15	18.0
	AA	Mo	Be	0.6	0.04 Pb	28	640	45	11.86	14.8
E	Min-R	W	Be	1-2	0.6 Al+1.0 Al	25	45	46	0.55	9.3
	M	W	Be	1-2		25	1200	46	13.50	13.1
	AA	W	Be	1-2		25	400	46	4.51	10.0
	XRO	W	Be	1-2		44	300	36	0.90	12.7
F	Min-R	30%W, 70%Mo	glass	1-2	0.7 AL+0.5 Al	26	90	75	0.20	13.1
	M	"	"	1-2		22	1800	75	2.63	20.0
	AA	"	"	1-2		26	600	75	1.50	15.3
	XRO	"	"	1-2		48	180	75	1.38	12.4

*1-20 (best)

REFERENCES

1. Morgan, R. H., Bates, L. M., Rao, G. U. V. and Marinaro, A.: Frequency response characteristics of x-ray film and screens. Am. J. Roentgenol. 92:426-440, 1964.

2. Rossman, K.: Comparison of several methods for evaluating image quality of radiographic screen-film systems. Am. J. Roentgenol. 97:772-775, 1966.

3. Egan, R. L. and Fenn, J. O.: Phantoms for evaluating mammography techniques and roentgenographic detail. Am. J. Roentgenol. 102:936-940, 1968.

4. Snyder, R. S., Masterson, M., Miller, D., Kirch, R., Rothenberg, L., Hammerstein, G. and Laughlin J.: Image quality control and radiation exposure in mammography. Breast Carcinoma: The Radiologist's Expanded Role. W. W. Logen, Ed., 167-176. John Wiley and Sons, New York City. 1977.

5. Hevezi, J., Haus, A., Rothenberg, L., Stanton, L. and Wayrynen, R. The physics of mammography. In Radiologists' Guide to Detection of Early Breast Cancer by Mammography, Thermography and Xeroradiography. R. L. Egan, Ed. American College of Radiology, Chicago, Ill., 1976.

PHANTOM PANEL

Moderator, Phillip Muntz

Ed Sickles: I have a question for those members of the panel who have dealt
with the biological phantom, namely with breast tissue. As a clinician, I
find it much more meaningful to try to find objects on a background of the
anatomic structures of the breast rather than on a uniform background such
as one has with lucite or aluminum. When you use the uniform background you
see things that are much smaller than when you use breast tissue. For those
of you who have used breast tissue, how do you preserve it? How do you laminate it so that it stays whole and maintains its structure?

Dr. Egan: I thought it much better too, to go to biological tissue and that's
the reason I got away from grids and bars and things like that. This slide
shows a metal ring on the right and a plastic one on the left. These are the
closest I've come to being able to evaluate both film and xeromammography.
This slide shows plastic broken up into chips, embedded in varying amounts of
paraffin, which corresponds very closely to fibroglandular tissue in the breast.
This is the closest thing nonbiologic I have been able to find that would
assimilate the actual breast tissue.

Michael Friedrich: Our phantom is now 2-3 years old and we keep it frozen,
very thoroughly. Originally, it was fixed in a very dilute formalin, to
sterilize, but the water content was not changed too much. We embedded it in
plastic in a very simple mold to obviate water losses, and we have deep frozen
it. I'm not sure if it would preserve at normal temperature. We keep it
frozen only because we are anxious to prevent water loss, not decomposition.

Dr. Egan: I have some 1956 tissue still intact. I took a large block of
fresh tissue and fixed it. Then I radiographed it again, and found no difference in the density. As Dr. Friedrich, we didn't fix it very well, but enough
to keep it preserved, and then encased it in the plastic.

Dan Miller: We fixed the tissue in our phantom that I showed for 3 or 4 weeks
in formalin. To fix it in place in the phantom is a multistep process. We
place the specimen in a machine-made hole in a tissue equivalent block. We
then use a deaerated epoxy resin (an epoxy resin that's been mixed under vacuum
to get all of the air bubbles out). We pour that over the specimen, put it in
a bell jar and again re-evacuate it for about a half hour or so to further remove trapped air. We weight it down with some teflon gloves and let it cure
overnight (these teflon gloves are slick enough so that you can pull them right
out of the hardened epoxy). Following that we top it up again with an overnight application of epoxy, and machine off the top surface. With respect to
the question of visibility of objects against a clear background, I think that
is a great limitation of non-tissue phantoms. That's one of the limiting
factors of phantoms which contain simple objects, where you simply count the
number that you can see, or score the smallest one that's visible. A more
sophisticated analysis of single tissue equivalent test objects is called for,
and this is a subject we are going to look into.

Dr. Egan: Ed, my red book by Williams and Wilkins goes into great detail on how to do this, how to prepare the plastic mold, and how to prepare the tissue.

Bob Wagner: Dan, can you say whether you anticipate any commercial availability of a phantom like what you're working with?

Dan Miller: Well, it's possible. I think that the physics test strip portion of it can certainly be mass produced very reliably. There are very definite limitations with respect to the use of human tissue. At Memorial Sloan-Kettering we cannot use human tissue except for research purposes. I don't see any way that we can get around that or even that we would want to.

Leonard Stanton: I would just like to briefly comment on the use of uniform phantoms as test objects. This is covered much more fully in a paper that we published in Investigative Radiology in the July-August 1979 issue. I won't take the time to go into the argument here except to say that the absence of parenchymal detail is certainly a limitation of the phantom. This allows you to evaluate contrast and resolution of the entire system, including the eye, but it does not take into account the noise introduced by the anatomy. It is analogous to the use of MTF for measuring nonbiologic systems, before we were able to measure noise, which is a much more sophisticated measurement.

Michael Friedrich: Another comment on biological phantoms: standardization of biological phantoms is almost impossible.

Dr. Egan: I've had the same problem with the breast tissue. I've made probably 3 or 4 dozen of them and no two of them have been the same, as much as I've tried. The nonbiological ones, we were able to standardize.

Dr. Cameron: We should give credit to Leonard Stanton who really did the preliminary work on these test objects with the fibrils and specks. We modified them, and made them randomizable. We did it to make them available commercially. There are now about 50 of them around the world. I think they are reasonably consistent from one to the other in terms of size of the objects, uniformity of the nylon fibers, speck size, and the masses. I think they satisfy to a large extent the need for standardization, and we're thus grateful to Leonard Stanton. We didn't think the Kodak Pathe phantom was suitable. Just because you can see through clear plastic does not mean it is suitable for mammography imaging. I think its been an unfortunate thing to have wire mesh available for naive people to look at and say "gee I can see all this nice wire mesh so clearly. I guess that means my mammography equipment is working fine" - I don't worry about the experts; the people in this room are of no worry at all. But many of you now realize there is need for improvement out in the field. A simple standardized phantom could help cure this problem.

Roger Schneider: I would like to follow up a little bit on your last comment and your earlier discouragement of use of the Kodak Pathe phantom and the BENT program. I think that it's important that people realize that the improvements in image quality being effected by the BENT program that were referred to by Dr. Lester yesterday are not coming about as a result of fine tuning of systems and sophisticated facilities. They are coming about as a result of cleaning up of some pretty unsophisticated facilities. We have found the Kodak Pathe phantom to be more than adequate for that. In fact the opportunity it affords for direct comparison between a visual presentation and a radiographic presentation have quite an impact on radiographic facilities. Many people using poor practices in low work load facilities have elected to stop the practice of mammography when that has been demonstrated to them.

Phil Muntz: I think there are two purposes for a phantom. One is to progress the state of the art, and one for quality control.

Wende Logan: I have compared the Kodak Pathe phantom with others. One thing I like about it is the variable size of calcifications. I've compared it with the Sloan-Kettering phantom and felt that it correlated very well, in the degree of increased visualization of smaller calcifications with improved images. The only thing to keep in mind, is that in order to simulate a clinical situation, the Pathe phantom should be placed on top of three 1 cm high lucite blocks. When you are evaluating a gradation of images you reach your end point very quickly if you use the phantom by itself. The reason the phantom should be on top of the lucite blocks, is to evaluate geometric unsharpness problems. Also, the combined thickness of the Pathe phantom and 3 lucite blocks more closely simulates the thickness and density of an average breast.

Dr. Muntz: Bernie, would you like to defend the Kodak phantom?

Bernie Roth: I had the same reaction to the phantom when I first looked at it, that John Cameron did. However when I read the directions, I realized that the wire mesh was there for one purpose only and that was to look at the geometric aspects of the system and not to look at the recording system.

Dr. Cameron: I agree with that. In fact it's a very useful thing to have. Naive people may misunderstand possibly.

Emil Kaegi: I'd like to make one critical comment on the Kodak Pathe phantom. I first worked with the early numbered series, under 200, which had a very fine pattern of calcifications in it. Later we worked with some in the 300 series and now I've seen some in the 900's, and the fine calcifications have gradually grown larger and larger.

PART III

THE STATE OF THE ART

PRACTICAL ASPECTS OF GOOD QUALITY
FILM/SCREEN MAMMOGRAPHY
Mary Ellen Masterson, M.S. and Daniel W. Miller, Ph.D.
Memorial Hospital
1275 York Avenue
New York, New York 10021

Prior to the introduction of film/screen systems for mammographic examination, radiologists relied on fine grain, double emulsion, direct films, such
as Kodak AA (Figure 1). These films were associated with relatively high
patient exposure, and the long exposure times necessary with some equipment may
have led to motion unsharpness. Not uncommonly, images were purposely overexposed to take advantage of the increased contrast at higher densities which
characterized these films.

Radiographs shown in this paper were taken using a phantom[1] developed
jointly by the Northeast Center for Radiological Physics and D.R. White of St.
Bartholomew's Hospital, London. As shown in Figure 2, the phantom consists of
a largely intact mastectomy specimen embedded in a plastic matrix which is
equivalent to 50% mammary gland - 50% adipose tissue with respect to radiation
interaction properties in the mammographic energy range. The phantom also contains an interchangeable test strip for quantitative analysis based on microdensitometric scans.

Figures 3 through 5 are phantom images obtained with film/screen combinations. The introduction of the vacuum packed combination (called Lo Dose) as
developed by Dupont was first reported upon by Ostrum, Becker, and Isard in
1973[2]. These detector systems generally consist of a single emulsion film kept
in intimate contact with a single screen by placing both in a plastic bag and
evacuating it. There are two commonly used bagging systems -- the Picker
bagger with disposable polyethylene envelopes, and the E-Z-Em reusable bags.
Based on test results obtained at 0.34 mm Al HVL, the Picker bags transmit 25%
more radiation to the screen than the E-Z-Em bags. Recently Kodak has marketed
a rigid cassette for use in mammography which produces approximately the same
attenuation as the E-Z-Em bags and achieves the intimate film/screen contact
required for good resolution.

The intensifying screens used for mammography are either conventional
calcium tungstate or rare earth oxysulfide. The recently developed rare earth
screens differ from $CaWO_4$ in the mammographic energy region because of significantly higher x-ray to light conversion efficiencies. Terbium activated
lanthanum oxysulfide has a conversion efficiency of 13%, that of terbium activated gadolinium oxysulfide is 18%, while that of $CaWO_4$ is only 4%[3,4,5].

As opposed to the blue light emitted by $CaWO_4$, the rare earth screens emit
primarily green spectra to which the spectral response of the film should be
optimally matched. Since the film for use with rare earth screens is green
sensitive, darkroom safelights must be redder than the standard safelight to
minimize fogging.

The radiographic conditions which give good image quality for mammographic
film/screen systems have become quite standardized in the radiologic community.
The molybdenum target with a 30μ molybdenum filter, a combination which passes
the characteristic lines of Mo, is most commonly used. Operating around 26 to
30 kVp, this gives half value layers in the range 0.30-0.36 mm Al. Figure 3
compares Lo-Dose 1 images taken with Mo and W/Mo alloy targets. Note the de-

gradation in contrast in the alloy target image, attributable, at least in part, to the continuous W bremstrahlung spectrum.

Dupont Lo-Dose II screen/film system (Figure 4) was introduced in 1976. The film is the same as that used in the Lo-Dose I system, but the screen is a faster version of $CaWO_4$. As shown in Figure 4, the new screen effects approximately 40% reduction in skin exposure over the Lo-Dose I system.

Kodak Min R (Figure 5) is a rare earth screen/film combination introduced in 1976. It provides increased soft tissue contrast over Lo-Dose II at approximately 15% less exposure.

According to W.W. Logan[6] the most vigorous compression that can be tolerated by the patient should be applied during the mammographic examination. This procedure minimizes geometric unsharpness by decreasing the object - detector distance; improves contrast by diminishing scatter; diminishes motion unsharpness; provides more homogeneous film density from chest wall to nipple; and reduces dose.

In addition to the choice of detector system and the radiographic and positioning techniques employed, processing conditions will have a significant effect on mammographic image quality and patient dose. Work done at the NECRP last year examined the dependence of mammographic film/screen systems on the type of developer chemistry employed and the temperature of the developer solution[7]. Four film/screen receptor systems were investigated including Dupont Lo-Dose I, Lo-Dose II, Kodak Min R, and 3M Trimax. (Trimax is a rare earth screen mated with a double emulsion film). Two developer chemistries - Kodak XRP and Dupont XMD were sequentially studied in the same processor. Developer temperatures ranged from 84-107°F. The results of this study argue that each mammographic installation should carefully investigate processor effects since for some systems it is possible to reduce patient dose without producing significant degradation of image quality at elevated developer temperatures.

A caveat is appropriate at this point since potential long-term processor effects such as increased evaporation and chemical decomposition, coupled with a possibly significant increase in quantum mottle, suggest that a program of frequent monitoring accompany significant increases in developer temperature. Even aside from deliberate changes in processing conditions, a daily quality control program on the mammographic system will avoid many cases of unnecessary patient exposure.

Recently, we and others, have been examining images resulting from mixing and matching films and screens. As examples, phantom images from the Min R film/Min R screen combination exposed at Memorial require 555mR at the position of the surface of the breast. Using Min R screen and Kodak NMB film requires 444mR and produces a slightly more contrasty, slightly more noisy image. The Min R screen in association with Dupont MRF31 film requires 400 mR. The Min R screen combined with Agfa MR3 film requires 148mR. Again, however, caution must be exercised in judging the trade off between image quality and exposure. Of course, one can take mammograms with exposures approaching 0 Roentgens, but if they are not of diagnostic quality, the patient has been unduly exposed. As an example, with the Min R - Agfa combination (148mR) mottle is increased significantly and resolution is sacrificed.

Finally, in order to examine common clinical techniques, Figure 8 shows exposure and absorbed dose data from the 29 NCI Breast Cancer Detection Demonstration Projects. The data were collected by all six Centers for Radiological Physics. The left side of the figure shows average surface exposures (Roentgens) for Xerox and film. In 1975, some screening centers were using

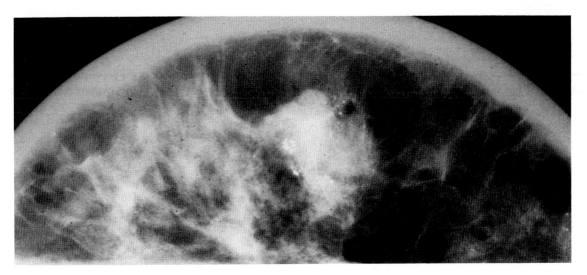

Figure 1. Phantom image and associated technique settings for Kodak AA film.
CGR Senographe Molybdenum Target .03 mm Mo filter, 8.29 R skin
exposure, 28 kVp, 35 mA, 6.0 s Beryllium window: 1 Phase, Focal
spot size: 0.8x0.9 mm. Target-skin distance: 34 cm 0.36 mm Al
1st HVL, 0.40 mm Al 2nd HVL. Kodak M4B Processor, Developer
temperature: 79° F, Drop time: 13 min.

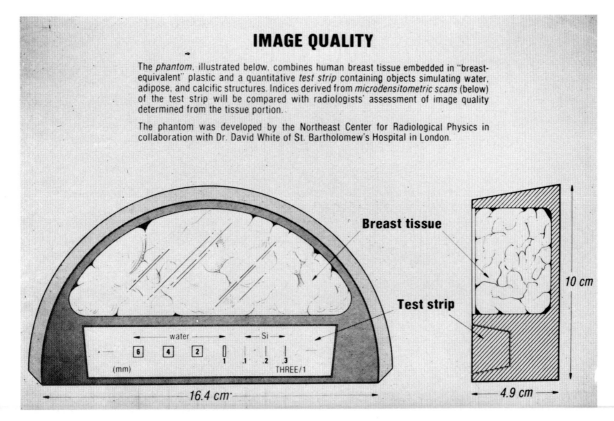

Figure 2. Sketch of Memorial/Barts Mammographic Imaging Phantom.

331

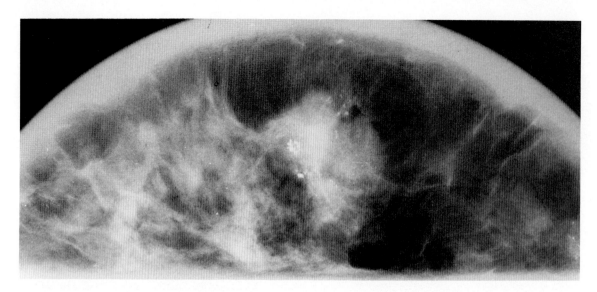

CGR Senographe Molybdenum Target .03 mm Mo filter, 1.48 R skin exposure,
28 kVp, 30 mA, 0.8 s Beryllium window: I Phase, Focal spot size:
0.8x0.9 mm Target-skin distance: 28 cm 0.36 mm Al 1st HVL, 0.40 mm Al 2nd
HVL. Kodak M-6 Processor Developer temperature: 90° F, Drop time: 90 s.

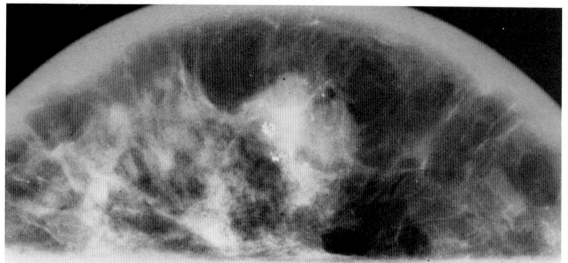

GE MMX Tungsten-Molybdenum Target .03 mm Mo filter, 1.35 R skin exposure,
31 kVP, 200 mA, 0.4 s Beryllium window: 1 Phase, Focal spot size:
3.2x2.7 mm Target-skin distance: 57 cm 0.30 mm Al 1st HVL, 0.38 mm Al
2nd HVL. Kodak M-6 Processor Developer temperature 89° F, Drop time: 90 s.

Figure 3. Dupont Lo-Dose I images obtained using a molybdenum target/
           molybdenum filter combination (above) and using a tungsten -
           molybdenum target and molybdenum filtration (below).

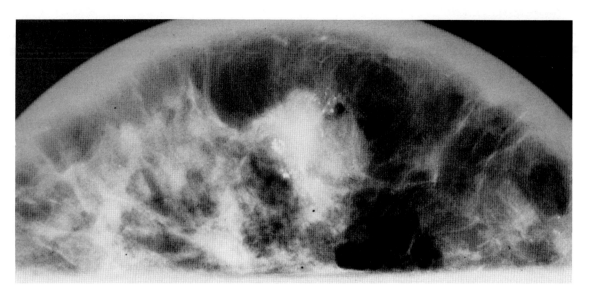

Figure 4. Dupont Lo-Dose II phantom image and associated technique settings. CGR Senographe Molybdenum Target .03 mm Mo filter, 0.84 R skin exposure, 28 kVp, 30 mA, 0.45 s Beryllium window: 1 Phase, Focal spot size: 0.8x0.9 mm Target-skin distance: 28 cm 0.36 mm Al 1st HVL, 0.40 mm Al 2nd HVL. Kodak M-6 Processor Developer temperature: 90° F, Drop time: 90 s.

non-screen film which raised the average surface exposure. Use of direct film was abandoned, and as new film/screen combinations were introduced, the average surface exposure fell to about 750 mR in 1976. The corresponding midbreast doses - based on our work at the NECRP[8] reported elsewhere in this book by G.R. Hammerstein - are shown on the right hand side. As can be seen, midbreast doses for film/screen systems are currently running at about 40 mrad per view - 9 times less than Xerox - and 25 times less than the previously used figure of 1 rad/view employed by the Upton sub-committee.

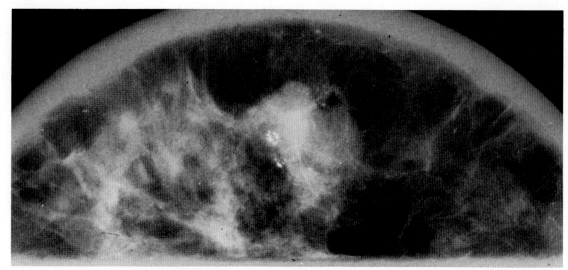

CGR Senographe Molybdenum Target .03 mm Mo filter, 0.74 R skin exposure,
28 kVp, 30 mA, 0.4 s Beryllium window: 1 Phase, Focal spot size:
0.8x0.9 mm Target-skin distance: 28 cm 0.36 mm Al 1st HVL, 0.40 mm Al
2nd HVL. Kodak M-6 Processor Developer temperature: 90° F, Drop time: 90 s.

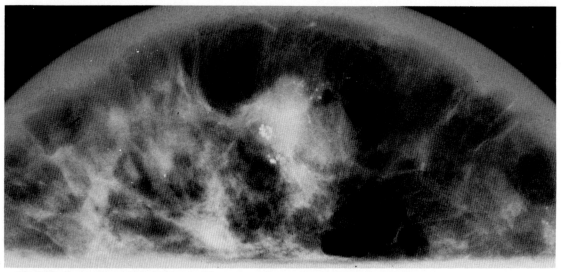

GE MMX Tungsten-Molybdenum Target .03 mm Mo filter, 0.99 R skin exposure,
30 kVp, 200 mA, 0.3 s Beryllium window: 1 Phase, Focal spot size:
3.2x2.7 mm Target-skin distance: 57 cm 0.29 mm Al 1st HVL, 0.36 mm Al
2nd HVL. Kodak M-6 Processor Developer temperature: 89° F, Drop time: 90 s.

Figure 5.   Phantom images using Kodak Min-R film/screen combination
obtained on Mo/Mo and alloy/Mo target/filter units.

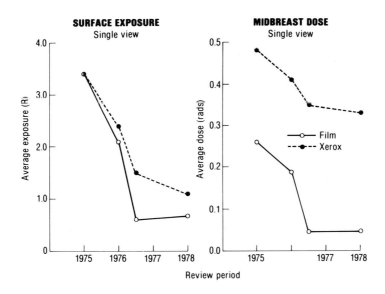

Figure 6. Left: Average surfaces exposure data collected by the six Centers
for Radiological Physics at the 29 Breast Cancer Detection Demonstration Projects (BCDDP's) for film (solid line) and Xerox
(dotted line) systems 1975-1978. Right: Average dose to glandular
tissue at 3cm depth in a breast composed of 50% adipose tissue -
50% mammary gland calculated from BCDDP exposure and HVL data,
1975-1978.

REFERENCES

1. Masterson, M.E., Miller, D.W., White, D.R., Snyder, R.E., Rothenberg, L.N.,
    Kirch, R.L.A., Laughlin, J.S., A New Mammographic Test Object. Works-in-
    Progress. RSNA, Chicago, 1976.

2. Ostrum, B.J., Becker, W., Isard, J., Low Dose Mammography. Radiology,
    1973, 109, 323-326.

3. Buchanen, R.A., Finkelstein, S.I., Wickersheim, K.A., X-ray Exposure
    Reduction Using Rare Earth Oxysulfide Intensifying Screens. Radiology,
    Oct. 1972, 105, 185-190.

4. Bril, A., Klasens, H.A., Intrinsic Efficiencies of Phosphors Under
    Cathode Ray Excetation. Philips Research Reports. Dec. 1952, 7,
    401-420.

5. Coltman, J.W., Ebbinghausen, E.G., Altor, W., Physical Properties
    of Calcium Tungstate X-ray Screens. J. Appl. Phys. 1947, 18, 530-544.

6. See Logan's chapter on Proper Screen/Film Techniques.

7. Masterson, M.E., Miller, D.W., Snyder, R.E., Caley, R., Keegan, A.F.,
    Dobrin, R., Berkovitz, L., Schimpf, J.H., Effects of Film Processor
    Conditions on Mammographic Image Quality and Patient Exposure.
    Presentation, paper 274, RSNA, Chicago, 1977.

8. Hammerstein, G.R., Miller, D.W., White, D.R., Masterson, M.E., Helen Q.
    Woodard, Laughlin, J.S., Absorbed Radiation Dose in Mammography.
    Radiology 130: 485-491, February, 1979.

ELECTRON RADIOGRAPHY TECHNIQUES AND EXPOSURES

Emil M. Kaegi

Standard X-Ray Co.
Xonics, Inc.
Van Nuys, Ca. 91406

INTRODUCTION

In electron radiography image quality depends not only on the x-ray beam characteristics but on the type of imaging gas and the properties of the toner developer system. While these are analogous to screen and film characteristics in the silver halide process, there is a degree of flexibility and a new system of constraints which must be understood. This paper discusses the role of these parameters in light of experience gained with the Xonics mammography system (XERG). A description on the operation of this equipment is presented, and the techniques investigated to achieve clinically acceptable mammograms are reviewed.

Electron radiography (1,2,3), an electrostatic imaging technique, uses an imaging chamber to form a layer of high atomic number gas (under pressure) over a thin sheet of dielectric. The x-ray photons passing through the subject and into the chamber are absorbed in this layer. Part of their energy is converted into positive and negative ions. An electric field across the chamber causes the negative ions to be collected on the dielectric sheet. The resulting latent electrostatic image is then developed in a processer by allowing positively charged toner particles to be attracted to the sheet.

Clinical application for mammography was begun by Xonics in the Fall of 1975. These systems had a 14.1 x 25.7 cm. cassette on available commercial mammography x-ray stands. Xonics then built their own stands using a micro focal spot tube. The cassette was increased to its current 20 x 28 cm. size, and the first units employing a 10 mA fixed anode tube were installed in hospitals during June 1977. These were subsequently replaced with units having a 50 mA rotating anode tube. The operation of this current generation equipment is described below.

DESCRIPTION OF THE EQUIPMENT

Figure 1 is a photograph of the stand. The image chamber or cassette is rigidly mounted on the arm. This particular unit has a movable platform for magnification studies. In the background is a table with removable inserts. This is positioned around the cassette for the retro or recumbent lateral views. The dispenser (background Fig. 2) provides the discharged receptor ready for insertion into the cassette. The processor (foreground Fig. 2) develops and fixes the image. The base provides storage for consumables and also houses a small cooling system for maintaining the toner at a constant temperature.

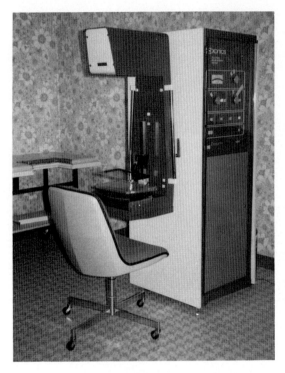

Fig. 1. Photograph of stand and table.

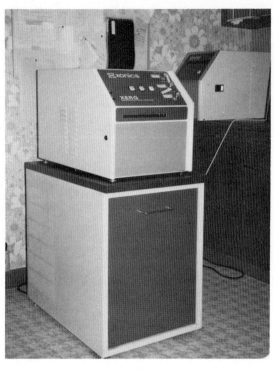

Fig. 2. Photograph of processor and dispenser.

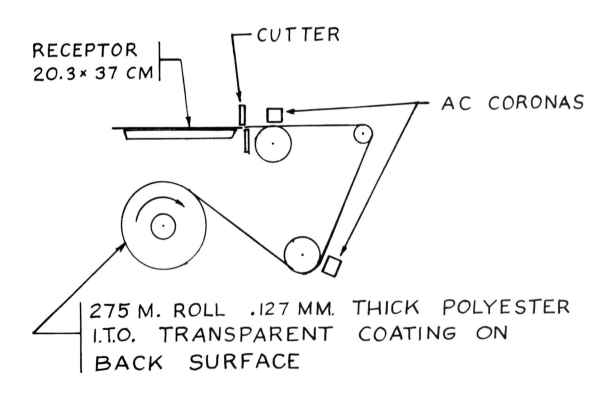

Fig. 3. Schematic of the dispenser operation.

Figures 3, 4, and 5 are schematics that describe the operation of the equipment. The dispenser (Fig. 3) contains the supply roll of receptors, enough for over 700 images. The film is .127 mm thick polyester with a transparent Indium tin oxide coating one side to provide a conductive backing. From the roll the film passes under 2 AC coronas. These discharge the surface to less than 1 volt. It is then cut to a 37 cm length and is ready for use. Cycle time is less than 30 seconds.

The first production stands (Fig. 4) use a battery and a 400 Hz square wave driver and inverter system in the generator. This fully rectified signal produces virtually a DC potential on the tube. It also permits operation off a 110 V. 20 A. wall outlet. The subsequent versions have a more standard 60 Hz single phase, fully rectified generator with higher kVp and mA capability. The tube has been tilted to provide a strong "heel effect" at the chest wall. The imaging chamber has a graphite composite top. Spherical electrodes aligned with the tube permit an 11 mm thick gas layer to be used without causing image unsharpness.

In operation, the discharged receptor is inserted into the cassette, and the "close" cycle is initiated. A hydraulic system closes the cassette. It is then flushed with CO_2 to rid the system of trapped air. Next, it is pressurized with the imaging gas. This occurs in less than one minute. When the exposure is initiated, the anode is brought up to speed and the 14 KV potential is placed across the electrodes to attract the negative ions to the receptor. The exposure duration is controlled either by timer or one of two radiation sensors located near the chest wall edge (for craniocaudad and medio-lateral views) or close to the center of the cassette for retro-lateral views. Following exposure, the imaging gas is returned through a purification stage to the reservoir bottle. A second flush of CO_2 scavenges the last atmosphere of gas from the cassette. The baralyme absorbs the CO_2 from the gas, and the drierite, a disiccant, removes the water formed by the CO_2 absorption reactions. Total time of this cycle is under two minutes. There is a sufficient quantity of the consummables for over 500 cycles between servicing. A new strategy currently being field tested eliminates the second flush and simply replaces from an additional supply the gas not recovered. This has been shown to increase the operation between servicing to 1300 cycles for the CO_2 and 1800 cycles for the rest.

The exposed receptor with its latent image is inserted into the processor (Fig. 5). It is then transported under a DC corona, which can be used to "clip" high, unwanted background signals from the image without affecting the low level information. The function of this corona is to act as a "density limit" on the processing. The developer stage consists of a 4 liter reservoir of toner, a pump, and a fountain. The latter produces a very smooth flow of toner into which the film is dipped. The toner is attracted in proportion to the available charge. By biasing the fountain with respect to the image, voltage or charge available for developing may be varied. This permits the overall image "contrast" to be changed. This will be discussed in more detail later. A turbidity meter monitors the toner concentration and automatically replenishes the system. The developed image next passes through a drying stage and then is laminated on one side. There is sufficient laminating material on a roll for about 500 images. The entire sequence takes about four minutes, but a second image can be started after two minutes.

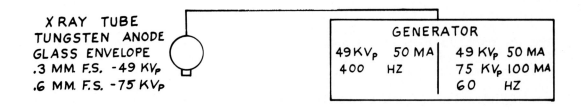

X RAY TUBE
TUNGSTEN ANODE
GLASS ENVELOPE
.3 MM. F.S. -49 KV$_P$
.6 MM. F.S. -75 KV$_P$

GENERATOR

49 KV$_P$ 50 MA	49 KV$_P$ 50 MA
400 HZ	75 KV$_P$ 100 MA
	60 HZ

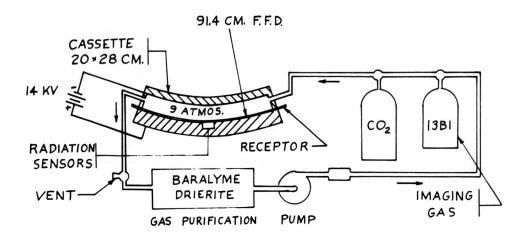

91.4 CM. F.F.D.

CASSETTE
20 × 28 CM.

14 KV

9 ATMOS.

RADIATION
SENSORS

RECEPTOR

CO$_2$ 13BI

VENT

BARALYME
DRIERITE

GAS PURIFICATION   PUMP

IMAGING
GAS

Fig. 4.   Schematic of the stand operation.

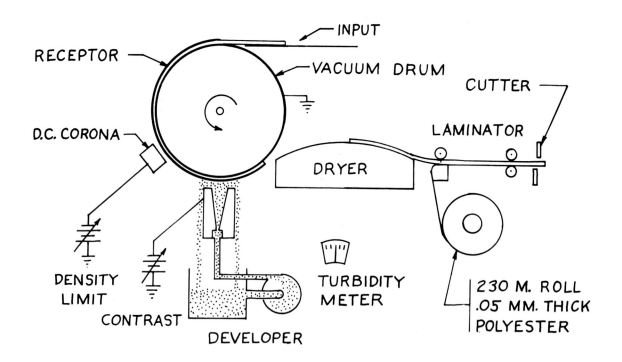

INPUT

RECEPTOR

VACUUM DRUM

CUTTER

LAMINATOR

D.C. CORONA

DRYER

DENSITY
LIMIT

CONTRAST

DEVELOPER

TURBIDITY
METER

230 M. ROLL
.05 MM. THICK
POLYESTER

Fig. 5.   Schematic of the processor operation.

THE EFFECTS OF PROCESSOR SETTING

To better understand the processor settings consider Fig. 6. The drawing at the upper left is a representative of an image. The image voltage distribution along A-A is shown below it. By adjusting the "density limit," high background voltages can be removed without affecting the low signal information. This reduces the toner usage, since optical densities greater than 4 are unnecessary. One must, however, use this density limit judiciously, as it can affect information at the skin line.

The "contrast" control simply biases the developer fountain with respect to the image potential. The difference between the image potential (or the "density limit" setting in the case of the background) and the "contrast" of the optical density distribution (shown at the right). The use of "contrast" thus increases local contrast in the information area and offers a means of reducing the effects of uniform scattered radiation from the image (3,4).

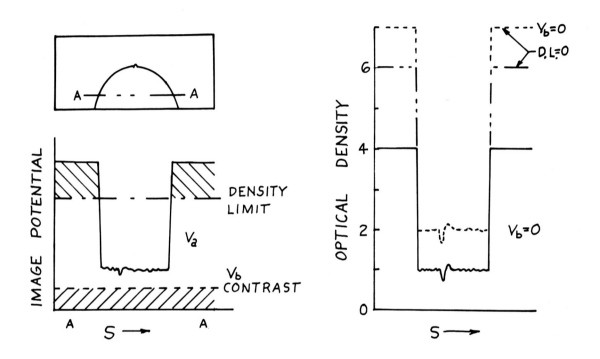

Fig. 6. The effects of processor settings on the development process.

SYSTEM PARAMETERS INFLUENCING ERG TECHNIQUES

The techniques used to achieve acceptable image quality require careful consideration of all the system parameters. In electron radiography new variables are introduced with degrees of flexibility constraints that must be understood. The practicality of optimization strategies must be weighed in terms of hardware limitations. Table 1 lists the parameters available in the current Xonics system.

Table 1. Imaging System Parameters

X-Ray Beam

kVp: 30-46
mAs: 10-100
HVL: .5-1.5 mm Al.

Magnification

1.05 - 1.3

Cassette

Pressure: 8.2 - 10.5 Atmos.
Gas: Xenon, Krypton, 13B1

Processor

Toner Speed ($\Delta V/\rho$): 15-50
Image Neutralization ($\Delta V/V_a$): 8-70%
Contrast (fountain bias): 20-400 V
Density Limit: None - O.D. = 4

The lower limits on kVp are dictated by radiation output rates (governed by maximum tube currents possible with the small focal spots and on exposure time limits to avoid patient motion problems) and inherent window filtration. The small focal spot makes magnification feasible. An upper bound of 1.3 is dictated by practicable considerations of cassette width.

The quantum efficiency of the system depends on the type of gas related to the x-ray beam properties and its concentration in terms of gas layer thickness and pressure. With regard to cassette geometry ion recombination and fringing field effects limit the electrode gap (or gas layer thickness). Structural considerations, the design trade-off in minimizing the absorption versus strength dictate maximum operating pressures. The type of imaging gas can drastically alter sensitivity and image quality. The noble gases xenon and krypton, with their K edges at 34 and 14 keV, respectively, and the bromine-freon compound (13 B1) are available. Their relative sensitities will be discussed later.

The processor properties are very flexible. The inherent speed of the toner ($\Delta V/\rho$, the volts required to produce an optical density of 1.0) and the degree of image signal neutralized by the toner ($\Delta V/V_a$, a function of the fountain geometry and the transport rate) combine to define the overall "developer speed." The degree of neutralization affects the amount of edge enhancement. High values (greater than 40 or 50%) produce an undesirable lack of sharpness. Very low values present artifact problems. Contrast settings (fountain bias) affect latitude and exposures. This will also be discussed later.

IMAGING GAS SENSITIVITIES

The effects of different imaging gases on system sensitivity are shown in Fig. 7. The volts measured on the receptor (per milliroentgen of exposure) are plotted against beam half value layer for different tube

voltages. While pure xenon exhibits the highest sensitivity, it requires
the addition of a getter SF$_6$ to reduce scattering and improve resolution.
The krypton with 3% 13B1 (acting in a similar capacity as the SF$_6$) is slightly
less sensitive, and 13B1 is the least. By simply varying gases equivalent
image voltages can be obtained with a 60% change in exposure. It is then
necessary to match up the processor parameters to these image voltages.

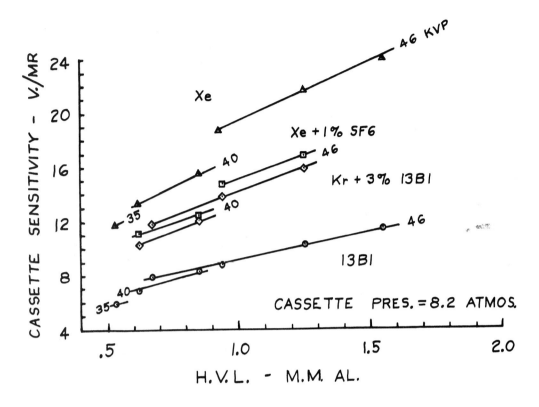

Fig. 7. Imaging gas sensitivities for different beam energies.

DEVELOPER PROPERTIES

To gain a better insight into the developer parameter, consider Fig. 8.
Here some typical H-D curves are shown as a function of the "developer speed"
and "contrast" (V_b). Net optical density is plotted against receptor image
voltage. Overall "developer speed" is a function of the inherent toner
speed, the degree of neutralization, and a factor F (to correct for losses
in density during the fixing process). Then, for a "speed" of 150 V to
achieve a density of 1, a toner $\Delta V/\rho$ of approximately 25, a developer
process neutralizing about 20% of the available signal, and F = .85 are
required. Obviously, there is a whole family of combinations possible to
obtain the same speed. Conversely, with the same toner ($\Delta V/\rho$) the speed can
be varied by changing ($\Delta V/V_a$) (by changing the processor transport rate, or
fountain configuration, or toner concentration). Three speeds are shown
plotted for the same "contrast" setting (150 V). Speed and contrast affect
the system latitude. By reducing the contrast (for the same speed, S = 150 V,
and V_b from 150 V to 20 V) the latitude is increased. Obviously, higher
"developer speeds" and higher contrast settings require more exposure to
achieve equivalent optical densities.

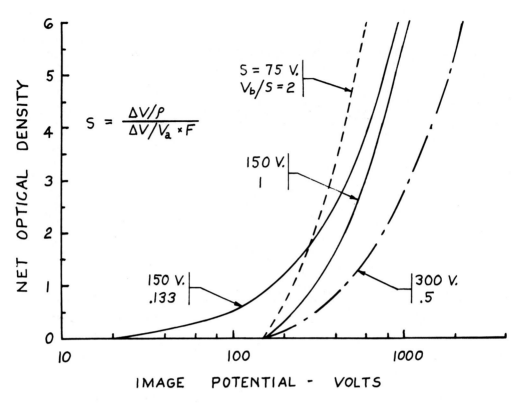

$$S = \frac{\Delta V/P}{\Delta V/V_a \times F}$$

Fig. 8. Representative developer H-D curves.

TABLE 2 SUMMARY OF TECHNIQUES

TIME PERIOD	EQUIP. VIEW	KVp	HVL	IMAGING GAS	PROCESSOR CONTRAST-V	SKIN EXPOSURES-Mr
1975	(1)CC-	40 50	1.0 1.2	X_e+1%SF_6 "	50	60
	(2)CC-ML	48-54	1.7	"	100-350	100
1976	(3)CC-ML	46	.94,1.24	"	100	150
	Retro ML	46	1.24	"	5	100
1977	(4)CC-ML	40	.85	(Kr),13B1	150	(180), 210
	CC-ML	46	.94,1.24	" "	150	(150), 200
	Retro	46	1.24	" "	20	(100), 160
1977-78	(5)CC-ML	38.8	.87	13B1	150	210
	CC-ML	44	1.3	"	150	170
	Retro ML	38.8	.87	"	20	230
Current	(5)CC-ML	36	.81	"	150	250
	Retro ML	36-38.8	.71-.77	"	20	280

(1) 3Ø Moly. Anode
(2) 1Ø Tungsten Anode
(3) X.M.S. 5 MA. Tungsten Anode
(4) X.M.S. 10 MA. Tungsten Anode
(5) X.M.S. 50 MA. 400 Hz Tungsten Anode

CLINICAL TECHNIQUES

The techniques currently being used with the Xonics system can best be understood by reviewing those investigated earlier. These are summarized in Table 2.

Initial efforts in 1975 were with a commercially available stand having a three-phase generator and molybdenum target tube. Considerable aluminum filtration was added so that HVL's were 1.0 and 1.2. Based upon our earlier work in general radiography (5), xenon was used as the imaging gas. Rather dramatic images were obtained at 60 mR with a laboratory model processor (6).

The use of even harder beams was investigated with another stand. Attempts to compensate for the loss in contrast due to the smaller differences in absorption coefficients by operating the processor with higher "contrast" (bias) levels resulted in latitude problems. There was also a growing concern by the radiologist on the visual noise (due to quantum mottle).

The introduction of our own stand in mid 1976 required strategies geared to the lower output tube. A technique for the retro or recumbent medial-lateral view was developed. These required lower contrast settings and harder beams to obtain sufficient latitude.

In 1977 other imaging gases and still softer beams for some views were investigated. These reduced the quantum mottle at the expense of dose. This effort established 13B1 as the prime gas for use on soft tissue. In September, 1977, the 50 mA rotating anode tube units were introduced. Initially the kV's were adjusted to match the HVL's used with the stationary anode system. Softer beams for the retro views were found necessary to improve image quality.

This trend toward softer beams has continued to the present. Tube voltages have been reduced to 36 kVp with some installations across the country running as low as 32 kVp. Typical skin exposures are about 250 mR for the CC and ML views and somewhat higher for the retro views (where there is less compression). The difference in HVL's reflect beam hardening due to the compression paddle.

SUMMARY

The parameters affecting image quality and sensitivity in electron radiography have been discussed. From clinical experience with the Xonics mammography system a series of techniques have evolved. Currently the best imaging gas for soft tissue is 13B1 with beam HVL's ranging between .7 and .8 mm Al. The average skin exposures are about 250 mR.

ACKNOWLEDGMENTS

The author gratefully acknowledges the assistance and cooperation of Dr. Evelyn Wilkinson and Dr. E. Phillip Muntz, Los Angeles County-University of Southern California Medical center and Dr. Saar Porrath, Santa Monica Hospital Medical Center.

REFERENCES

1. Muntz EP, Lewis J, Azzarelli T, et al: On the characteristics of electron radiographic images in diagnostic radiology. (In) Medical X-ray Photo-Optical Systems Evaluation, 56:208, SPIE Seminar Proceedings, October 21-23, 1974.

2. Proudian A, Carangi RL, Jacobson G, and Muntz EP: Electron radiography: a new method of radiographic imaging. Radiology 110:667-671, March 1974.

3. Muntz EP, Jacobson G, Kaegi EM, et al: Electronic grids for electro-static imaging systems. Radiology 121:197-204, October 1976.

4. Muntz EP, Welkowsky M, Kaegi E, et al: Optimization of electrostatic imaging systems for minimum patient dose or minimum exposure in mammography. Radiology 127:517-523, May 1978.

5. Stanton L, Brady LW, Szarko FL, et al: Electron radiography, a new x-ray imaging system. Appl. Radiology 53, March/April 1973.

6. Muntz EP, Meyers H, Wilkinson E, Jacobson G: Preliminary studies using electron radiography for mammography. Radiology 125:517-523, November 1977.

DOSE REDUCTION IN XEROMAMMOGRAPHY

Gopala U.V. Rao and Panos P. Fatouros
Radiation Physics Division, Medical College of Virginia
Richmond, VA 23298

Xeroradiography is perhaps the most commonly used modality in modern day mammography in the United States. Edge enhancement is the primary mechanism responsible for image formation in this modality. Extended areas are depicted in a xeromammogram with no significant change in density resulting in a characteristic curve that is very nearly flat (Figure 1). For this reason, xeromammography has a much larger "recording latitude" than film mammography and makes possible the simultaneous visualization of the skin line, the nipple, ducts, micro calcifications, tumor masses, and the chest wall in a single image. Surface exposures with this technique are of the order of 0.5 to 2.0 rads. These are about a factor of 2 larger compared to the surface exposures with single screen - single emulsion type image receptors such as Dupont Lo-dose and Kodak Min R. Surface exposures with non-screen films are 10 to 20 times larger.

In this paper, various means and potential means for reducing dosage in xeromammography will be explored.

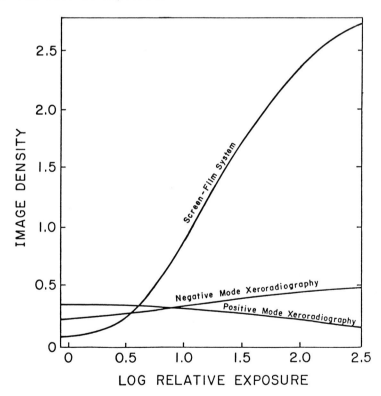

Figure 1   Typical characteristic curves for xeroradiography and film screen - film radiography.

Beam Quality

Single screen single emulsion type image receptors require about 20 to 50 mR for optimal exposure while a xeroradiographic plate used in the positive mode requires about 150 to 250 mR depending on beam quality. Surface exposures however are of the same order of magnitude with both systems since it is customary to use higher beam qualities and tungsten targets with the latter. In other words, beam penetration is larger in the case of xeromammography. The use of higher beam qualities is possible in xeromammography because the loss in image contrast resulting from a decrease in subject contrast is not as severe as in the case of film-screen systems. Indeed Wolfe (1) believes that a molybdenum anode x-ray tube does not produce as good a xeromammogram in a very dense dysplastic breast as a tungsten target tube does.

In most institutions, xeromammography is performed using 35-45 kVp, with the only filtration being that inherent in the tube (between 0.5 to 0.8 mm Al). All exposures are made with a fixed tube current (usually 300 mA). The time of exposure is also usually the same (1 sec.). Van De Riet and Wolfe (2) have recently shown that clinically acceptable mammograms can be obtained at reduced entrance exposures by increasing the total filtration up to 3.2 mm of aluminum. If the mAs is kept constant, this will mean that the technologist has to use a much higher kilovoltage for similar breasts. This necessarily results in reduced contrast in the image. Van De Riet and Wolfe have found that some of the lost contrast can be restored by reducing the positive bias voltage during development from the usual 2000 volts to 1425 volts.

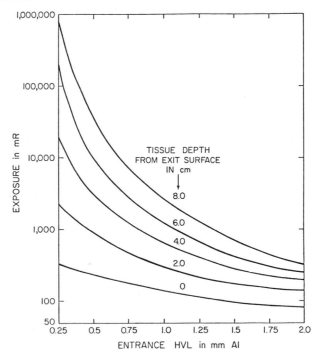

Figure 2   Diagram illustrating the exposure required at various depths from the exit surface for optimal image in negative mode xeroradiography.

Use of higher quality x-ray beams as a rule results in reduced entrance exposures. It must be remembered however that this does not necessarily mean that the same factor of dose reduction occurs throughout the breast tissue (Figure 2). This is because, the larger beam quality, the larger the penetration and the larger the percentage of skin exposure that reaches the deeper layers of the breast.

Use of Negative Mode

The use of negative back bias is another way of achieving reduction in dose. Many authors (1,3) have shown that at a given beam quality, entrance radiation exposures are 20 - 30% lower in the negative mode. The negative mode is also believed to offer greater resolution for calcifications. The negative bias potential currently used in the Xerox 125 System is 3350 volts. It may be possible to increase this to restore some of the contrast reduction that occurs at higher qualities.

Compression

Compression of the breast reduces the overall thickness, reduces scatter, brings anatomical details closer to the image receptor and reduces geometric unsharpness. It also helps to reduce motion unsharpness, and reduces radiation exposure. From a clinical point of view, it makes it possible to make an accurate assessment of the relative densities of the masses and tissue details. It must be remembered however that the compressing device should not be coincident with the end of the collimating cone. If it is, then the posterior aspect of the cone should be cut out. In the case of xeromammography, balloon compression is preferred. Dr. Logan however believes that even in the case of xeromammography, vigorous compression using other means may improve image quality.

Focus to Skin Distance

For the same thickness of the breast, the larger the FSD, the less the difference between the entrance and exit exposures because of inverse square law. Furthermore, the larger the FSD, the less the penumbra due to the focal spot. However, the larger the FSD, the larger the exposure time and hence the larger the motion unsharpness. With 0.6 to 1.6 mm focal spots, focus to skin distances of the order of 65 to 75 cm are currently considered optimal.

Receptor Sensitivity

About 2 years ago, we reported (4) that the amount of edge enhancement δ in xeromammography is related to the exposure R transmitted through the object being imaged through the equation:

$$\delta = \delta_0 \; \frac{e^{CR/R_0}}{1 + \frac{V_b}{V_0} \, e^{R/R_0}}$$

within the breast. Many radiologists consider this to be more important
than the visualization of the skin line. Skin thickening, according to
them, is easily determined by palpation and furthermore is present only
in advanced cancers which are easily reocognized anyway from other radiographic features.

Figures 3 and 4 taken from bulletins 7 and 8 issued by the Xerox Company
illustrate this point. Notice that the parenchymal detail is superior
in what are labeled by the Xerox Company as under exposed images.

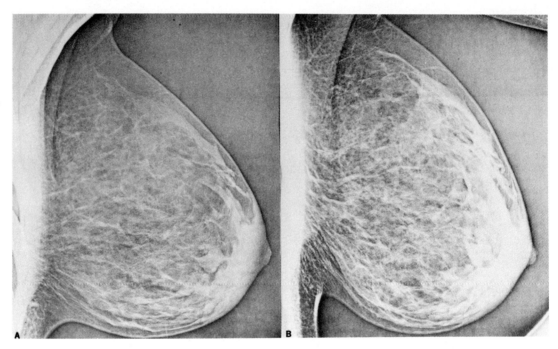

Figure 3   Examples of negative mode xeromammograms. A is considered to be a
           properly exposed image and B is considered to be underexposed accord-
           ing to the Wolfe criterion of a 1 mm halo at the skin line. Notice
           however that the parenchymal detail is superior in B.

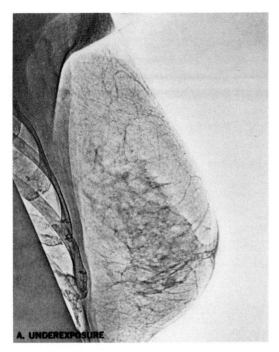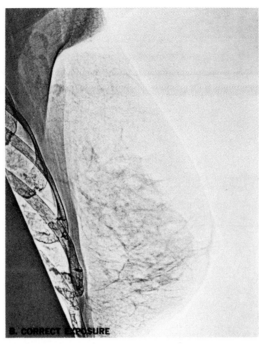

Figure 4   Examples of positive xeromammograms. A is considered to be an underexposed image and B a correctly exposed image according to the
Wolfe criterior of a 1 mm halo at the skin line. Notice however
that the parenchymal detail is superior in A.

Use of Red Filters for Viewing

A common photographic technique for enhancing cloud patterns against a
blue sky is to use a red filter. A red filter absorbs blue light and thus
increases the contrast between clouds in the sky. Based on this reasoning,
Kalisher (7) reported last year that the perception of xeromammographic
images can be markedly enhanced by viewing them with deep red goggles.
Alternately, the image can be viewed with a bright red photographic safe
light.

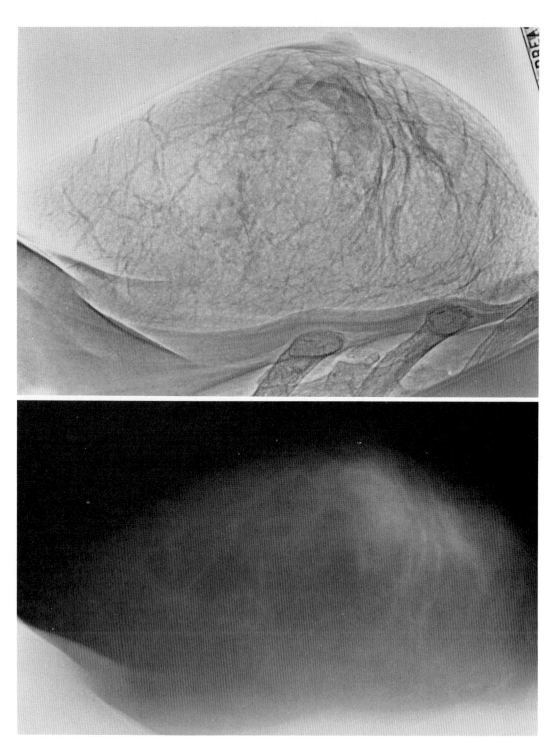

Figure 5 Diagrams illustrating the potential of simultaneous xero-film
mammography Top: A xeromammogram Bottom: A film mammograph
made simultaneously.

where C is the subject contrast, V_b is the developer bias potential, V_0 is the selenium plate charging potential and R_0 the selenium plate discharge constant. R_0 is defined as the exposure required to reduce the charging potential from V_0 to V_0/e, since it is known that $V = V_0e^{-R/R_0}$. δ_0 is a constant of proportionality that depends on the design of the development chamber, the configuration of the various baffles and grids and the proper-ties of the aersol powder used. We (4,5) have further shown that in the case of low contrast structures, there exists an optimal transmitted x-ray exposure which results in a maximum value of δ. At this optimal exposure, the visibility of low contrast details is at its best. On the basis of the above equation and additional theoretical studies (6), we have firmly established that the optimal receptor exposure in positive mode xero-mammography is 1.2 R_0. In the case of negative mode, it will be between 20 to 30% less. In either case, if R_0 can be reduced by improvements in the photoconductive layer, reduced patient exposures will be possible. Furthermore there exists the possibility of increasing δ_0 itself by im-provements in the design of the development chamber and the associated components.

The constant R_0 depends on the nature of the photo-conductive material used, its thickness and the quality of the x-ray beam impinging on it. In the case of selenium, the maximum sensitivity is known to occur at a thick-ness of about 130 microns. This is the thickness used in commercial selenium plates. The lowest curve in Figure 2 represents the values of R_0 at dif-ferent half-value layers in the case of present day selenium plates used in the negative mode. Notice that the higher the beam HVL, the smaller the value of R_0, another reason for the reduction in dosage at higher beam qualities.

From the equation given in the preceding paragraph, it is also seen the smaller the ratio V_b/V_0, the larger the edge enhancement for a given subject contrast C and a given exposure R. This implies that the bias voltage should be as small as possible and the charging voltage should be as high as possible. In practice, however these are limited by the design charac-teristics of the development chamber.

Automatic Exposure Termination

Based on the finding that there exists an optimal transmitted x-ray ex-posure which produces maximal edge enhancement of soft tissue details within the breast, we (4,5) have been advocating the use of automatic exposure ter-mination (AET) in xeromammography for the last 2 years. One of the initial difficulties in adopting AET on a practical basis was the presence of a sup-porting metal bar on the back side of the xeroradiographic cassette. The Xerox Company since then has developed a modified cassette which eliminates this problem. It should now be possible for commercial vendors to incorpo-rate provisions for xeromammographic AET in their equipment.

The introduction of AET will go a long way in reducing repeat studies. It must be pointed out however that the AET based on delivering an exposure equal to 1.2 R_0 to the plate in the case of the positive mode and 20 - 30% less in the case of the negative mode, may not always correspond to the Wolfe criterion of a 1 mm halo at the skin line. On the other hand, it re-sults in reduced patient exposure and optimal visualization of the parenchyma

Scattered Radiation

Scatter is known to degrade image quality to a significant degree in the case of film screen mammography. To what extent scattered radiation affects image quality in xeromammography is not clearly understood at this time. However, the restriction of beam size and the interposition of a small air gap between the breast and the xero cassette may have some influence on the improvement of image quality due to the elimination of scattered radiation even in the case of xeromammography.

Simultaneous Xero Mammography

Table 1 shows the optimal exposures required at receptor surface for different image receptors. Notice that Kodak type MA non-screen film and Xerox 125 casssettes both require about 125 mR. This implies that it should be possible to simultaneously expose both the image receptors with the film placed between the patient and the xerox cassette. In practice the film is taped to the xerox cassette. This technique has the potential of yielding two images with no additional exposures, a film mammogram highlighting soft tissue densities and a xeromammogram highlighting microcalcifications, vasculature and ductal patterns.

TABLE 1

OPTIMAL EXPOSURES REQUIRED AT RECEPTOR SURFACE

(Exit HVL 3.0 mm Al)

IMAGE RECEPTOR	OPTIMAL EXPOSURE REQUIRED (mR)
Kodak Type M	400
Kodak Type MA	125
Xerox 125 (+Ve mode)	125
Dupont Lodose I	20
Kodak Min R	16
Dupont Lodose II	10

Figure 5 shows that the technique has potential. The fact that the film was laid above the xerox cassette did not contribute in any way to the deterioration of the xeroradiographic image itself.

Ideally, it would be nice if a single film, single screen combination of the same order of sensitivity as the Xerox 125 system were available. It is of course important that the film screen combination does not absorb a large percentage of the x-ray energy incident on it. With such a system, the film image will have better contrast than is possible with a non-screen film. Adopting some of these ideas, we feel that it should be possible to design a combination xero-film system which would require less exposure than is currently being used with xeroradiographic systems alone.

Single View Mammography

Buchannan et al (8) claim that no reduction of diagnostic accuracy occurs if only the mediolateral view is taken instead of the usual two projections. While this point of view is not shared by many, it should not be overlooked as a possible approach for dose reduction at least in screening procedures.

Conclusion

In conclusion, one can only say, where there is a will, there is a way. Radiologists should be genuinely interested in reduced dose mammography. As far as xeromammography is concerned the use of higher beam qualties, use of negative mode, good compression, and increased FSD are currently accepted means of dose reduction. Red goggles may be tried as a means to increase detail perception. Manufacturers should make xeromammographic AET possible with their equipment. Future efforts should be directed towards exploring the potential of simultaneous xero film mammography, increasing receptor sensitivity and electronic read-out of the charge distributions on the plate.

ACKNOWLEDGMENTS

This research was funded by Grant 7R01 FDO 1004-01 from the U.S. Department of Health, Education and Welfare.

Our thanks are due to Miss Inez Wasicki for her secretarial assistance.

REFERENCES

1. Wolfe, J.N.: Mammography, Radiologic Clinics of North America, Vol. XII, No. 1, Apirl 1974.

2. Van De Riet, W.G. and Wolfe, J.N.: Dose Reduction in Xeroradiography of the breast, Am. J. Roentgenol 128: 821-823, 1977.

3. Osterman, F.A., Zeman G.H., Rao, G.U.V., Gayler, R., Kirk, B.G. and James, A.E.: Negative Mode Soft Tissue Xeroradiography, 124, 689-694, 1977.

4. Zeman, G.H., Rao, G.U.V. and Osterman, F.A.: Evaluation of Xeroradiographic Image Quality. Radiology, 119, 689 1976.

5. Zeman G.H., Osterman, F.A., Rao, G.U.V., Kirk, B.G. and James A.E.: Xeromammographic Automatic Exposure Termination, Radiology, 126: 117 (1978).

6. Fatouros, P.F. and Rao, G.U.V.: On Optimizing the Xeromammographic Image, Medical Physics Physics (In Press).

7. Kalisher, L.: Enhancement of Xeroradiographic Image Contrast Using Red Filtration, Radiology, Vol. 119, No. 2, 477, 1976.

8. Buchanan, J.B. and Jager, R.M.: Single View Negative Mode Xeromammograph: An approach to reduce Radiation Exposure in Breast Cancer Screening. Radiology, 123: 63, 1977.

CENTRAL AXIS DEPTH DOSE CALCULATIONS IN MAMMOGRAPHY

Gopala U.V. Rao, Panos P. Fatouros and Alfred M. Strash
Radiation Physics Division, Medical College of Virginia
Richmond, VA 23298

Information concerning the absorbed dose distribution within the breast during a mammographic examination is of interest to radiologists, statisticians and physicists alike. Figures 1,2 and 3 show central axis depth dose data applicable to mammography. In Figure 1, a breast composition of 50% glandular tissue and 50% adipose tissue is assumed. In Figure 2, the breast is assumed to be composed predominantly of fatty tissue. In Figure 3, it is assumed to be composed predominantly of glandular tissue. Notice that in these figures, relative exposure is expressed as a function of tissue depth from the exit surface and beam quality (entrance half-value layer). Notice also that the data is normalized with respect to the exposure at zero depth from the exit surface. These figures are applicable to any type of mammography. They have been generated on the basis of central axis depth dose information provided by Hammerstein et al (1) and Morgan and Nickoloff (2). Rigorously speaking, they are valid only for large skin distances (so that the effect of inverse square law is negligible), large breast thicknesses so that a finite relationship exists between the entrance HVL and the exit HVL as shown in Figure 5 , a tungsten target and narrow beam geometry (so that the data is independent of field size). In practice however, the variations in relative exposure due to changes in target material, field size and focus to skin distance are small compared to differences due to varying breast compositions.

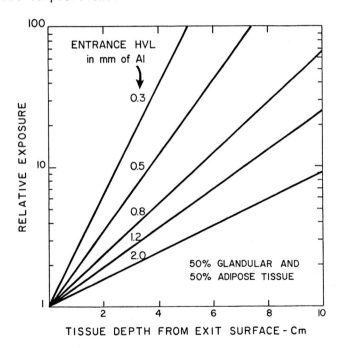

Figure 1 Normalized central axis depth data for breast tissue composed of 50% glandular tissue and 50% adipose tissue.

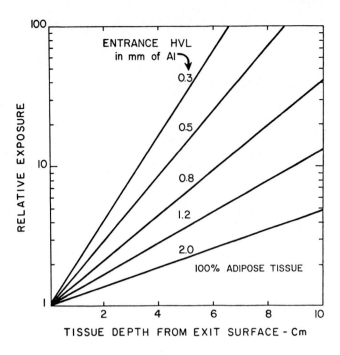

Figure 2   Normalized central axis depth dose data for breast tissue composed mainly of adipose tissue.

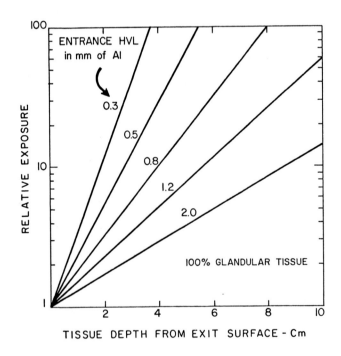

Figure 3   Normalized central axis depth dose data for breast tissue composed mainly of glandular tissue.

358

The best way to describe the usefulness of Figures 1, 2 and 3 in practice is by means of a specific example. At the Medical College of Virginia in Richmond, a certain patient was radiographed at 40 kVp, 300 mAs. The image receptor was a xeroradiographic cassette used in the negative mode. The total filtration in the beam was 2.8 mm Al. From Figure 4 prepared on the basis of data published in references 3 and 4, it can be seen that the entrance HVL must have been 1.5 mm Al. From Figure 5, it can be seen that the exit HVL is about 3.0 mm Al. The air exposure at the end of the cone and balloon with this unit was 400 mR at 40 kVp (Line 2, Table 1). Adding 25% for back scatter, it follows that the surface exposure must have been 500 mR and the surface dose 400 millirads (assuming a roentgen to rad conversion factor of 0.8). If the entrance HVL had been below 0.5 mm Al, the measured air exposure would have been increased by only 10% to account for backscatter. If it had been between 0.5 mm and 1.0 mm Al, a figure of 20% would have been more appropriate. For entrance half-value layers in excess of 1.0 mm Al, a backscatter correction of 25% is more reasonable (5).

At an exit half-value layer of 3.0 mm Al, a xeroradiographic plate requires about 100 mR in the negative mode for optimal exposure. The ratio of surface to receptor exposures, was therefore 500/100 or 5.0. Knowing this ratio, an equivalent breast thickness can be estimated from Figure 1. At an entrance HVL of 1.5 mm Al, the equivalent breast thickness for the case on hand is seen to be 6 cm. The mid-line exposure, that is 3 cm within the breast is seen to be 2.25 times the exposure at the cassette or in other words 225 mR. If glandular tissue is present at the mid-line, the dose will be 225 x 0.8 = 180 millirads. If adipose tissue is present, it will be 225 x 0.5 = 112.5 millirads. In a similar manner, the dose at any other depth can be determined. For example, at 1 cm from the entrance surface or 5 cm from the exit surface, the relative exposure is seen to be 4.0. Tissues located at this depth would therefore have an exposure of 4 x 100 = 400 mR. The absorbed dose to these tissues will again depend upon the nature of the tissues present at that location. If it is glandular tissue, the absorbed dose would have been 400 x 0.8 millirads. If it is adipose tissue, it would have been 400 x 0.5 millirads.

Table 1 shows a typical calibration report based on calculations outlined above. If the breast is significantly more glandular or significantly fattier than the 50/50 composition assumed in Figure 1, either Figure 2 or 3 would have been used as appropriate.

In summary, the procedure described above provides a quick and reliable way of estimating the dose at various locations within the breast with any given image receptor. The only experimental data needed is the air exposure for the machine in question at the tip of the cone or compression device.

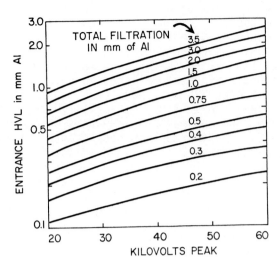

Figure 4 Relationship between kVp, total filtration and half-value layer for full-wave rectified units.

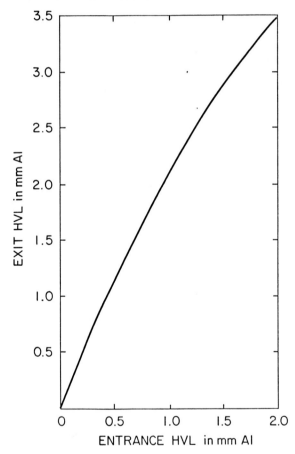

Figure 5 Relationship between entrance HVL and exit HVL for breast thickness in excess of 4 cm. Narrow beam geometry is assumed.

TABLE 1

SUMMARY OF CALIBRATION DATA FOR A TYPICAL MAMMOGRAPHIC UNIT

Focus to Skin Distance: 28.8 inches

Total Beam Filtration: 2.8 mm Al

KVP Set	HVL (mm Al)	AIR EXPOSURE For 300 mAs (mR)	SURFACE EXPOSURE For 300 mAs (mR)	SURFACE DOSE For 300 mAs (mrad)	MID LINE DOSE FOR 300 mAs (mrad)* Glandular Tissue	Adipose Tissue
35	1.4	200	250	200	121	75
40	1.5	400	500	400	180	113
45	1.8	640	800	640	225	140
50	1.9	1000	1250	1000	304	190

*Breast Composition Assumed: 50% Glandular and 50% Adipose

Breast Thickness Assumed: 3 cm for 35 kVp, 6 cm for 40 kVp, 8 cm for 45 kVp and 10 cm for 50 kVp

Rad/R Factors Assumed: Glandular Tissue 0.8 (Reference 1)
Adipose Tissue 0.5 (Reference 1)

361

REFERENCES

1. Hammerstein,G.R., Miller, D.W. White, D.R., Masterson, M.E., Woodard, H.Q. and Laughlin, J.S.: Radiation absorbed dose in mammography. Radiology (In Press).

2. Morgan, R.H. and Nickoloff, E.: Depth dose data for mammography presented at NCI Workshop, Bethesda, Maryland Aug. 8-9, 1978.

3. Cohen, M., Jones, D.E.A. and Greene D.: Central axis depth dose data for use in radiotherapy. Brit. J. Radiol., Suppl. 11, 1972.

4. NCRP Handbook 33: Medical x-ray and gamma-ray protection for energies up to 10 MeV-Equipment design and use.

5. Dubuque, G.L., Cacak, R.K. and Hendee, H.R.: Backscatter factors in the mammographic range. Medical Physics, Vol. 4, No. 5, 397-399, 1977.

ACKNOWLEDGMENTS

This research was funded by Grant 7R01 FDO 1004-01 from the U.S. Department of Health, Education and Welfare.

Our thanks are due to Miss Inez Wasicki for her secretarial assistance.

SYSTEM SPECIFICATIONS FOR REDUCED DOSE MAMMOGRAPHY

Melvin P. Siedband
University of Wisconsin

ABSTRACT :

In order to take advantage of the newer methods of exposure reduction, the design of mammographic systems must incorporate certain elements. These include constant potential operation, selection of beam filters, small focus tubes, very low off-focus radiation, proper geometry and proper patient positioning. At this time, few, if any, commercial machines have all of these necessary features. Many commercial machines are so designed that modification to incorporate these features is impractical. In other cases, the use of simple filtering capacitor circuits, tube replacement and the modification of key mechanical parts can result in significant improvements of image quality and reduction of exposure to the patient. The use of purchasing specifications to list immediate requirements and anticipate future developments can assure the radiologist of high quality images at low levels of exposure.

ELEMENTARY NOISE CONSIDERATIONS

During the early years of television when new types of television camera tubes were being developed, the ultimate sensitivity of camera tubes was a subject of intensive research. The development of night vision tubes and the x-ray image intensifier followed closely the development of the new camera tubes. Psycho-physical experiments, such as those performed by Coltman[1] and Rose[2] and others[3], demonstrated the existence of a photon limit, that is, the number of photons required to produce a particular image. If the light level falls below a certain bound, there is no way to produce an image without errors of perception. The writer developed an approximation formula for the number of photons required per image[4] and, thus, the minimum exposure per image in the diagnostic range, based on the experiments of Coltman and extended this to a simple formula useful for estimating minimum exposure requirements to produce a conventional radiographic image, given the contrast and pixel size. While this formula has not been modified to give correct values in mammography, it is shown because the basic principles are still correct.

$$R/EXP \simeq \frac{2 \times 10^{-7}}{\left(\begin{array}{c}\text{Detection}\\\text{Efficiency}\end{array}\right)\left(\text{Radiolucency}\right)\left(\begin{array}{c}\text{Pixel}\\\text{dia. in mm}\end{array}\right)^2 \left(\text{Contrast} -0.05\right)^2}$$

The general exposure requirements are related to the inverse square of the contrast. As the contrast approaches say 5%, exposure rises dramatically. If the resolution requirements are doubled, the exposure requirements are quadrupled. If the quantum detection efficiency is increased, exposure requirements are decreased. Because exposure requirements increase so dramatically for objects near the assumed visibility limit of 5%, image contrast is of paramount importance. Efforts to reduce extra focal radiation will increase the transmitted beam modulation and means for the reduction of scatter detected by the film-screen combination are almost always worth the effort.

It might seem possible to operate below a noise threshold by spatial filtration means. In general, such techniques involve the use of circuits or optical filters tuned-in to particular features of the image. Such circuits resonate with portions of the image to complete that image feature. For example, if the image of three-fourths of a circle appears, the circuit completes the circle. Unfortunately, such circuits for spatial filtering may also draw circles when the image of random noise is presented to them. A spatial filter tuned in to gallstones, when set to the highest sensitivity, will proclaim every patient the victim of gallstones.

A four quadrant Bayes analysis of any image anomaly can be made.[5,6] An event is called true, given that it is true, or an event is called false, given that it is false and those two diagnoses will be correct. But an event can also be called false given that it is true, in which case the diagnosis is called a false-negative; or the event can be called true, given that it is actually false, in which case the event is called a false-positive. It is not enough to obtain images of reasonable clarity and low noise; it is also required that the number of false-positives and false-negatives in sets of such images be held to rather low levels.

As the thickness of the body part increases, the modulation of the trans-mitted x-ray beam by an object of a given size within that body part will decrease, scatter will increase, beam penetration decrease. Since the modula-tion decreases, the contrast of the final image will also decrease. The fluctuation number of the background photons caused by the random or Poisson distribution is equal to the square root of the mean number of background photons per pixel and can be assumed to be the minimum noise of the system and the modulation of that background a reasonable value for the signal level. Thus, the signal-to-noise ratio will decrease with increasing thickness for constant input exposure levels. Obviously, the radiation level must increase with increasing body part thickness to maintain a constant signal-to-noise ratio. Alternatively, penetration can be increased by raising kVp so that peak signal-to-noise ratio may increase with increased kVp except that modula-tion decreases with increased kVp. Thus, it is apparent that at low energies where the absorption is higher, the modulation of the exit photons is greater; but the number of exit photons is diminished because of the increased absorp-tion. At the higher energies, the number of exit photons increases and the modulation diminishes. It is obvious there is an optimum value of energy as a function of tissue thickness for a given signal-to-noise ratio. Figure 1 shows the results of a simple study[7] showing relative exposure for a constant signal-to-noise as a function of patient thickness for mammography. Operation above or below these values will result in either loss of contrast or excessive patient exposure, particularly for those cases where the image contrast, resolu-tion and noise are far in excess of what is required for a diagnosis with a reasonable probability of false-positive or false-negative results. The key point in the selection of apparatus for reduced dose mammography is that it is certainly possible to get a better picture if patient exposure is increased, but the objective is to obtain an acceptable image at the lowest possible exposure.

BEAM ENERGY DISTRIBUTION

The curve of Figure 1 assumes a monochromatic energy distribution. At present there are only two methods commonly used for obtaining near mono-chromatic energies in the x-ray region. For crystallography, one can direct a beam of x-rays at the surface of a single crystal of known atomic spacing, so that the reflected beam will have a peak in the distribution of wavelengths related to the atomic distances of the lattice. This crystalline "diffraction grating" method can produce very narrow energy distributions of the resulting x-rays of low intensities. Such beams are useful for crystallographic

Figure 1.

Exposure vs Photon Energy.
Note that optimum energy
is a function of the thickness of the breast and that
the value of this optimum is
the same for the two phantoms
studied. This data must be
compared to the energy
response of the detector to
obtain a <u>system</u> optimum.
While close to optimum for
film-screen systems, it is
about 8 keV low for Xerox
systems.

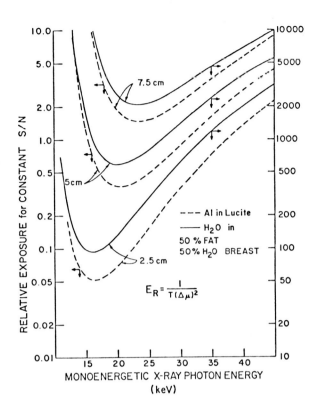

analysis but would require long hours of exposure for taking even the simplest
mammogram due to the low beam intensity.

A second method for producing nearly monochromatic beams would be to use
the k-shell or characteristic radiation of the appropriate anode material
filtered by a thin foil of the same material or of a material of slightly lower
atomic number. In the mammographic range, anodes would have to be chosen to
cover the energy range of 15 keV for thin breasts, to 25 keV for thick breasts,
so that anodes would have to be made of molybdenum, Z=42, through cadmium, Z=48,
to have the range of energies required. Molybdenum was used with molybdenum
foil in many of the earlier systems and produced an image of extremely good
contrast and moderate exposure for thin breasts. Figures 2, 3, and 4 show the
operating characteristics of molybdenum anode tubes with molybdenum foil
filters. The k-alpha radiation appears to dominate the input spectra; however,
the exit spectra of a 5 cm plexiglass phantom shows that the higher energies
are not as well attenuated as the lower energies and can exit to irradiate the
screen.[8,9]

When the screens are designed appropriately, they absorb the higher
energies less efficiently so that the transmitted energy above the k-edge has
a lesser effect than Figure 3 would imply, particularly for the tube operated
at 30 kVp. At 35 kVp, however, the energy above the k-edge dominates so that
the value of such methods for producing high contrast films remains within
acceptable limits only when the tube is operated at low anode potentials. If
the molybdenum anode tube is operated above 35 kVp, the use of the molybdenum
foil filter becomes impractical. It is often thought necessary to operate such
tubes at say 45 kVp, with an aluminum filter as thick as 2 mm (plus the inherent
filtration of the tube assembly) for use with Xerox systems. An unfortunate

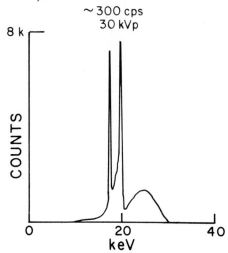

Mo-ANODE TUBE

25μm Mo FILTER + 5cm LUCITE

~300 cps

30 kVp

Figure 2
Mo-Mo, 30 kVp

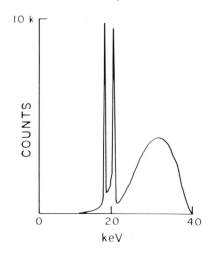

Mo-ANODE TUBE

25μm Mo FILTER + 5cm LUCITE

~1 k cps

40 kVp

Figure 3
Mo-Mo, 40 kVp

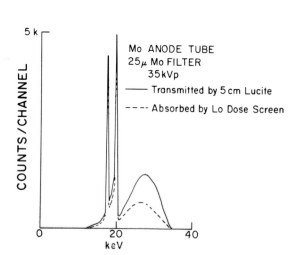

Mo ANODE TUBE
25μ Mo FILTER
35 kVp
—— Transmitted by 5cm Lucite
----- Absorbed by Lo Dose Screen

Figure 4
Mo-Mo, 35 kVp, Screens

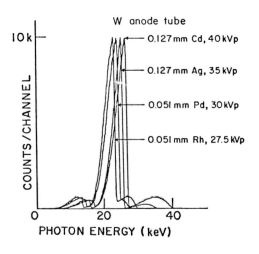

W anode tube

← 0.127mm Cd, 40 kVp

← 0.127mm Ag, 35 kVp

← 0.051mm Pd, 30 kVp

← 0.051mm Rh, 27.5 kVp

Figure 5
W Anode, Thin Foils

effect in using the molybdenum tube under these conditions is that the characteristic radiation is totally absorbed by the patient and contributes nothing to the film.

However, it is possible to use a tungsten anode tube to produce beam energies having a distribution selectable as a function of patient thickness. Figure 5 shows the results of using a tungsten anode x-ray tube with filters of rhodium, palladium, silver and cadmium. When necessary to use the tungsten anode tube up to 55 kVp with an aluminum filter, high levels of characteristic radiation (the k-shell binding energy of tungsten is about 68 keV) are not present so that there is a significant reduction of patient exposure when compared to a molybdenum tube in the same energy range. Further, the bremsstrahlung output of the x-ray tube is proportional to the atomic number of the anode material so that tungsten (Z=74) will have a greater output than molybdenum (Z=42). The increased output of the tungsten anode tube per unit of energy in the form of electrons impinging at the anode means that the tungsten anode tube can have a smaller focal spot or that exposures can be made in a shorter time.

As Figure 6 illustrates, a filter of aluminum can be used with the tungsten anode tube to produce a relatively narrow energy distribution. However, when the aluminum is sufficiently thick to produce a narrow energy distribution, the anode may be severely loaded in that the overall efficiency of x-ray production is far less than that achievable with a thin metal foil filter having its k-edge below the energy corresponding to the voltage applied to the anode of the x-ray tube. The advantage of the thin metal foil filters is not only that they produce narrow energy distributions of the beam to the patient, but that they do so with a higher level of efficiency than the conventional aluminum filters so that the tubes may be operated more efficiently, focal spots can be smaller, and exposure times reduced.

In a broad energy distribution, the lower energies are mostly absorbed-- some are transmitted very well modulated. The higher energies are mostly transmitted rather poorly modulated. Thus, lower patient exposures can be achieved with narrow energy distributions.

The energy distribution is also a function of the anode voltage waveform. Figure 7 shows a tungsten anode x-ray tube operated at constant potential and operated with unfiltered single phase rectified voltage pulses. Because of the fraction of time that the lower voltages are applied to the x-ray tube, there is an increase in the low energy radiation exiting the tube. Since this is absorbed by the patient, there is an obvious increase in the patient exposure. Further, bremsstrahlung production is proportional to the square of the voltage applied to the x-ray tube, but anode dissipation is linear with that voltage. Efficiency of x-ray production is also diminished for single-phase full-wave rectified operation when compared to constant potential operation. In the diagnostic range at 80 kVp at 1 meter, the output of constant potential machines is about 6.5 mR/mAs, and for single-phase machines, about 4.0 mR/mAs. In the mammographic range, for close-spaced tubes (referring to the distance between cathode and anode) of tubes specifically designed for mammography, the output and energy distribution are affected as described. However, when conventional or wide-spaced tubes are used in the mammographic range, e.g., the situation when using a conventional overhead tube for both general radiography and mammography (by removing the filter), the electron beam emission of the tube is reduced during that fraction of the time when the anode voltage is at the lower portion of the sine wave cycle. However, as in the case of all single phase generators, there will be a significant reduction of output permitted from such tubes simply because of the unequal distribution around the periphery of the

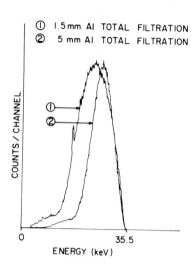

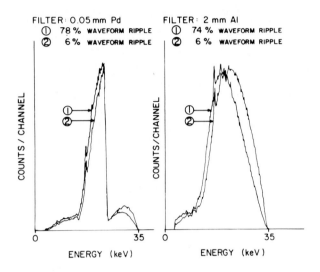

Figure 6   Figure 7

rotating anode. Such reductions of efficiency force the designer to use substantially larger focal spot dimensions than would otherwise be the case for polyphase or constant potential operation of the tubes.

The compromise in the design of low exposure mammographic systems is made between tube loading (therefore, focal spot size and exposure times), energy distribution of the beam and the characteristics of the required filter. The use of other than constant potential applied to the anode of the tube will broaden the energy distribution and cause an increase of tube loading for the same output. It is essential for efficient operation that only constant potentials be used, obtained by means of polyphase x-ray generators or by the use of single-phase systems with filter capacitors to smooth the voltage waveform applied to the anode.

SCATTER AND OFF FOCUS RADIATION

Measurement of the ratio of scattered to primary radiation in the mammographic range shows little dependence on kVp.[10] As kVp increases, the probability of occurrence of a Compton scattered photon increases as photo-electric absorption decreases and beam penetration increases at almost the same rate as the production of scattered photons. For a point on the base of a test object located in the center of the beam, primary radiation to that point will remain constant while scattered radiation reaching that point will increase in proportion to the diameter of the beam until such time as the diameter is equal to the thickness of the test object (this is a useful approximation). When the detector is in close contact with the object, the effect of scattered radiation and the resulting degradation of image contrast can be minimized by compression and by minimizing the field diameter.

The wavelength change of a Compton scattered photon is given by $\Delta\lambda = 0.241$ $(1 - \cos\theta)$ Å. For a mean arriving photon energy of 25 keV and a scattering angle of 30°, the maximum energy loss is only 1.5 keV, far less than the width of the energy distribution of the arriving beam in most cases. Since in the center of the beam, the scattering angle is usually less than 30° to that point, the energy loss of a single Compton scatter reaction will be less than 1.5 keV. For that reason, energy discrimination methods as a means for the reduction of scatter have not been very successful. Such methods considered the use of special phosphors or filters involving k-edge discrimination techniques as part of the detection mechanism. The use of grids as a means for the reduction of scatter based on the geometry of the system, the scattered photons are not paraxial with the primary beam, has had a better measure of success. However, the interspacing material of grids, when made of aluminum, offers increased attenuation so that patient exposure must be increased to compensate. A 3 mm grid using aluminum interspace material will attenuate the beam about four times. Fiber interspaced grids attenuate the primary beam far less than the aluminum, but so far the fiber interspaced grids do not have the homogeneity and uniformity of the aluminum grids and may produce image artifacts. Stationary grids show harmonic patterns when the spatial frequency of the grid corresponds to that of the striae or spicules in the image. The use of moving grids results in magnification due to the necessity of space for mechanical apparatus. Scanning slit devices have similar and additional problems. The benefit of the scanning slit results only when two slits are used, one to form the sheet beam, and the second to act as a focal plane shutter in order to exclude scattered radiation from outside of that volume of tissue being surveyed at a given instant. Without the focal plane shutter-slit, the time integral of a slit scanned image is exactly the same as that of a single "flash" exposure. Slit techniques offer the possibility of a great reduction of exposure but increase the burden on the tube anode; the tube loading must increase by the ratio of slit width to field diameter. Since the scattered radiation reaching a point is related to the solid angle of irradiated tissue volume subtended by that point, increasing the distance between the detector and the volume of tissue irradiated is an effective way of reducing the scattered radiation reaching that point without affecting the primary beam. Such techniques, variously called magnification or air gap techniques, also place a burden on the tube in that only small focal spots can be used for this purpose. Considering the air gap or magnification technique using the same terminology often used in radiology, that is, in terms of K, the contrast improvement factor, and B, the bucky factor, versus magnification for the geometry shown, we see a significant increase in contrast improvement factor up to a magnification of about 1.3 times as shown in Figure 8. A further increase

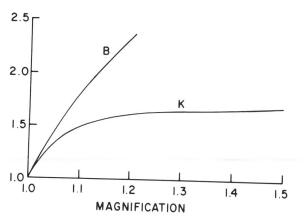

Figure 8.

Contrast Improvement Factor K, and Bucky Factor B vs Magnification (FFD 70 cm, Field 12 cm dia.).

369

in magnification results in no further real improvement. However, the exposure must continue to increase to result in the same film darkening. However, consideration of resolution-sensitometry relationships for film means that a lower resolution film could be substituted, images optically reduced for the same visual characteristic for ever-increasing magnifications, another way of saying that no further improvement results. A practical mammographic system to maximize contrast should be designed to permit a modest amount of image magnification, not for magnification per se, but magnification to have the capability for the improvement of image contrast.

Off-focus radiation is defined as x-radiation appearing from within the x-ray tube from a point other than the defined focal spot. The principal cause of off-focus radiation is the poor geometry of the primary electron beam source.* Many x-ray tubes use a simple tungsten filament mounted in a trough. The trough serves the same purpose as the reflector of a common headlight bulb. Electrons from the front side of the filament and from the rear side of the filament are focused to form a sheet or two adjacent sheets of electrons which strike the anode to produce a single line or a pair of adjacent lines of impact at the surface of the anode. Since the anode is angled, from the point of view of the patient these lines of impact are foreshortened and form the "line focused focal spot." However, as many as 30% of the primary electrons are simply projected in the general direction of the anode, where they are equally effective in producing x-radiation as the line focused sheet beam of electrons. For rotating anode x-ray tubes, it is possible for x-rays produced by these off-focus electrons to exit the tube port if not properly masked. For simple fixed-anode x-ray tubes, a shield structure around the tungsten insert can reduce the efficiency of off-focus x-ray production and so reduce the magnitude of the off-focus radiation, or the shape of the anode itself can mask the off-focus radiation so that it cannot exit the tube. If the anode is made in the shape of a needle or fine point, the primary electrons can only land at the point of the needle causing it to incandesce and produce a beam with almost no off-focus radiation. Needles are small and the rating of such tubes is very low. Such tubes have been made by the Comet Corp. and used by Westinghouse in the Panoramix generator and have measured foci of .07 mm dia. but have a maximum rating of only 75 watts and maximum exposure times of 2 seconds. For rotating anode x-ray tubes, it is important that a lead cone be fitted into the tube port to restrict the exit angle of the x-ray beam to that portion of the anode containing the line focused focal spot. Adjustable collimators must have lead fingers or an iris diaphragm fitted into the tube port. For dedicated mammographic systems, the use of the fitted lead cone is superior to the adjustable collimator.

Until recently, experiments on x-ray tubes having oxide coated filaments or other cathode structures other than a pure tungsten helix were not very successful. Positive ion bombardment caused by the ionization of residual gas in the tube by the electron beam limited the tube life. Arcing within the tube caused by the inductive effects of the high voltage transformer and the discharge of the energy stored in the cable capacity destroyed flimsy metal structures used for beam shaping and trimming. However, new tubes

* There exists some controversy over the cause of off-focus radiation. It is not caused by the action of secondary electrons. The production of secondary electrons uses the energy of the primary electrons. The average energy of the secondary (or back scatter) is less than a third of that of the primary beam electrons.[11],[12] Since measurements of the energy distribution of the off-focus radiation show almost the same values as the radiation from the focal spot, the off focus radiation cannot be caused by secondary or back scattered electrons.

have recently appeared which use various beam trimming structures so that the "floodlight" to "spotlight" ratio of the electron beam is reduced, resulting in a corresponding decrease in the off-focus radiation output of such tubes.

SYSTEM GEOMETRY

We can make several assumptions about the distribution of objects within the breast. The first assumption will be that objects of interest can occur at any point within the breast so that the limiting resolution of the system must be defined as the worst resolution measured at any point within the breast. When the ratio of distance between the focal spot to distal surface of the breast and focal spot to proximal surface of the breast is very large, inverse square law considerations dictate that surface exposure must increase by the square of that ratio. This is illustrated in Figure 9. Systems having small focus film distances, therefore, necessarily result in higher patient exposure and will have variations of resolving power for objects at different levels within the breast. Obviously, systems of low FFD should not be used. If we establish the arbitrary criterion that the ratio of exposure should result in a less than 20% increase, then a minimum FFD for a 5 cm thick breast under compression should be 50 cm, and for a larger breast under slight compression, 75 cm would be a more practical value.

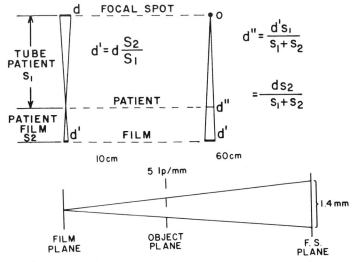

Figure 9.

Focal spot effect on estimate of the MTF of the focal spot:

$$MTF = 1 - \frac{S_2 a}{0.7\,S_1}$$

where a is the nominal dimension of the focal spot.

An easy mnemonic for the effect of tube focal spot size is to project from a point on the detector surface through one line pair in the plane of interest of the object to the plane of the focal spot. When so projected, so that one line pair within the object exactly matches the linear dimension of the focal spot then that object just disappears in the image plane. For example, let us assume we wish to image objects of 0.1 mm diameter, 0.1 mm apart in the breast, and let us assume that the system geometry is such that there is a 10 cm distance between that plane of the object and the film and a 60 cm distance between that plane of the object and the focal spot in the tube. Then the projected image of the 0.1 mm object and the 0.1 mm space in the plane of the focal spot is (0.1 + 0.1) x 7 so that a tube having a focal spot diameter of 1.4 mm would just _not_ resolve those objects. A 1.0 to 1.2 mm focal spot tube (actual size) would, however, resolve them. On the other hand, suppose it is desired to image such that the distal surface of the breast must be magnified 20% in order to reduce the effects of scatter and the breast is 7.5 cm in thickness, then the 70 cm system would require a focal spot of 0.67 mm to just _not_ resolve the objects, or a practical focal spot of less than 0.5 mm actual size. It must be pointed out that actual sizes of small focus x-ray tubes in their largest dimension are about double the nominal values. Thus, in the previous example, to be able to resolve objects of 0.1 mm in diameter throughout the breast for the geometry described would require a nominal focal spot of 0.3 mm or smaller. If the focal spot is made much smaller than this, the tube loading limitations would mean that exposure times would have to increase so that patient motion may be a problem in image resolution.

TUBES AND GENERATORS

In order to accommodate the requirements of narrow energy distribution, matching the required distribution to breast thickness for a minimizing exposure versus thickness and minimizing tube loading, x-ray generators which provide constant anode potential during the exposure are most practical. Another consideration of x-ray tube design for operation in the mammographic range is concerned with the filament structure. Filament emission is described by the limiting effects of two equations, the Richardson-Dushman equation, and the equation of Childs law. Figure 10 illustrates these effects.

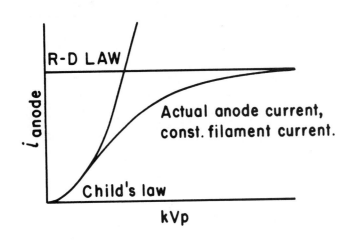

Figure 10.

Richardson Dushman:

$$J_1 = A_1 T^2 e^{-u/kT}$$

Childs Law:

$$J_2 = A_2 V^{3/2} / d^2$$

J is current density,
T is filament temp.,
V is anode voltage,
d is anode-cathode dist.

Conventional x-ray tubes are temperature limited diodes, so that a given filament setting should produce almost the same output current independently of variations of kVp. It is imperfect so as the kVp is changed at the x-ray generator, a compensating current is added in the filament circuit to maintain constant anode current. In the diagnostic range, the magnitude of this "space-charge compensation" is small. When wide-spaced tubes are used in the mammographic range, the tubes are far more sensitive to small changes of kVp than in the diagnostic range. In many cases, small focus wide-spaced tubes will not have adequate emission at normal filament temperatures in the mammographic range. For that reason, the use of fractional focus tubes shared between mammography and conventional radiography may be limited by filament emission at low anode kVp's, and is often impractical. Reducing the spacing between anode cathode to two-thirds of its wide-spaced value will permit operation at reasonable values of filament emission down to about 28 kVp. However, the reduced spacing puts a high voltage limit on such tubes of about 110 kVp and so limits performance in the diagnostic range. However, such tubes exist and are a practical compromise.

In chest radiography, automatic exposure termination or phototiming (phototiming used here is not limited to those circuits involving photomultiplier tubes, but is broadened to include all methods of automatically terminating the photographic exposure including ion chambers, solid state devices,

scintillation pickups, etc.) is a necessary circuit element because the fraction
of air space relative to patient thickness may not be known in a particular
patient. Wide variations of exposure to produce an image of a given density
are anticipated. For mammography, a trained operator can observe the differences in density of the breast by palpation and a simple scale to determine
thickness permits an operator to set the machine with assurance that films
will be of proper density. Phototiming sensors placed between the patient and
the detector will result in some attenuation of the beam. Phototiming detectors
placed after the image detector are subject to vagaries of performance as a
result of variations in beam attenuation by the detecting system. Additionally,
the energy response of the phototiming detector may be different from that of
the imaging detector and must be compensated in the circuitry. While phototiming detectors can be made to function quite well, the range of application
may be narrow and they must be used carefully.

Tungsten anode x-ray tubes must be used. Figure 11 compares the operation
of systems using a tungsten tube and 0.5 mm of aluminum filtration with operation with 1 mm and 5 mm of aluminum, and 1 and 2 thicknesses of palladium
foil. These computer-determined measurements have been spot-checked by means
of measurements on a phantom and illustrate the effects on tube loading,
patient exposure and image contrast. A figure of merit, exposure divided by
the square of the contrast, is minimized for the best system. However, the
limitations of tube loading must also be considered. Examination of the
tabulated data demonstrates the value of one or two thicknesses of palladium
foil when used at the appropriate anode voltage.

kVp	Filtration	Entrance Exp. $(mR-Cm^2)$	E/E_{Ref}	C/C_{Ref}	W/W_{Ref}	E/C^2
25	0.5 mm Al	2.561×10^7				1.179×10^{-8}
	1 mm Al	1.694	0.661	0.986	1.276	0.802
	5 mm Al	1.262	0.493	0.913	34.04	0.697
	0.075 mm Pd	1.474	0.576	0.983	4.120	0.702
	0.038 mm Pd	1.671	0.652	1.006	1.436	0.760
30	0.5 mm Al	2.100				2.073
	1 mm Al	1.849	0.880	0.982	1.462	1.881
	5 mm Al	1.347	0.641	0.888	14.64	1.685
	0.075 mm Pd	1.478	0.704	1.338	4.940	0.814
	0.038 mm Pd	1.713	0.816	1.235	1.950	1.104
35	0.5 mm Al	1.803				3.196
	1 mm Al	1.574	0.873	0.979	1.557	2.790
	5 mm Al	1.416	0.647	0.868	9.633	3.334
	0.075 mm Pd	1.265	0.702	1.386	5.098	1.168
	0.038 mm Pd	1.564	0.867	1.141	2.355	2.128
40	0.5 mm Al	1.596				4.506
	1 mm Al	1.387	0.869	0.977	1.244	4.101
	5 mm Al	1.167	0.731	0.852	6.02	4.101
	0.075 mm Pd	1.167	0.787	1.147	6.60	2.697
	0.038 mm Pd	1.543	0.967	1.017	2.75	4.212

Inherent Filtration: 0.5 mm Al in W-tube.
Phantom: 5 cm lucite with 50 mg cm^{-2} Ca as contrast.
Equal energy at detector.

Ref (0.5 mm Al).

Figure 11

SPECIFICATION OF THE SYSTEM

Before purchasing an x-ray system for mammography, consideration must be given to whether a dedicated system will be used or whether an overhead tube or other apparatus will be time-shared. Will the system be used for research? Will it be used with Xerox detectors or film screen detectors? Can the necessary modifications of anode waveform, beam filtration, reduction of off-focus radiation and patient positioning be accommodated in the proposed system? Is apparatus on hand to make frequent checks of equipment performance, patient exposure and proper use of apparatus by the technologists? Are phantoms available to evaluate the system to be certain that optimum operating conditions are used to minimize patient exposure and to maximize image contrast and to produce films of the highest diagnostic quality? In examining prospective suppliers, will they have service available in the area and is a product specialist available at the manufacturer's home office from whom good consulting advice can be obtained? Will the apparatus be used for other purposes than mammography? For example, studies of the peripheral bones can also be made on mammographic apparatus because of the need for high resolution and the relative thinness of body parts being examined. Is there a need for special requirements such as specimen analysis or other research activities? When all the considerations of this type have been listed, then a specification can be written for the purchase of the apparatus. The specification should define the apparatus, where it is to be used, when it is to be installed, the responsibilities of the institution and the supplier regarding shielding, electrical and physical requirements. A certain fraction of the purchase price should be withheld until the unit has been inspected to some recognized standard of performance. Penalty clauses are a two-edged sword; the supplier may add an insurance factor to his bid costs if the performance penalties are excessive. A rail strike, failure of one of his suppliers to deliver or the random failure of a critical component can delay the installation. It is best to pick a supplier of good reputation and not have to rely on penalty clauses. The apparatus can be defined in terms of the needs of the institution. It is a sound idea to consult with several suppliers prior to writing the specifications, and further to write the specifications in such a way that suppliers can offer what is requested and yet offer optionally items which they feel may improve the configuration of the apparatus and its use. An example used at the University of Wisconsin is listed below.

MAMMOGRAPHIC X-RAY SYSTEM (Example Only - Conventional Mammo)

I. General

This specification describes a mammographic x-ray system consisting of a close-spaced tungsten anode tube, special cones, cassette and film holders, rotating support arm, positioning apparatus, generator and filter holders. The supplier will inspect the room plan of the hospital and propose necessary modifications to assure proper installation and adequate working areas. The hospital will be responsible for the preparation of the room including shielding, electrical and physical requirements. Minimum requirements are listed. Exceptions may be allowed and should be described by bidders. Complete service instructions and manuals will be provided. All apparatus will meet the standards of BRH-DHEW and UL. The bidder will list all items not listed in this specification but obvious and required, e.g., x-ray cables, control boxes, power supplies. The hospital will be the sole judge of acceptability and may accept/reject all or part of proposals submitted. Bidders must indicate whether items proferred meet these specifications or list exceptions and/or alternative items. The hospital reserves the right to withhold payment of 20% of the total amount until all items have been accepted, tested to reasonable standards of performance (e.g., proposed AAPM, BRH or University of Wisconsin methods) to limit listed in this specification.

In the event of award, the bidder will provide information on technical changes, improvements, cost of such "updates" and other information of use to users of this type of apparatus.

II. X-Ray Generator

General Ratings: 55 kVp/200 mA max., 25 kVp/50 mA min., 0.5 kVp adj., 50/100/200 mA (selection of focal spot), capacitor smoothing, filter interlock, standard speed anode rotation.

A. Power Input: 208/220 VAC, 60 Hz, 60 A. (may be 2 Ø of 3 Ø line). Safety ground. 100 A mains. 2.5% V.R.

B. kVp Range: 25 to 49 and 25 to 55 (filter interlocks).

C. Timing: 0.1, 0.2, 0.3, 0.4, 0.6, 0.8, 1.0, 1.25, 1.5, 2.0, 2.5, 3.0 sec.

D. Tube Current: 50 S, 100 S or L, 200 L mA.

E. Tube Protection: If the factors chosen are outside the rating, an "overload" light will be energized, the generator will be interlocked so that an exposure cannot be made. The protection circuits must permit operation above 85% of single exposure tube KWP ratings and not above 100%.

F. Filament Boost: Tube filament must be such that emission will be below 3% of set anode current if anode voltage were applied rotor on-time plus 2.0 seconds.

G. Rotor Start: 60 Hz, starting voltage to permit 1.0 sec start time; run voltage to be less than 65 VAC.

H. X-Ray Tube: The tube will be a close-spaced 100 mm dia. anode tube having small focus less than 0.3 mm nom. and large focus between 0.6 and 0.8 mm nom.

I. Collimator and Cones: The collimator assembly will be supplied with 6 cones: 100 x 70 mm, 140 x 95 mm, 185 x 120 mm, 235 x 155 mm, 54 mm dia. and a compression cone of 180 x 300 mm (to be specified after installation and 30 days use). Filter tray to permit the use of 5 types of beam filters with interlock to the generator. Small proximal cone must be used in tube port to reduce OFR.

J. Voltage Filter: A capacitor of 0.25 to 0.50 mfd rated 60 k VDC with impedance limitations and protective bleeder resistors will be incorporated in the tube cathode lead. This will cause a fixed mR/mAs error as a function of kVp at all timing stations equivalent to an exposure of less than 5 mAs at any kVp.

III. Positioning Apparatus

General Description: Isocentric arm assembly on telescopic tube attached to floor to ceiling suspension. Controls for locks, field illuminator, distance scales, cassette (film and Xerox) holders and breast compressor will be provided. The cassette holder must swing away for recumbant (table) use.

A. Tubestand Movements:

1. Rotational: + 90° min
2. Compression: 20 cm excursion (min), flat, up to 10 kg force
3. Film plane at 0°: 60 to 100 cm (from floor)
4. Tilt (toward/away from patient): + 10°
5. Lateral (along the wall for storage): + 120 cm.

Note: Except for lateral motion, indicating scales are required, 70 cm min. FFD.

B. Receptor Holders:

1. Film-Screen in plastic envelopes, Kodak or Plastilix Cassettes
2. Provision for use of moving grids (future)
3. Xerox Cassettes
4. Swing-away feature (recumbant patient)

C. Cone Holder and Tube Mount:

1. Provision for 5 filters (supplied by U.W.H.)
2. Slide-in or other illuminator
3. Port coning (to match largest field)
4. Control of locks
5. Cone holders (See II-I) with interlocks

D. Patient Chair:

An hydraulic chair similar to (supplier name) will be provided.

IV. Special Note

This system will be used for clinical work and must incorporate certain features developed in the course of research programs at U.W. Essential items are:

1. Close control of kVp and mA.
2. Use of special beam filters as a function of breast size.
3. Near-constant potential.
4. Use of small focus tube with tungsten anode.
5. Reduction of off-focus radiation.
6. Reduction of exposure to patients.
7. High repeatibility and reliability.
8. Interchangeable components for film-screen, film, Xerox cassettes.
9. Use of experimental grids.
10. Production of outstanding radiographs.

ACKNOWLEDGEMENTS

The work of graduate students, Cupido Daniels, in making many of the measurements and determinations of equipment performance, and David L. Ergun, in the development of a computer program for determination of tube loading, patient exposure, and image contrast is acknowledged. Their work was vital in the studies of tube and circuit performance in mammography. The assistance and advice of Dr. Raul Matallana in reviewing films prepared with these new methods and his demonstrated faith in purchasing a unit designed to meet the specification is also appreciated.

REFERENCES

1. Coltman, J.W., The Scintillation Limit in Fluoroscopy, Scientific Paper #1815, Westinghouse Research Labs., Pittsburgh, PA, 1954 (Also, Radiol. 63:867, 1954).

2. Rose, A., Vision: Human and Electronic, Plenum Publishing Co., New York, 1973.

3. Biberman, L.M., Perception of Displayed Information, Plenum Press, New York, 1974.

4. Siedband, M.P., Holden, J.E., Medical Imaging Systems (from Medical Instrumentation, Webster, Ed.), Houghton Mifflin, Boston, 1978.

5. Goodenough, D.J., et al, Radiographic Applications of Receiver Operating Characteristic (ROC) Curves, Radiology 110:89, 1973.

6. Feller, W., An Introduction to Probability Theory and Applications, Wiley, New York, 1968.

7. Siedband, M.P., Improvement of X-Ray Contrast (Final Report NCI Contract NO1-CB-53914), Medical Physics, U.W. Medical School, Madison, WI, Feb. 1978.

8. Siedband, M.P., Jennings, R.J., Eastgate, R.J., Ergun, D.L., X-Ray Beam Filters for Mammography, SPIE Conf., Boston, October 1977 (Vol. 127, Optical Inst. in Med. IV).

9. Siedband, M.P., Beam Filtration in Diagnostic Radiology, NBS Symposium on Real-Time Radiologic Imaging, Gaithersburg, MD, May 1978.

10. Barnes, G.T., Brezovich, I.A., Contrast-Effect of Scattered Radiation (from Breast Carcinoma, Logan, Ed.), Wiley, New York, 1977.

11. Sternglass, E.J., Backscattering of Kilovolt Electrons from Solids, Phys. Rev., Vol. 95, No. 2, 345-358, July 1954.

12. Darlington, E.H., Backscattering of 10-100 keV Electrons from Thick Targets, J. Phys. D: Appl. Phys., Vol. 8, 1975.

CONTROLLED EVALUATIONS OF IMAGE QUALITY AND DIAGNOSTIC ACCURACY OF LOW-DOSE MAMMOGRAPHY SCREEN-FILM SYSTEMS

Edward A. Sickles, M.D.
Department of Radiology
University of California School of Medicine
San Francisco, CA 94143

In 1973 the DuPont Lo-dose screen-film system was introduced, to offer a lower-dose alternative to both xeromammography and direct exposure film mammography (1,2). More recently, several new mammography screen-film combinations have been developed, purporting to allow for further reduction in radiation dose without substantial degradation of image properties.

We designed a clinical study to choose the optimal screen-film combination for use in our mammography suite, i.e., that combination which allowed for the highest accuracy of diagnostic interpretation at the lowest radiation dose. First we conducted parallel laboratory and clinical studies to compare the image quality (resolution, noise, contrast) of four lower-dose recording systems to DuPont Lo-dose (3). The second portion of the study evaluated the abilities of the various recording systems to portray the clinically relevant features of the mammographic image: visibility of breast architecture, mass lesions, calcifications, and most importantly, overall accuracy of diagnostic interpretation (4). This paper is based on the data from both image quality and clinical evaluations, and emphasizes the interrelationships between the physical and anatomic properties of the mammographic image.

MATERIALS AND METHODS

The five screen-film combinations tested are listed in Table I. Each was loaded into light-tight plastic envelopes from which almost all the air was then evacuated to ensure intimate and uniform screen-film contact. All radiographs were taken by the same technologist using the same x-ray tube (CGR Senographe, which has a molybdenum anode, beryllium window, 30 μm molybdenum filtration, and a nominal focal spot size of 0.8 mm). All exposures were taken at a 33 cm focus-film distance, using 35 kVp and 0.4 sec. Only the tube current (mA) was adjusted, to allow for differences in object thickness and density. The first half-value layer under these conditions is 0.35 mm Al. All films were developed in the same Kodak X-omat automatic processor (91° F, 24 sec immersion time, Kodak chemistry). Radiation exposure (entrance skin dose) was measured for the first 40 patients by thermoluminescent dosimetry, using polyethylene capsules containing lithium fluoride (Radiation Detection Co., Sunnyvale, CA); absorbed dose was calculated according to the method of Hammerstein et al (5).

Table I. Screen-Film Combinations Tested

Screen	Film	Name of Combination
DuPont Lo-dose	DuPont Lo-dose	Lo-dose
DuPont Lo-dose-2	DuPont Lo-dose	Lo-dose-2
Kodak SO-299	Kodak SO-442	Min-R
Kodak SO-299	Kodak SO-179	Min-R/Nuclear Medicine
3M Alpha-4	Kodak SO-442	Alpha-4/Min-R

We studied 100 consecutive patients undergoing routine mammography, which we perform for a variety of indications from suspected cancer to baseline examination. After completion of conventional mammography (with DuPont Lo-dose) informed consent was obtained and four additional craniocaudal projection mammograms were taken of one breast, using each of the lower-dose screen-film combinations. Generally we selected the breast which was more symptomatic or which appeared more abnormal on the Lo-dose mammograms. Clinical evaluations were then performed on the five craniocaudal projection mammograms from each patient. All interpretations were done in single-blind fashion, with two radiologists working independently, neither knowing the identity of the screen-film combinations or the patients whose mammograms they were interpreting (films were evaluated in random order, with all distinguishing features removed). All films were interpreted under standard viewing conditions, including the use of a 2X magnifying lens. Criteria for evaluation are listed in Table II.

Table II. Criteria for Evaluation (Random-Order Interpretation)

Physical Parameters	Anatomical Parameters
Overall Film Quality - Optimal - Adequate - Poor, but diagnostic - Unacceptable	Internal Breast Architecture (breast tissue, blood vessels, trabeculae) - Optimally visualized - Adequately visualized - Poorly visualized, but diagnostic - Not visualized

Film Density
- Optimal
- Adequate
- Poor, but diagnostic
   Too dark or too light
- Unacceptable
   Too dark or too light
	Skin - Nipple - Areola
	- Optimally visualized
	- Adequately visualized
	- Poorly visualized, but diagnostic
	- Not visualized

Noise (mottle) - No noise visible - Minimal noise - Noisy, but does not interfere with diagnosis - Noise interferes with diagnosis	Breast Mass(es) - Optimally visualized - Adequately visualized - Poorly visualized, but diagnostic - Not visualized

Contrast
- Optimal
- Adequate
- Poor, but diagnostic
   Too gray or too black/white
- Unacceptable
   Too gray or too black/white
	Breast Macrocalcifications (1 mm +)
	- Optimally visualized
	- Adequately visualized
	- Poorly visualized, but diagnostic
	- Not visualized
	Also count # macrocalcifications seen

Detail (resolution) - Optimal - Adequate - Poor, but does not interfere with diagnosis - Lack of detail, interferes with diagnosis	Breast Microcalcifications (<1 mm) - Optimally visualized - Adequately visualized - Poorly visualized, but diagnostic - Not visualized Also count # microcalcifications seen Diagnosis - Benign - Equivocal - Malignant

The second phase of the study involved evaluation-by-rank of all the films. The random order of screen-film combinations was maintained, but the five films from each patient were grouped together for ranking, using the parameters listed in Table II, and according to criteria ranging from "best visualized" (rank 1) to "most poorly visualized" (rank 5). For rankings of image quality, rank 1 represented least noise, most contrast, and greatest resolution (detail).

RESULTS

DOSIMETRY

Thermoluminescent dosimetry documented a twofold-to-threefold reduction in radiation dose for each of the new, faster screen-film combinations, as shown in Table III. Our measurements for the Lo-dose system are in close agreement with those reported elsewhere, using the same x-ray tube and similar exposure factors (6).

Table III. Measurements of Radiation Dose Per Exposure (40 Consecutive Patients)

Screen-Film Combination	Entrance Skin Dose*	Mid-Breast Dose[†]	Mean Dose to Glandular Tissue[†]
Lo-dose	1.26 R	0.093 rad	0.146 rad
Lo-dose-2	0.64 R	0.047 rad	0.074 rad
Min-R	0.57 R	0.042 rad	0.066 rad
Min-R/Nuc Med	0.52 R	0.039 rad	0.060 rad
Alpha-4/Min-R	0.37 R	0.027 rad	0.043 rad

* Measurement includes backscatter.

† Calculated according to data of Hammerstein et al (5), assuming an average compressed breast thickness of 5 cm and an average breast composition of 50% glandular-50% adipose tissue. Among the various parameters of dose measurement, mean dose to glandular tissue should correlate most closely with radiation risk.

NOISE

Subjective single-blind evaluations of noise were complicated by the presence in some of the mammograms of processor artifacts much more noticeable than the noise pattern itself; however, attempts were made to evaluate noise independent of these processor artifacts. These results are presented in Table IV. The random-order evaluation showed that only a few (6-12%) of the Lo-dose-2 and Min-R system films were judged more noisy than the top-rated Lo-dose system films. However, a substantial number of the Alpha-4/Min-R (36%) and Min-R/ Nuclear Medicine (60%) images were found to have higher levels of noise. Rank evaluation produced results showing the same rank order, with even sharper distinctions among the five screen-film combinations.

Table IV. Subjective Single-Blind Evaluation of Noise (Mottle)

Screen-Film Combination	Random-Order Evaluation			Rank Evaluation*	
	Optimal	Adequate	Poor, but Diagnostic	Mean Rank Score	Rank
Lo-dose	6	92	2	1.06	1
Lo-dose-2	1	96	3	2.11	2
Min-R	1	84	15	3.06	3
Min-R/Nuc Med	0	38	62	4.83	5
Alpha-4/Min-R	0	62	38	3.94	4

* Rank 1 represents least noisy images, rank 5 most noisy images.

CONTRAST

Subjective single-blind evaluations of the 500 mammograms showed the contrast of the five screen-film combinations to be, in increasing order: Lo-dose, Lo-dose-2, Alpha-4/Min-R, Min-R, and Min-R/Nuclear Medicine (Table V). Little difference was found between Lo-dose and Lo-dose-2 systems, and between Min-R and Alpha-4/Min-R systems, suggesting that contrast was more dependent on the type of film than on the screen. The random-order evaluation indicated clinically noticeable differences between the highest-contrast and lowest-contrast combinations in 23% of the films.

Table V. Subjective Single-Blind Evaluation of Contrast

| Screen-Film Combination | Random-Order Evaluation | | | Rank Evaluation* | |
	Optimal	Adequate	Poor, but Diagnostic	Mean Rank Score	Rank
Lo-dose	5	70	25	4.39	5
Lo-dose-2	5	77	18	4.17	4
Min-R	21	72	7	2.22	2
Min-R/Nuc Med	28	67	5	1.56	1
Alpha-4/Min-R	15	76	9	2.67	3

*Rank 1 represents highest contrast; rank 5 lowest contrast.

RESOLUTION

The evaluating radiologists tried as best they could to judge "detail" as resolution alone rather than as a combination of resolution, noise, and contrast. These evaluations, summarized in Table VI, showed similar resolution for all of the screen-film combinations, except for the Alpha-4/Min-R combination, which was judged poorer in 25% of the films in the random-order evaluation. Of the four similarly-rated combinations, Lo-dose was judged to be best.

Table VI. Subjective Single-Blind Evaluation of Resolution (Detail)

| Screen-Film Combination | Random-Order Evaluation | | | Rank Evaluation* | |
	Optimal	Adequate	Poor, but Diagnostic	Mean Rank Score	Rank
Lo-dose	39	55	6	2.44	1
Lo-dose-2	37	56	7	2.89	4
Min-R	36	58	6	2.56	2
Min-R/Nuc Med	35	58	7	2.67	3
Alpha-4/Min-R	15	75	10	4.45	5

* Rank 1 represents greatest resolution (sharpest detail); rank 5 represents poorest resolution (detail least sharp).

NORMAL BREAST STRUCTURES

All five screen-film combinations portrayed the skin, nipple, areola, and internal breast architecture with approximately equal clarity. Random-order and rank evaluations of the visibility of these anatomic structures showed variations in ratings of only 1-4%. The Lo-dose system was rated best in both types of evaluation, although the differences involved were minimal.

BREAST MASSES

Masses were found in 22 of the 100 patients. The masses were identified on all 5 films for 21 of 22 patients. In the case of the remaining patient, the breast mass was located close to the chest wall and was not included on one of the 5 images. Results of the random-order and rank evaluations are shown in Table VII. These data show the differences among Lo-dose, Lo-dose-2, and Min-R systems to be minimal, with slightly poorer ratings for the Alpha-4/Min-R and Min-R/Nuclear Medicine combinations.

Table VII. Subjective Single-Blind Evaluation of Breast Mass Visibility

| Screen-Film Combination | Random-Order Evaluation | | | | Rank Evaluation* | |
	Optimal	Adequate	Poor, but Diagnostic	Not Seen	Mean Rank Score	Rank
Lo-dose	2	14	5	79[+]	1.91	2
Lo-dose-2	3	14	5	78	1.89	1
Min-R	2	15	5	78	2.34	3
Min-R/Nuc Med	0	15	7	78	4.64	5
Alpha 4/Min-R	0	15	7	78	4.22	4

* Rank 1 represents breast mass best visualized; rank 5 represents breast mass most poorly visualized.

+ In one patient, a breast mass located close to the chest wall was not included on the Lo-dose image.

CALCIFICATIONS

Macrocalcifications (1 mm or larger) were identified in 16 of the 100 patients. The same number of calcifications was counted on each of the 5 films for each of these patients, and the random-order and rank evaluation of macro-calcification visibility showed minimal differences among the screen-film combinations.

Slightly more variability was seen in the analysis of microcalcifications (smaller than 1 mm). Three or more calcifications were identified on all 5 films in 36 of the 100 patients. Calcifications were identified on all films for each of these patients, but the counts varied by as much as 6 calcifications among the films of patients with more than 15 microcalcifications. However, overall analysis of calcification counts showed only minor differences among the screen-film combinations. Random-order and rank evaluations of micro-calcification visibility also showed these differences to be small (Table VIII), with the Alpha-4/Min-R combination rated slightly lower than the others.

Table VIII. Subjective Single-Blind Evaluation of Microcalcification Visibility

| Screen-Film Combination | Random-Order Evaluation | | | | Rank Evaluation* | |
	Optimal	Adequate	Poor, but Diagnostic	Not Seen	Mean Rank Score	Rank
Lo-dose	2	27	7	64	2.37	1
Lo-dose-2	0	28	8	64	3.06	4
Min-R	1	28	7	64	2.75	3
Min-R/Nuc Med	0	28	8	64	2.70	2
Alpha-4/Min-R	0	25	11	64	4.12	5

* Rank 1 represents microcalcifications best visualized; rank 5 represents microcalcifications most poorly visualized.

DIAGNOSTIC IMPRESSION

There was striking consistency in the diagnostic impressions of both radiologists for the several films of each patient. These are listed in Table IX. In only one patient was there any difference in final diagnosis among the five screen-film combinations, due to failure to include a spiculated mass, representing carcinoma, on the Lo-dose system film. Pathological proof of diagnosis was obtained for 19 patients. Carcinoma was found in all 8 patients whose mammograms were judged "malignant"; three of these cancers were so small that they could not be palpated by experienced examiners even in retrospect. Four other carcinomas were found, two of which came from patients whose mammograms were read by both radiologists as "equivocal" for malignancy; the other two represented palpable masses that were not detected on any of the films by either radiologist.

Table IX. Random-Order Evaluation of Diagnostic Impression

Screen-Film Combination	Radiologist A			Radiologist B		
	Malignant	Equivocal	Benign	Malignant	Equivocal	Benign
Lo-dose	7*	5	88*	7*	9	84*
Lo-dose-2	8	5	87	8	9	83
Min-R	8	5	87	8	9	83
Min-R/Nuc Med	8	5	87	8	9	83
Alpha-4/Min-R	8	5	87	8	9	83

* In one patient, a spiculated mass located close to the chest wall was not included on the Lo-dose image (see Table VII); therefore, the Lo-dose image was interpreted as "benign" but the other four images were judged "malignant".

DISCUSSION

Recent reports concerning the possible radiation hazards of screening mammography (7,8) have caused great public concern, and a clamor for methods of reduced-dose mammography. One encouraging result of this publicity has been a substantial nationwide dose reduction for both screening and diagnostic mammography examinations (9-11). However, while reduction in radiation dose is a worthwhile goal, we must ensure that decreased dose is not achieved at the expense of the currently high level of diagnostic accuracy.

This prospective, controlled study of low-dose screen-film combinations demonstrates that substantial dose reduction can indeed be obtained without sacrifice in diagnostic accuracy. Although dose reduction is accompanied by slightly poorer resolution and varying amounts of increased noise, as judged subjectively, these minor degradations in image quality are apparently not of sufficient magnitude to interfere with the overall accuracy of diagnostic interpretation.

Comparing results of the image quality and clinical studies, we find that the data from our analyses of breast mass visibility (Table VII) closely parallel those for noise (Table IV), whereas the microcalcification visibility data (Table VIII) are strikingly similar to those found for resolution (Table VI). This is not surprising, since it has been postulated for many years that radiographic detection of round, low-contrast objects is relatively more dependent on noise, while detection of linear or punctate objects of high contrast is more dependent on resolution (12).

FOLLOW-UP STUDY

More recently, the use of even faster screen-film combinations has been proposed, in an attempt to achieve further reductions in radiation dose. To assess the clinical value of these ultra-fast screen-film combinations, we began another controlled single-blind study, identical in design to and using the same equipment as that of the initial study. Five new screen-film combinations were evaluated (Table X), with the DuPont Lo-dose 2 system acting as the standard for comparison. Entrance skin exposure was measured for 10 consecutive patients, using thermoluminescent dosimetry, as described above.

Table X. Screen-Film Combinations Tested in Follow-up Study

Screen	Film	Name of Combination
DuPont Lo-dose-2	DuPont Lo-dose	Lo-dose-2
Kodak SO-299	Kodak Ortho-G	Min-R/Ortho-G
DuPont Par	DuPont Lo-dose	Par/Lo-dose
DuPont SP	DuPont Lo-dose	SP/Lo-dose
DuPont Hi-Plus	DuPont Lo-dose	Hi-Plus/Lo-dose
DuPont Lo-dose-2	Kodak RP	Lo-dose-2/RP

Dosimetry documented considerable further dose reductions for the new screen-film combinations, as much as a three-fold reduction for the fastest system (Table XI). However, because the image quality of the ultra-low-dose mammograms was so noticeably worse than that of the Lo-dose-2 system (reduced resolution, increased noise), a random-order clinical evaluation was carried out after only 30 of the projected 100 patients were studied. Results showed a substantial reduction in visibility of microcalcifications for all of the faster screen-film combinations. Most importantly, two non-palpable carcinomas containing clustered microcalcifications could not be seen on the ultra-low-dose images, even in retrospect, although they were easily visible on the Lo-dose-2 mammograms. This demonstration that the ultra-fast screen-film combinations do not routinely permit detection of small breast cancers led to the prompt termination of the follow-up study.

Table XI. Measurements of Radiation Dose Per Exposure
(10 Consecutive Patients)

Screen-Film Combination	Entrance Skin Dose*	Mid-Breast Dose[†]	Mean Dose to Glandular Tissue[†]
Lo-dose-2[‡]	0.64 R	0.047 rad	0.074 rad
Min-R/Ortho-G	0.55 R	0.041 rad	0.064 rad
Par/Lo-dose	0.52 R	0.039 rad	0.060 rad
SP/Lo-dose	0.41 R	0.030 rad	0.047 rad
Hi-Plus/Lo-dose	0.31 R	0.023 rad	0.036 rad
Lo-dose-2/RP	0.21 R	0.016 rad	0.024 rad

* Measurement includes backscatter.
† Calculated according to data of Hammerstein et al (5). Refer to similar footnote, Table III.
‡ Measured on 40 consecutive patients in the initial study (Table III).

Several different ultra-low-dose screen-film combinations have recently been developed, demonstrating substantially increased contrast, similar resolution, but considerably increased noise compared to currently acceptable screen-film systems (Fig. 1). Prospective controlled clinical evaluations are being mounted, but until they are completed, these new screen-film combinations should be considered insufficiently tested to be suitable for general use.

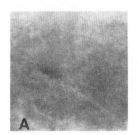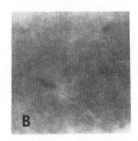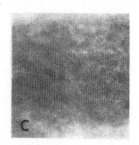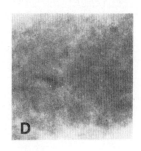

Fig. 1. Radiographs of a whole, fresh (unfixed) breast removed from an adult female cadaver, using several low-dose screen-film combinations. Five 0.35 mm aluminum oxide specks have been placed between specimen and recording system to simulate the appearance of breast microcalcifications.

A. Lo-dose-2 system, demonstrating all five simulated microcalcifications.

B. Hi-Plus/Lo-dose combination. Decreased resolution and increased noise are evident. The aluminum oxide specks cannot be seen.

C. Lo-dose/RP combination. Decreased resolution and a further increase in noise are evident. The specks cannot be seen.

D. Experimental ultra-low-dose screen-film combination. Resolution is similar to the Lo-dose-2 image, permitting visualization of all five specks. The contrast is substantially increased, as is the background noise.

CONCLUSIONS

Our initial study shows that four low-dose mammography screen-film combinations produce images of quality comparable to that of the original DuPont Lo-dose system, without any loss in diagnostic accuracy. Routine mammography with any of these screen-film combinations appears preferable to use of DuPont Lo-dose, except that some radiologists may find objectionable the relatively high noise levels of the Min-R/Nuclear Medicine combination. The follow-up study, on the other hand, indicates some impairment of diagnostic accuracy with four other lower-dose screen-film combinations, which therefore are not recommended for mammography despite the additional dose reduction they allow.

In the strictest sense, these results apply only to screen-film mammography as it was performed in this study, although it is likely that the same conclusions apply to other commonly used techniques having minor differences in kVp, focal spot size, and focus-film distance. As these differences become greater, however, such as for x-ray tubes of different anode composition or for microfocal spot magnification mammography techniques (13-17), different results may well be found. Similar controlled trials will be necessary to evaluate reduced-dose screen-film combinations for use in these situations, as well as for high-filtration versus standard xeromammography techniques.

REFERENCES

1. Ostrum BJ, Becker W, Isard HJ: Low-dose mammography. Radiology 109:323-326, Nov 1973.
2. Weiss JP, Wayrynen RE: Imaging system for low-dose mammography. J Appl Photogr Engineer 2:7-10, Winter 1976.

3. Sickles EA, Genant HK, Doi K: Comparison of laboratory and clinical evaluations of mammographic screen-film systems. In Application of Optical Instrumentation in Medicine VI. Bellingham, WA, Society of Photo-Optical Instrumentation Engineers, 1977, Vol 127, pp 30-35.

4. Sickles EA, Genant HK: Controlled single-blind clinical evaluation of low-dose mammographic screen-film systems. Radiology, in press.

5. Hammerstein GR, Miller DW, White DR, et al: Radiation absorbed dose in mammography. Radiology, in press.

6. Rothenberg LN, Kirch RLA, Snyder RE: Patient exposures from film and xero-radiographic mammographic techniques. Radiology 117:701-703, Dec 1975.

7. Bailar JC III: Mammography: a contrary view. Ann Intern Med 84:77-84, Jan 1976.

8. Breslow L, Thomas LB, Upton AC: Final reports of the National Cancer Institute ad hoc working groups on mammography in screening for breast cancer and a summary of their joint findings and recommendations. J Natl Cancer Inst 59:473-541, Aug 1977.

9. Lester RG: Risk versus benefit in mammography. Radiology 124:1-6, Jul 1977.

10. Gold RH: Mammography: Where are we? Where did we come from? Where are we going? In Margulis AR, Gooding CA, eds: Diagnostic Radiology 1978. San Francisco, University of California Press, 1978, pp 483-500.

11. Dodd GD: Dosage with current mammography techniques. Presented at Annual Conference on Detection and Treatment, National Conference on Breast Cancer, San Francisco, March 6, 1978.

12. Rossmann K: Comparison of several methods for evaluating image quality of radiographic screen-film systems. Am J Roentgenol 97:772-775, Jul 1966.

13. Sickles EA, Doi K, Genant HK: Magnification film mammography: image quality and clinical studies. Radiology 125:69-76, Oct 1977.

14. Logan WW: Overview of the radiologist's role in breast cancer detection. In Logan WW, ed: Breast Carcinoma. The Radiologist's Expanded Role. New York, Wiley, 1977, pp 343-365.

15. Gorski JW, Skucas J, Logan WW: A comparison of conventional and magnification mammography. Presented at Annual Meeting of Radiological Society of North America, Chicago, Dec 1, 1977.

16. Arnold BA, Eisenberg H, Bjarngard B: Low-dose magnification mammography. Presented at Annual Meeting of Radiological Society of North America, Chicago, Dec 1, 1977.

17. Sickles EA: Microfocal spot magnification mammography using xero-radiographic and screen-film recording systems. Presented at Annual Meeting of Radiological Society of North America, Chicago, Nov 28, 1978.

XERG MAMMOGRAPHY
A REVIEW OF SIXTEEN MONTHS EXPERIENCE PLUS A COMPARISON WITH XEROMAMMOGRAPHY

Saar A. Porrath, M.D.
Department of Radiology
Santa Monica Hospital Medical Center

In June of 1977, Santa Monica Hospital Medical Center obtained a 10-MA XERG Mammography unit with a microfocus, tungsten target, stationary anode with beryllium window.

The system, which has been described earlier in this meeting, uses a gas process to produce a latent electrostatic image on a polyester sheet. The image is then developed with liquid toner and laminated with polyester, so that a permanent record is obtained.

There was a certain breaking-in period which was necessary with the new unit. The initial images were of very poor quality and rather poor detail. Part of this was due to the film itself, which was a gold-coated polyester sheet, but most of the problem was due to technique, experimentation with types of gases, and inconsistency of the toner. Krypton gas was originally tried but was found to have too much sensitivity to allow adequate visualization of skin and soft tissues at the same time that calcium deposits were visualized. We eventually settled on a bromated Freon, which was somewhat slower than the original gas. At the end of approximately one month, image quality had improved markedly.

It became apparent that the 10-MA unit was not sufficient to obtain quality images at a time interval short enough to prevent motion artifacts. The XERG unit was subsequently changed to a 50-MA tungsten target glass envelope unit with a measured focal spot of 0.21 mm.

At 38.8 kVp the HVL is 0.87 mm Al. Exposure to the breast at the surface of the breast, including backscatter, ranges from 48 mR at 0.1 seconds to 434 mR at 1 second.

By the beginning of September 1977, approximately 2 months later, the image quality had reached a relative consistency, so that more than 75% of the images were of reasonable quality.

It was decided at that time to collect 40 consecutive, technically satisfactory cases, which had both xeromammogram and XERG films on the same patient. At that time we were still performing the xeromammograms on a Senographe molybdenum target unit, with only a small proportion of the examinations on the XERG unit. The xeromammography was performed with a molybdenum target, 40-MA, 50 kVp unit; the average exposure was above 2R (as determined by the State of California Testing Device), with many images of even higher dose. Because we had found it impossible to obtain good quality xerox images on the Senographe using a higher filtration, the XERG images were compared with the high dose, high contrast proven xeromammography technique rather than a highly filtered low dose, low contrast technique. In addition, the XERG system was still undergoing some initial shakedown.

Forty cases were obtained with the comparison mammograms and shown to 10 mammographers from different areas of the United States. The bias of the mammographers was approximately equal, with half of the radiologists being film mammographers and half being xeromammographers. There were nine carcinomas scattered among the 40 cases. In addition, there were atrophic breasts, breasts with minimal as well as marked mammary dysplasia, benign fibroadenomas and cysts, and cases with prosthetic devices.

The miss-rate of diagnosing carcinomas was approximately the same with both systems. Nine carcinomas times the 10 observers would have made 90 times that the carcinomas should have been diagnosed. There were 5 misses with xeromammography and 4 with the XERG system. In addition, a very rough grading system was used to determine the amount of information present on the films. The observer was asked to review the films a second time, after having made his or her initial observation to determine the diagnostic quality of the film. If the diagnostic quality of the XERG and xeromammography was approximately equal, a 0 (zero) was given. If the xeromammograms were somewhat better, a -1 (minus one) was assigned; if the xeromammograms were much better, a -2 (minus two) was assigned. If the XERG images were better, a +1 (plus one) was assigned; and if the XERG images were much better, a +2 (plus two) was given. This would allow a maximum swing of 2 points per case or 40 cases X 2 points X 10 observers, which would be 800 possible points if one system were consistently much better than the other. Out of a possible 800 points, the rough grading system showed a deviation of 7 points, or less than 1% in favor of the high dose, high resolution xeromammograms.

There are a number of problems with this particular study in that it is not truly a good scientific study. Ideally, it would have been better to be able to have sent one of the sets to an observer, followed two to three months later by the set of the opposite mode of examinations. Unfortunately, time commitments did not permit this. In order to make this study as reasonable as possible, within the time frame, the cases were mixed so that the observers initially saw the xeromammograms on some of the cases and the XERG mammograms on the other cases, with the opposite mode being examined later in the same sitting. Ultimately, all 40 cases were seen, of both XERG mammography and xeromammography. A diagnosis was made on each case by each observer. In order to eliminate some problems in the grading system, all the images were constantly mixed for different observers. Despite these problems, and despite the fact that because of the necessity of obtaining technically satisfactory cases, not all cases were consecutive, we felt that the study did show us that the XERG images were essentially equal diagnostically, or almost equal diagnostically, to the high dose, high resolution xeromammogram images, with a marked reduction in dose from over 2R to approximately 150-200mR. Because of this finding at our institution, we converted to using XERG images for mammography. One of the assumptions that we made in this study, (although we could not prove) is that high contrast high dose xeromammography is of better diagnostic quality than low dose highly filtered low contrast xeromammography. Because of this assumption, a second test comparing XERG images and low dose, low contrast xeromammography was not done.

Comparison was done, however, using multiple test objects and phantoms. A Kodak phantom of the 400 series, abalone shell phantoms, made by Dr. Phillip Muntz, and calcium carbonate phantoms, made by Dr. Russell Morgan, were compared on the XERG system at Santa Monica Hospital Medical Center, and the highly filtered xeromammography system at Los Angeles County-University of Southern California unit with a half value layer of 1.75 mm of aluminum. The findings of these studies showed that the image quality resolution was approximately the same on the two systems, but that the dose varied from 3-4 times greater on the xeromammography system.

I would now like to try to share my feelings about the XERG system, compared to xeromammography. The essential advantages and disadvantages are shown on the accompanying tables.

TABLE I: TECHNICAL CONSIDERATIONS

	XERG	XEROMAMMOGRAPHY
Reliability:	equal	
Ease of Use:	equal	
Technologist Dependent:	equal	
Cost/film:	equal	
Cost of Machine:	more costly	
Maintenance Requirements:	equal	
Minor breakdowns fixed by technologist:		easier to fix

Table II: EXAMINATION QUALITY

	XERG	XEROMAMMOGRAPHY
Ease of Reading:	learning curve to read - once trained, equal	most Radiologists trained on system
Detection of soft tissue masses (edge effect):	masses seen slightly better	
Calcifications:	less than high dose xerography, equal or better than low dose xeromammography	
Skin Line:		better seen
Chest Wall	equal	
Light Used:	transmitted	reflected

Initially, the XERG unit was not nearly as reliable as the xeromammography unit, which in itself was never, at best, the most reliable unit. Over the last nine months, however, the reliability of the XERG unit is at least as good, if not better, than the xeromammogram unit. Changes have been made by the company in the transport system and in the film dispenser. In addition, there has been a marked improvement in the toner quality. Once the technologist has experience on either unit, the ease of use by the technologist is approximately the same, or perhaps minimally easier on the XERG unit. Both units continue to be technologist dependent in that a good technologist can obtain good films from either unit, whereas a disinterested technologist will tend to obtain poorer images even under ideal circumstances. Although the cost per film was approximately equal on either unit, the original cost of the XERG system is much more expensive than a xeromammography unit. The maintenance requirements are approximately equal. However, at the present time, it is easier to fix minor breakdowns on the xeromammography unit than on the XERG unit.

As for image quality and quality of the examination itself, there is a definite learning curve associated with a new system. Those who are trained on film mammography have an easier time adapting to the XERG system than those who are trained on xeromammography. However, once somebody is trained, I feel that the ease of reading is approximately equal. Detection of soft tissue masses is slightly to much improved with the XERG unit over xeromammography. Calcifications, however, present a real problem because the calcifications on the XERG unit are not nearly as well seen as on the high dose xeromammography. However, they are equal to or better delineated than the low dose, low contrast xeromammography. Because of problems with toner breakdown, the skin line is somewhat better seen on xeromammography than XERG, although this is improving recently with the XERG unit. The visualization of the chest wall is approximately equal. As for viewing, the XERG images use a transmitted light, whereas the xeromammography images are viewed with reflected light.

At this time, we have performed more than 1500 mammograms with the XERG unit. My partners and I are almost as comfortable reading the XERG images as we were with the previous high dose, high contrast xeromammogram images and much more comfortable than we were when we were reading the low dose, low contrast xeromammogram images. We have not yet obtained exact figures, but we feel that our false negative rate is approximately the same as our previous statistics under the prior system. There has been a continual improvement in the images over the 16 months that we have had the XERG unit. Improved compression devices have helped us in obtaining better XERG films than previously. There have been numerous cases in which microcalcifications have been as visible, if not more so, than they would be on a low dose, low contrast xeromammography image.

In summary, I feel that the XERG unit at this stage in its development, provides images which are diagnostically close to high contrast, high dose xeromammography and much better than low dose, low contrast xeromammograms, at lower breast glandular dose than the low dose xeromammograms. In addition, I would like to take this opportunity to add one other remark: when we compare systems, the true test of efficacy is what an individual mammographer can do with a particular system. It has been my experience that unfortunately a large portion of mammography is of very poor quality. It is just as important for us to realize that we must train mammographers well, as it is for us to continue to improve the equipment.

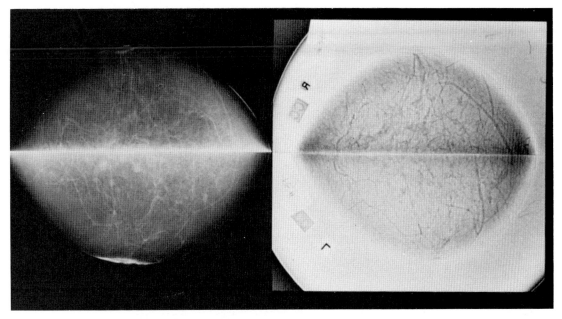

Figure 1: Atrophic breasts: XERG (Xonics) study on the left, compared with
a high dose high contrast xeromammogram on the right (same patient).

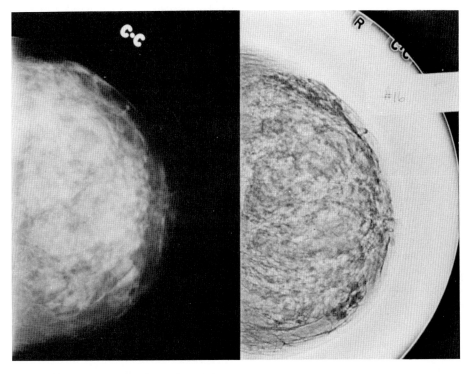

Figure 2: Moderate mammary dysplasia. XERG study on the left, compared to a
high dose high contrast xeromammogram on the right (both studies
on same breast).

REFERENCES

1. E.P. Muntz, H. Meyers, E. Wilkinson, and G. Jacobson, "Preliminary studies using electron radiology for mammography". Radiology 125, 2, 517-523, November 1977.
2. S. Blake, "Comparison of XERG and hard beam xeroradiography for mammography." Private communication, March 1978.
3. M. Friedrich, W. Hoeffken, and E. Kaegi, "Comparison of XERG and various other mammography systems." Private communication, April 1978.
4. S. Porrath, L.T. Avallone, S.K. Shearer: Low dose XERG mammography, A comparison with xeromammography. RSNA, Nov., 1977.

XERG AND LO-DOSE MAMMOGRAPHY:
A COMPARATIVE CLINICAL STUDY

Robert L. Hirschfeld, M.D.
Diagnostic Radiology Department
Greater Baltimore Medical Center

Since 1926 when Stafford Warren of Rochester, New York demonstrated the promise that breast radiography held (9), radiologists have struggled to discover methods that would increase the resolution while maintaining acceptable radiation dose levels. Simultaneously, Salomon in Germany described radiographic characteristics of breast diseases on approximately 3,000 amputated breasts. Despite a flurry of activity in the early 1930's, most of the authors were disappointed in the results and the poor quality of the radiograms. From Philadelphia, Gershon-Cohen (4) persisted in the belief that diseases of the breast could be demonstrated radiographically and began to publish in 1953 some of the early results of his work. Despite his early enthusiasm, Haagensen stated in 1956 that roentgenography had no place in the diagnosis of breast disease. During the mid '50's, Gilbert Fletcher and Gerald Dodd persuaded Robert Egan, then at M.D. Anderson Hospital in Houston, to pursue this field. By 1960, Egan's technique, using fine grain Kodak industrial film without screens was widely published (2) but dose levels were high with techniques that used 1,800 MAS. Despite initial enthusiasm in isolated segments of the country, it was not until the late 1960's, when xeromammography became available, that breast radiography began to achieve more popularity. Those men who became early champions of the technique were Ruzicka, John Wolfe, and John Martin (7,8,10,11). They compared film techniques with xeromammography, and were pleased with the improved resolution and wider latitude of xeromammography.

After several years of initial clinical trials, XERG mammography was made available in 1977 on a commercial basis. In this process, the x-ray image of the exposed breast is transmitted through a pressurized imaging gas which acts as an ionization chamber allowing the freed electrons to be collected on a clear mylar base which is backed with a conducting coating to enhance charge transfer. The magnitude of the charge is directly proportional to the incident x-ray exposure so that the resultant pattern is analagous to the latent image of the breast.

Development is accomplished by presenting a positively charged toner to the film. The developed density is proportional to the electrostatic charge. Edge enhancement, due to the interaction of the toner and the negatively charged mylar film, is not as pronounced as that produced in xeromammography where strongly fringing electrostatic fields result in a decrease or absence of powder on the plate where there is high subject contrast. Enough latitude is present in the XERG system so that a large difference in exposure does not necessarily result in a great difference in density. Therefore, over- and under-exposure does not usually result in non-diagnostic films.

Breast radiography using Egan's high mAs technique was begun at the Greater Baltimore Medical Center in 1966. The introduction of the DuPont Lo-Dose I screen-film combination in 1975 reduced the radiation dose considerably, and a further 50 percent decrease occurred with the availability of the Lo-Dose II screen in 1977. In September, 1977, we received delivery of a 50 mA XERG unit in our private office.

Since then, a series of changes have been made by Xonics Corporation and our local distributor, Standard Medical Systems, to make this system reliable (see Kaegi's article in this volume). New gas filters and a second baralyme bag for greater absorption have been added to make the x-ray generator the most dependable portion of the system. After a second film discharge unit was added to the film dispenser in June of 1978, no problems have been encountered with it. The processor has caused the greatest amount of downtime. Initially, replenishment was required every three days and toner smearing was a major problem. The addition of a self-contained cooling system and a liter replenisher allow 300-500 images to be processed before servicing. It would not be possible, however, to schedule a large number of patients for examination without the addition of a second processor. Initial film problems have been eliminated. The imaging qualities of the film now appear quite satisfactory. Initially, we used a gas mixture of 98 percent krypton and 2 percent bromated Freon; while this produces satisfactory images at an entrance exposure of less than 100 mr for the average breast, the cost of the imaging gas was significant. The gas mixture was then changed to 50 percent Freon and 50 percent xenon with an increase to approximately 120 mr per average breast exposure. Currently, we are using 100 percent bromated Freon as the imaging gas and have a surface exposure of approximately 160 mr. This has allowed us approximately the same ionization at 1/10 the cost.

STANDARD PROCEDURES

In our hospital practice screen-film studies are performed thusly: two initial exposures are made with the patient sitting using the General Electric MMX unit, with the DuPont Lo-Dose II, screen-film combination contained within E-ZM Vacuum cassettes. The positioning is identical for the XERG craniocaudad view.

The upright medial lateral view is difficult to perform and will often fail to visualize the retromammary fascia. In our office practice, we have overcome this by a special cut-out table that allows filming in the recumbent position. We use a cone compression device utilizing a balloon similar to that used in xeromammography, designed by Doctor Vernon Croft of Baltimore. We feel the standing craniocaudad position is superior to the sitting position as it allows for the greatest amount of breast tissue to be compressed. This lateral view positioning is identical for both screen-film and XERG studies.

The addition of a third view tangential to the outer quadrant and axillary tail is made if:

1. The patient's complaints are referable to this area,

2. If there is any abnormality noted in this area in viewing the initial study, or

3. Is requested by the radiologist who examines each patient.

The keys to good breast radiography are positioning and good compression.

The fatty breast offers no problem with any modality used; images are easy to obtain and interpret. It is in the dense, fibrocystic breasts where the greatest improvement with XERG mammography is seen. Penetration is easier. Nodular changes are simpler to display using the transmitted light source. Lo-Dose and other film techniques often produce an underpenetrated, conglomerate, underpenetrated image that obscures calcification or increase in tissue density (see Fig).

Radiation dose depends on both the x-ray system (characteristics of the beam and recording media) and the breast size and composition. Although diagnostic films can be obtained using the Lo-Dose techniques, the number of repeat films with the dense dysplastic breast may increase the dose per examination. We have found that the use of high filtration results in a reduction in the overall contrast, with subsequent loss of detail which is not justified by the dose reduction. We have, therefore, abandoned high filtration techniques on all but the post-menopausal and fatty breasts.

The average techniques for our Lo-Dose studies on the MMX unit are summarized in Table 1. The HVL is equal to approximately 0.4 mm Al with low filtration, at 30 kVp, with a fixed 60 cm TFD. For a Lo-Dose I-cronex single emulsion film study, the typical breast surface exposure is 0.51R at 35 kVp with high filtration, and 2.5R at 35 kVp with low filtration. The dose is reduced by approximately 50 percent with Lo-Dose II screen-cronex film studies.

The XERG unit has a HVL equal to 0.75 mm Al at 45 kVp and a fixed 94 cm TFD. The typical breast surface exposure is between 130 mR to 210 mR for 40 to 50 kVp. Our usual breast exposures are summarized in Table II.

RESULTS

Review by diagnosis of 430 cases performed on the XERG unit reveal that 80 percent have predominantly fibrocystic structures, 6 percent fatty structure, and 11 percent post-menopausal or atrophic breasts. Four percent have had biopsy-proven carcinoma. The more dysplastic breast structure of our patients, when coded by Wolfe criteria, is also reflected in that 59 percent of 154 patients categorized have DY structure while distribution for other types is fairly equal (Tables III, IV).

The average patient seen in our office practice is young, 24 percent being from age 31 to 40, as compared to 13 percent at the hospital. In the office, 83 percent of the patients are between the ages of 30 to 60, whereas 63 percent are in that age group at the hospital and 36 percent fall above 61 (Table V). The referral pattern by specialty is shown in Table VI.

CONCLUSIONS

Clinical evaluation, comparing our experience with Lo-Dose screen-film mammography and the newer XERG mammography, leads us to conclude that we are achieving our goal of satisfactory resolution and decreased radiation dose. The latitude of the process allows us to image the entire breast spectrum without undue difficulty or significant repeat studies. The acceptance of this technique by our colleagues has been slow but seems to be gaining. An initial reluctance was noted because of the familiarity with xeromammography and a preference for viewing studies with reflected light. Although we feel that on the average XERG mammography offers greater accuracy because of its ability to easily penetrate the dense dysplastic breast, it is too early for us to determine whether this method will significantly increase the number of malignancies detected.

Table I

Typical Exposure Average Breast and
Estimated Dose to Mammary Glands
Lo-Dose II - GE MMX Unit

CC - 30 kVp	60 mAs	336 mR (Lo Filtration)	
		75 mR (Hi Filtration)	
LAT - 35 kVp	100 mAs	187 mR	
		68 mR	

HvL = 0.4 mm Al (approx.)

Table II

Exposure to Average Breast XERG 50 mA Unit
Surface and Mean Absorbed Dose

CC - 38 kVp	16 mAs	136 mR	28.5 millirad
LAT - 44 kVp	16 mAs	204 mR	42.8 millirad

HvL = 0.75 mm Al

Table III

Patient Distribution
by Breast Type
(430 Cases)

Fibrocystic structure:	80%
Proven carcinoma:	4%
Fatty structure:	6%
P.M./Atrophic breasts:	11%

Table IV

Classification According
to Wolfe Criteria
(154 cases)

P1 - 14%
P2 - 12%
DY - 59%
N1 - 15%

Table V

Age Distribution

		Office Practice (694 Pts)	GBMC Practice (132 Pts)
Ages:	20 to 30 - 45	6%	
	31 to 40 -165	24%	13%
	41 to 50 -207	30%	17%
	51 to 60 -200	29%	34%
	51 & up - 77	11%	36%

Table VI

Source of Referral
(694 pts)

Doctors:		
	Gen Prac 16	2%
	Surgeons 180	26%
	OB/GYN 390	56%
	Other 46	7%
	Internist 63	9%

GBMC 1973 Survey
(133 pts)

Surgeons	40%
OB/GYN	50%
Internists	8%
Other	2%
Out Patients	90%

A minimal filtration lateral screen-film mammogram on the left, compared to a XERG (Xonics) lateral mammogram on the right, on the same patient, at one-third the average glandular dose of the screen-film study.

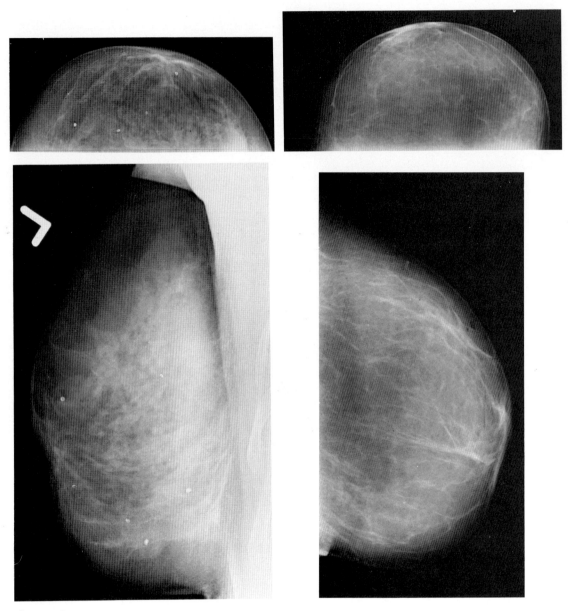

Figure 1

| LU | I. | cc view | RU | O. | cc view |
| LL | I. | lateral view | RL | O. | lateral view |

M.I.

    Dysplastic breast with secretory
calcifications. Xonics demonstrated
duct dilatation. Uniform penetration
achieved with compression. No halo
effect noted surrounding calcifications.

P.O.

    Young fatty breast--well defined
septations and fatty lobules. This
type of breast studied well with all
modalities. Here achieved with dose
levels around 160-200 millirad.

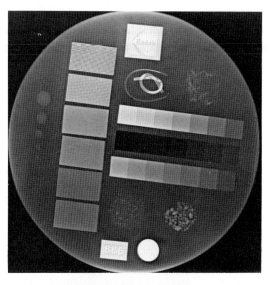
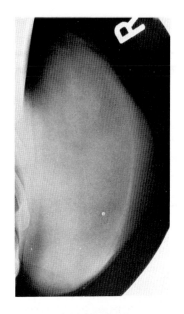
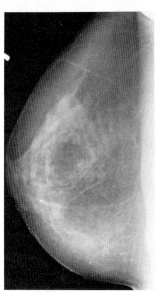
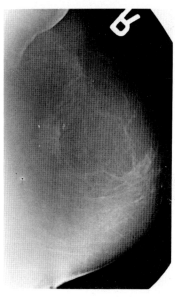

Figure 2

(M.C.)

a. LU   Kodak   phantom   b. RU   C.   lateral view
c. LL   S. (G.S)   lateral view d. RL   G.   lateral view

a. Kodak phantom demonstrates wide range of resolution possible with Xerg
    mammography.

b. M.C. 45y/o with diffuse cystic breast structure--uniform pattern with
    good penetration.

c. G.S 52 y/o asymptomatic with "lumpy breasts"--nodular umbilicated 6 mm.
    mass lying centrally inferior to nipple--ductal carcinoma.

d. (AG) 68 y/o typical scirrhous carcinoma pattern.

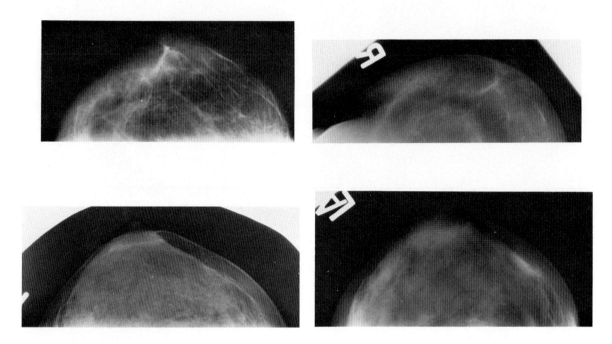

Figure 3

a.	LU	T.	Xonics	b.	RU	T.	Lo Dose I
c.	LL	S.	Xonics	d.	RL	S.	Lo Dose II

a. 29 y/o Xergmammography illustrates superb delineation of lobulation and small cyst detail while

b. Lo Dose I gives washed out detail of fine structure.

c. 39 y/o dense cystic structure uniform Xerg appearances versus

d. difficult to penetrate grey-white clouds of Lo Dose II.

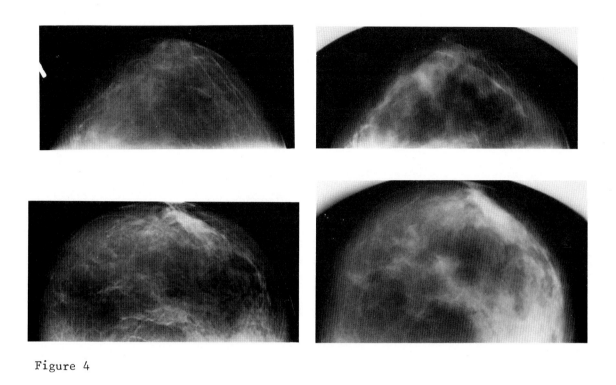

Figure 4

| a. | LU | M. | Xonics | b. | RU | M. | Lo Dose I |
| c. | LL | N. | Xonics | d. | RL | N. | Lo Dose II |

a. 40 y/o easily palpable discrete cyst inner quadrant

b. Lo Dose II similar appearance of cyst but less uniform penetration of dense fibrocystic stroma of outer quadrant.

c. 60 y/o with large post-menopausal but dense dysplastic pattern; small nodular pattern shown on Xerg study is lost on

d. Lo Dose II which does not give uniform penetration and obscures outer quadrant with dense pattern.

Summary

A direct comparison of our film screen studies with Xerg mammography is difficult because of varying technical factors resulting in the lack of comparable exposures in many cases. Those made on the G.E. MMX unit were often underexposed with photo timing particularly in the dense cystic breast and particularly when high filtration techniques were employed. The upright lateral position necessitated by the unit although comparable to that position on Xonics unit was decidedly inferior to the lateral recumbent view afforded by the use of a specially designed stretcher and balloon compression device.

In addition to a dose reduced to 1/4-1/5 that normally used with film-screen combinations, Xerg mammography allows greater uniform penetration of the dysplastic large breast, improved ductal demonstration, more discrete enhancement of calcifications and a greater latitude in the technical factors thus reducing the number of repeat exposures. Although equipped with photo timing the experienced technologist has no difficulty in employing her own techniques with greater consistency. Finally, patient acceptance with the lower dose has been a definite factor in overcoming initial resistence to radiation exposure.

*Acknowledgements:

    Ginette Johnson, R.T., for technical assistance;
    Gary Sterner for photographic reproductions.

References

1. Asbury, D.L. and Barker, P.G.: Radiation Dosage to the Breast in Well-Woman Screening Surveys. Brit. J. Radiol. 48:963-967, Dec 1975.

2. Egan, R.L.: Experience with Mammography in Tumor Institution. Radiology 75:894-900, Dec 1960.

3. Egan, R.L.: Mammography. Charles C. Thomas, Springfield, Ill., 1964.

4. Gershon-Cohen, J.: Technical Improvement in Breast Roentgenography. Am. J. Roentgenol. Rad. Ther. Nucl. Med. 84:224-226, Aug 1960.

5. Morgan, R.: Correspondence, September 4, 1977.

6. Ostrum, B.J., Becker, W. and Isard, H.J.: Low Dose Mammography. Radiology 109:323-326, Nov 1976.

7. Ruzicka, F.F., Kaufman, L., Shapiro, G., et al: Xero Mammography and Film Mammography, a Comparative Study. Radiology 85:260-269, 1965.

8. Van DeRit, W.G., and Wolfe, J.N.: Dose Reduction in Xeroradiography of the Breast. Am. J. Roentgenol. 128:821-823, May 1977.

9. Warren, S.L.: A Roentgenologic Study of the Breast. Am. J. Roentgenol. Rad. Ther. Nucl. Med. 24:113-124, August 1930

10. Wolfe, J.N.: Xeroradiography of the Breast. Geriatrics 29:67-73, April 1974.

11. Wolfe, J.N.: Risk for Breast Cancer Development Determined by Mammographic Parenchymal Patterns. Cancer 37:2486-2492, May 1976.

SCREENING FOR BREAST CANCER IN SWEDEN. A RANDOMIZED CONTROLLED TRIAL

L. Tabar*, A. Gad**, E. Akerlund+, B. Fors**, Departments of Mammography*, Pathology** and Surgery+, Central Hospital, Falun, Sweden.

G. Fagerberg*, L. Baldetorp**, O. Grőntoft+, and L.O. Lamke**, Institutions of Radiology*, Surgery**, Medical Microbiology and Pathology+, University of Linköping, Sweden.

Breast cancer screening with clinical examination and mammography has hitherto been the subject of one randomized controlled trial - the Health Insurance Plan (HIP study) in New York city in 1963. All data nine years after the start suggest a reduction in mortality from breast cancer in women over the age of 50 (1, 5). No such benefit effect of screening has so far been reported in women under this age.

Since the HIP study there has been a definite improvement in mammography. This includes the quality of the image as well as a reduction of radiation exposure to the breast tissue necessary to achieve this image. It seems reasonable to believe that the HIP study is not representative of what mammography today can offer to women.

In the present status of breast cancer screening many questions remain to be answered: Is mammography alone sufficient as a screening method? Can reduction in mortality rate be shown to include even women under the age of 50? What will be the proper interval between two consecutive screenings with mammography?

It is a well known fact that mammography can detect breast cancer before a palpable mass or other clinical signs of malignancy are present. However, the value of screening with mammography should also be seen in the light of its influence on the course of the disease and on the mortality from breast cancer. To achieve this within a reasonable period of time a randomized controlled trial of a sufficiently large population using mammography as a single screening procedure is mandatory.

The purpose of this paper is to announce the presence of such a study and to outline how it was organized, and to present the mammographic method used and the preliminary results of the first year.

ORGANIZATION

The Swedish National Board of Health and Welfare initiated a randomized controlled screening trial with mammography in two of Sweden's 24 counties, namely Kopparberg and Östergőtland. Screening started in Kopparberg on 3 October 1977 and in Östergőtland on 22 May 1978.

A total of 90,000 women above 39 years of age, with no upper age limit were invited to be screened. The control group included 70,000 women (age matched).

The total study population in each county was divided into blocks according to the area of residence. These blocks were further subdivided into two or
three smaller units according to the size of the block. One out of two or two
out of three of these units were randomly selected to form the active study
group. The remainder represents the passive study group ("control group").
The women in the active study group as well as the controls are recruited by
computer from the Swedish National Population Registry.

The active study group is to be examined twice in a period of five years.
The control group will not be screened under the study period.

METHODS

The screening method consists of low-dose film-screen mammography with
only one single view of each breast. The chosen projection is the so-called
oblique-view, described by Lundgren and Jakobsson (4).

Kodak Min-R screens vacuum packed in polyethylene bags in combination
with Kodak Nuclear Medicine-B films (single emulsion automatic processed) are
used.

The x-ray unit is a Philips Mammodiagnost. The tube has a molybdenum
target with a nominal focal spot of 0.6 mm and is equipped with a 0.03 mm
molybdenum filter. The beam HVL is 0.4 mm aluminium and the unit is operated
at 25 kVp. The film-focus distance is 45 cm. During examination the breast
is compressed by a plastic plate. The average thickness of the compressed
breast is 43 mm.

Skin entrance and exit doses per exposure, measured with thermolumines-
cence dosimetry (TLD) averaged: 5 mGy (500 mrad) and 0.12 mGy (12 mrad) respectively. This gives an average absorbed radiation dose of 0.72 mGy (72
mrad) per exposure.

A mobile screening unit especially designed for the purpose is used to
cover the widely separated rural areas of Kopparberg county (Fig. 1). Three
technicians do the screening work in this unit. The exposed films are sent
by mail to the Mammography Department at the Central Hospital of Falun, where
they are developed and interpreted by a radiologist. In the county of
Östergötland the screening is largely performed in stationary units. One-
hundred-110 women are examined per day at one screening unit in each county.

Those women whose single-view mammograms are interpreted as normal receive
their well-letters within 2-3 days after examination. Mammograms revealing
changes suspicious of cancer are selected from the single-view mammograms.
These cases are recalled for detailed mammography, after which a certain percentage of them are found to be normal. The remainder are subjected to further
clinical and cytological examinations. Ductography, pneumocystography or
surgical excision is performed as required.

All information gathered is computerized with special emphasis on data
which enable us to evaluate the effect of screening with mammography on life
quality and mortality in breast cancer cases.

RESULTS

A. Kopparberg County:

The population of Kopparberg county was 284,034 on 1 January 1978, of which 141,250 were women. The number of women above the age of 39 was 69,005. Forty-six thousand have been invited to be screened with mammography. The control group is composed of 23,000 women.

Participation rate: During the first 13 months, a total of 20,226 women have been invited; of these 17,516 accepted and were screened, an overall participation rate of 86.6%. Of women 40-49 years of age, 93.5% participated in the screening. Table I shows the age distribution of invited and participating women.

Table 1
Age Distribution of Invited and Participating Women

Age	Number of invited	Number of particip.	Attendence rate
40-49	4425	4184	94.6%
50-59	5433	5124	94.3%
60-69	5166	4742	91.8%
over 70	5202	3466	66.6%
Total 20,226		17,516	86.6%

Table II shows the age distribution of non-participants.

Table II.

Age distribution of non-participants

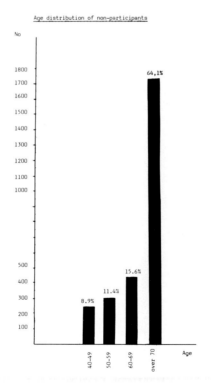

409

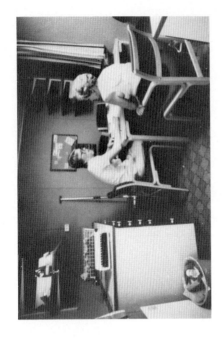

History

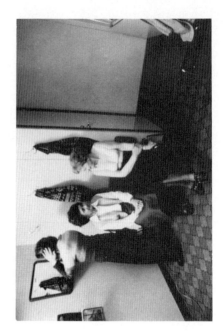

After the Mammogram

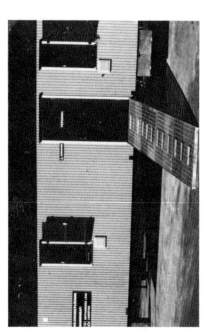

Portable Van for Screening

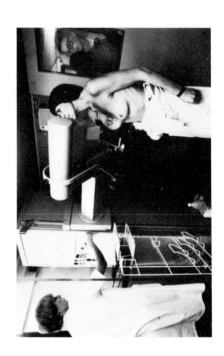

The Oblique View: Ave. Br. Compr. 4.3 cm.

410

Selection rate: Detailed examinations are done when the single-view mammography reveals suspicious findings. Of 17,516 participants, 718 (4.1%) were selected for detailed mammographic examinations. Three-hundred-thirty-three of these 718 selected women (46.5%) had breast abnormalities verified by additional radiographic evaluation.

Biopsy rate: (Table III) These 334 of 17,516 screened women (1.9%) were subjected to further clinical and cytological examinations. In 155 of 334 cases malignancy was excluded with the help of clinical examination, pneumocystography, and/or cytology. Combined pneumocystography and cytology have been helpful because most of the benign breast lesions have been cysts. All these cases have been kept under careful clinical and mammographic follow-up.

Table III
Selection Rate and Biopsy Rate
Number screened: 17,516

		% related to number of screened
Selected for further examination	718	4.1%
Number of lesions (benign and malign.)	334	1.9%
Referred to surgery and operated	179	1.0%
Number of detected cancers	118	0.67%

One-hundred-seventy-nine women were referred to surgery (1.0% of all screened). Referral in 147 cases was on the basis of mammographic findings suspicious for malignancy, and in 32 cases either because the cytology report was not decisive or because the patient requested removal of the lesion. All of the recommended operations have been carried out. In 118 out of 179 operated cases (65.8%), carcinoma was diagnosed histopathologically. This corresponds to 2 cancers in every 3 biopsied women.

Prevalence: One-hundred-eighteen cancers have been detected among 17,516 examined women (6.74 per 1000 examined women). Table IV shows the distributions of the detected cancers according to age, tumor diameters and presence of metastases.

Forty-nine of 118 detected cancers were 10 mm or less in size, and without metastases (41.5%). Eleven of 118 cancers (9.3%) were in women aged 40-49 years and 7 of them were 10 mm or smaller, and without metastases. Histologic examination of axillary lymph nodes and skeletal scintigraphy revealed metastases in 21 of the 118 detected cancer cases. In 82.2% of the cancer cases detected at screening, no metastases were detected.

The age-adjusted (40 year old and older) breast cancer incidence in Kopparberg county was 161 per 100,000 women in 1976. The prevalence of breast cancer in the first year of screening (674 per 100,000) was 4.2 times higher than the expected age-adjusted incidence. Table V shows the number of detected cancers as well as the cancer rates per 1000 examined women in different age groups.

Table IV
Distribution of Cancers According to Age and Tumor Diameters
as well as Occurrence of Metastases

Tumor size (mm)	Age					Metastases
	40-49	50-59	60-69	over 70	Total	
≤10	7	11	19	14	51	2
11-20	2	5	13	16	36	8
21-	2	6	12	11	31	11
	11	22	44	41	118	21

Table V
Age Distribution of Detected Cancers
As Well As Cancer Rates Per 1000 Examined Women

Age	Examined women number	Detected cancers number	Detected cancer rate per 1000 examined
40-49	4184	11	2.63
50-59	5124	22	4.29
60-69	4742	44	9.3
over 70	3466	41	11.83
	17,516	118	

Cost: According to our calculations, taking investments as well into consideration, the cost is as follows:

1. One examination costs 63.1 Swedish Kr (14.0 U.S. dollars)
2. One detected cancer costs 9,372.9 Swedish Kr (2,082.0 U.S. dollars)
3. One detected cancer without metastases costs 11,402.0 Kr (2,533.7 U.S. dollars)

B. Östergötland County:

In the county of Östeogötland 47,000 women over the age of 39 will be invited to screening, while the control group will number 44,000. By December 1978, a total of 7,578 women had been invited. Of these 6,347 accepted screening, an overall participation rate of 83.7%.

Forty breast carcinomas were diagnosed histopathologically, a prevalence of 6.3 per 1,000 women examined.

The grouping of carcinomas according to size, age and occurrence of metastases is shown in Table VI . All carcinomas reported were histopathologically infiltrating carcinoma.

Table VI
Grouping of Cancers According to Age, Tumor Diameters
and Occurrence of Metastases

Tumor size (mm)	Age					Metastases	
	40-49	50-59	60-69	over 70	Total	Axillary nodes	Extension beyond axillary nodes
≤ 10 mm	1	7	5	6	19	-	-
11-12	-	5	6	4	15	-	-
21-	1	1	1	3	6	2	2
Total	2	13	12	13	40	2	2

Sixty-three women were referred to surgery; thus 63.5% of the operated women had breast carcinoma. Axillary lymph nodes have in all cases been examined histopathologically, with metastases found in the nodes of two patients. The primary tumors in these two cases were large (24 and 40 mm respectively). All women with breast cancer undergo skeletal scintigraphy, chest x-ray, and cytological examination of the bone-marrow. No signs of distant metastases have been found so far.

SUMMARY

A randomized controlled breast cancer screening trial with mammography began in one of Sweden's 24 counties in October 1977, and in another one in May 1978. The main goal of this study is to evaluate the effect of screening mammography on the course of breast cancer, mortality rate, and the life quality of breast cancer patients. Single view screen-film low-dose mammography on women aged 40 and above is used. The average absorbed dose is 0.72 mGy (72 mrad) per exposure. The total number of the screened group is 90,000 women and of the control group, 70,000. The overall participation rate in the 2 counties is 85.8%. The cancer detection rate in one of the counties was 6.7

413

per 1000 examined women and in the other, 6.3 per 1000. The total number of cancers detected in both counties so far is 158. Of these, 68 were 10 mm or less in size, and without metastases. Thirteen cancers were found in women between 40 and 49 years of age. The detection of one cancer case cost 2082 U.S. dollars. The organization of the project, the screening method, and the results of the first year are described in detail.

APPENDIX

The following pathologists have contributed to the histopathologic and cytologic analysis of the material of Kopparberg county:

Larsson, E.L., R. Willen, H. Willen, S. Thorstensson

ACKNOWLEDGEMENT

We should like to acknowledge the skillful technical assistance of Barbro Ahlquist, Helen Ledin, Gunilla Lindström, Lillemor Lundström, Tommy Berglund, Birgitta Eldh and Sonja Svee of the Mammography Department, Falun, Kopparberg county, and of Gunnel Nyberg, Eva Liljemalm, Astrid Normark, Britha Oskarsson, Jan-Erik Svensk of the Mammography Department, Linköping, Östergötland county.

The experienced work of the technical assistance of the Department of Histopathology and Cytology is greatly appreciated.

REFERENCES

1. Breslow, L., Henderson, F. Massey, Jr., M. Pike, W. Winkelstein, Jr.: Report of NCI ad Hoc working group on the gross and net benefit of mammography in mass screening for the detection of breast cancer. J. Nat. Cancer Inst., 59, 2:475, 1977.

2. Fox, S.H., M. Moskowitz, E.L. Saenger, J.G. Kereiakes, J. Milbrath, M.W. Goodman: Benefit/risk analysis of aggressive mammography screening. Radiology 128:359-365, 1978.

3. Hutchinson, G.B., S. Shapiro: Lead time gained by diagnostic screening for breast cancer. J. Nat. Cancer Inst. 41:665-681, 1968.

4. Lundgren, B., S. Jakobsson: Single-view mammography: a simple and efficient approach to breast cancer screening. Cancer 38:1124-1129, 1976.

5. Shapiro, S.: Evidence on screening for breast cancer from a randomized trial. Cancer 39:2772, 1977.

6. Cancer Incidence in Sweden 1966-1972. National Board of Health and Welfare. The Cancer Registry, Stockholm, 1972.

7. NIH/NCI Consensus Development Meeting on Breast Cancer Screening. Preventive Medicine 7:269-279, 1978.

SCREEN-FILM MAMMOGRAPHY TECHNIQUE:
COMPRESSION AND OTHER FACTORS

Wende Westinghouse Logan, M.D.
Consultant, Roswell Park Memorial Institute
1351 Mt. Hope Ave., Rochester, NY 14620

Ann Westinghouse Norlund, R.T.
1351 Mt. Hope Ave., Rochester, NY 14620

Screen-film mammography has been performed since 1972.[1,2,3] The DuPont Lo-dose II screen-film system, and the Kodak Min-R screen-film system (NMB Kodak film can be substituted for the Min-R film), are those in most wide use at this time. The Agfa Gevaert Company has recently developed a similar rare earth screen-single emulsion film combination. I do not recommend the use of any screen-film systems which have less resolution, for routine work, although faster screen-film systems can be utilized for grid work or magnification work (see chapter on grid vs magnification, Logan). Use of faster systems is not necessary anyway, since average glandular dose with these present systems, is only approximately 200-300 millirads for a 2 view study.

Although the resolutions of these screen-film combinations (detector system resolutions) are considerably less than those of the direct exposure industrial hand processed films, their increased speed has created options of utilizing a low kVp (thus increasing image contrast), and increasing the focal spot to film distance (thus decreasing geometric unsharpness). Reduced exposure time has also resulted in less subject motion (thus reducing motion unsharpness). Use of the smaller focal spot now possible has also improved the aerial image of the breast tissue. Because of the potential for these improvements in the mammographic images, and because of the irradiation-induced breast carcinoma controversy (screen-film combination mammograms can be obtained at only one-third or less average breast glandular x-ray dose than that necessary for xeromammography or direct film mammography), many radiologists have replaced xeromammography or direct film mammography with screen-film mammography. The most important technical aspect of such a transition, and the one most commonly ignored, is that of proper compression (not moderate compression, but the most vigorous possible compression toler-ated by the patient). The remainder of this discussion describes problems encountered in the conversion to screen-film mammography, from various other methods of mammography.

XEROMAMMOGRAPHY

The considerable recording latitude of the xeromammography method enables the denser regions (such as the ribs), to be as equally well visualized as the nipple and skin (the penalty for this increased latitude is the inability to assess actual density of lesions). However the comparatively minimal recording latitude of the screen-film combination does not allow equal visualization of both of these areas. Either the rib areas will be under-penetrated, or the nipple-skin region will be over-penetrated. Bright lighting of single emulsion film does not enable as adequate visualization of these areas as does bright lighting of direct film images. Therefore the first step in conversion of the xeromammography method to the screen-film method is to realize that it is not realistic to expect a good diagnostic mammogram if the ribs are to be included in the study. The ideal soft x-ray beam necessary for a screen-film study should have a half value layer of .3 mm of aluminum or less, and it is not possible to adequately penetrate the rib area with this beam. Beam hardening allows rib penetration but diminishes the contrast necessary for calcium detection within the breast tissue. While many radiologists feel that rib visualization is necessary to be certain that all breast tissue is completely visualized, this is not so (see figure 1). If the technologist pulls the breast away from the rib cage as she positions the breast on the film, the glandular tissue is usually able to be totally visualized. The patient's arm should be kept to her side as close to the breast as possible for all positioning, since pulling the arm back or raising it, tightens the skin in the breast region, making it difficult for the technologist to pull the breast away from the chest and onto the film.

Approximately 5% of patients have axillary tail tissue which cannot be completely visualized on a routine 2 view mammogram (usually this is a patient with a medium to small breast size, who has had a 5 pound or more weight gain in the past few years. The skin around the recently enlarged breast hasn't had time to stretch, and it is often extremely difficult to pull the breast away from the ribs. It will also not be possible to see all of this patient's glandular tissue on a lateral xeromammogram view either - see figure 1). The clue to the presence of this situation is the visualization of a considerable amount of glandular tissue extending to the edge of the most posterolateral aspect of the cranial-caudad view (figure 1). An additional craniocaudad view, or oblique view (x-ray beam directed superomedial to infero-lateral) should then be performed with a lead shield covering the medial half of the breast, with the patient turned so that the axillary tail of the breast can be rotated onto the film. In situations where a one view (only) mammogram is ideal (for example a baseline study in a 32-year-old woman with a strong positive family history of breast cancer), the oblique view (but of the entire breast), is recommended, since this is the best single view for visualizing all of the breast tissue.[4] The angle of obliquity should be determined by placing the film lateral to the breast tissue, parallel to the pectoral muscle. In tall women, the pectoral muscle is almost vertical (this oblique view would be more similar to a lateral view), but in short stocky patients, the oblique view would be more similar to a craniocaudad view, since the pectoral muscle in this situation tends to be more horizontal in position. This oblique view allows the most posterior visualization of the breast tissue because the pectoral muscle is most compressible parallel to its lon-gitudinal plane of direction; therefore, if the breast is kept parallel to the pectoral muscle when it is placed on the film, compression will most efficaciously displace the breast anteriorly onto the film. In contrast, for a lateral view, compression "fights" the direction of the pectoral muscle, resulting in less compressed thickness, and incomplete anterior placement of the breast away from the ribs and onto the film. Anyone who has ever performed compression for a craniocaudad view knows how difficult it is to compress counter to the alignment of the pectoral muscle. Those who don't perform mammography can appreciate this problem by performing the following: pinch the skin in front of your biceps muscle in 2 ways - first, from side to side (equivalent to the oblique view). Next, pinch the skin from top to bottom (the craniocaudad view). Finally, pinch the skin obliquely to the muscle (as in the lateral view). When you see how much more tissue can be displaced away from the muscle on the side to side pinch, you can readily appreciate why more breast tissue can be positioned anteriorly when compression is per-formed in the same direction as the pectoral muscle. Since the position of the muscle differs from one patient to the next, the angle of the oblique view varies from 30° to 60°. It is important, of course, to compress both breasts at identical angles, for comparison, and to correctly label the angle of obliquity, for correct lesion location. I do not recommend the latero-medial view, since 70° of all carcinomas are in the outer half of the breast. Geometric unsharpness and scatter will make these carcinomas less obvious in this view, than they would be in a standard mediolateral view.

In my office, a routine mammogram consists of a craniocaudad view, followed by the oblique view as described above (rather than a lateral view).

A stiff compression device which is perfectly parallel to the film surface should be utilized, with no posterior sloping of the compression device at the base of the breast. Otherwise, relative underpenetration of the base of the breast will occur. The compression devices of many of the most widely used specialized mammography x-ray units fulfill this requirement (for example, the CGR Senographe, the Philips Diagnost-M, etc). However, at this time, the General Electric Mammex unit (in use in my office) compression devices all slope at the base of the breast, causing inadequate compression of the posterior aspect of the breast. This causes geometric unsharpness (the focal spot of the GE unit is a nominal 1 mm in size but measures larger), and relative underpenetration of the posterior aspect of the breast. At this time, the General Electric Company does not manufacture a stiff compression device which is perfectly parallel to the film, but this problem can be solved by removing their least sloped compression device and reattaching it backwards* (see figure 2). The reverse end serves as an improved compression device, and the posterior aspect of the breast is then well visualized (see figure 3). A further improvement has recently been made, by replacing the General Electric compression device with a 1 mm thick plastic Lexan[+] sheet (not the fire-retardant form) which has been bent at a sharp 85° angle at the posterior aspect of the breast. The 2 inch high plastic, angled upwards, pushes back the axillary fat fold which overlies the posterolateral aspect of the breast on the cranial-caudad view, and the sharp posterior angle allows the compression device to grip the posterior aspect of the breast tissue as it compresses it, rather than allowing it to slide out from underneath, as occurs with a more gently angled curvature compression device. A similar rigid compression device has also been devised for use with the Radiologic Sciences Inc. measured 150 micron tungsten target mammography x-ray unit[5] in use in my office (see figure 4).

If xeromammography is performed without the use of a dedicated mammography unit, conversion to the screen-film method should not be attempted. While it is possible to obtain a good image of breast tissue via xeromammography in this situation, the lack of edge effect of the screen-film combinations, and its minimal recording latitude, compared with xeromammography, are such that it is virtually impossible to obtain a diagnostic mammogram unless a special-ized mammography x-ray unit is utilized. Without the soft beam necessary for contrast, and without compression to reduce patient motion and geometric unsharpness, it is seldom possible to visualize the smallest calcifications and masses of the most easily treatable carcinomas (Fig. 5).

FILM MAMMOGRAPHY

Conversion of direct film mammography to screen-film mammography is possible without loss of information, if, and only if specialized mammography

---

*This modifcation was devised by Harvey Howe, General Electric engineer in Rochester, New York.

[+]Manufactered by General Electric

x-ray equipment is utilized, for several important reasons. A dedicated unit has 2 important contributions:

(1) Compression: vigorous compression with a stiff compression device (again, which is parallel to the surface on which the breast is placed) is the key to a smooth transition. The recording latitude of direct film is greater than that of the screen-film combinations (although not as great a latitude as xeromammography). Again therefore, homogeneous even compression must be obtained. There are other additional reasons why compression is important:

a. Geometric unsharpness: The larger the focal spot, the more important it is to compress the breast as much as possible, in order to minimize the effects of geometric unsharpness. The average breast in my office is compressed to 3.9 cm in thickness. The value of compression is carefully explained to each patient, and her co-operation is requested. I have examined over 3000 patients in this way in the past 3 years. No patient has ever refused to co-operate when the importance of compression has been explained to her. No instances of breast injury have been reported to me, either by the patients or their referring physicians. Explaining the importance of compression and eliciting patient co-operation often result in an additional one to three centimeters compression.

b. Contrast improvement: Compression improves contrast by diminishing scatter. Increased contrast enables improved calcification detection, and improved visualization of the outline of mass densities.

c. Diminished motion unsharpness: With vigorous compression, films should virtually never have to be repeated because of motion unsharpness. With adequate compression, even arterial motion should not occur. Without compression, or with only mild compression, motion unsharpness is a considerable problem, when superimposed upon the comparatively diminished detector system resolution of the screen-film systems, even with exposure times of .2 seconds. Vigorous compression times of 2-3 seconds can be tolerated by most patients.

d. Reduction of x-ray dose: A proportionately larger breast entrance exposure is necessary when a breast is only minimally compressed. Vigorous breast compression reduces this breast entrance exposure, and also reduces the average glandular dose (see figure 3).

e. Homogeneous film density: When the compression device is stiff and perfectly parallel to the film surface, vigorous compression enables the posterior aspect of the breast to be as well visualized as the anterior aspect. (With the minimal recording latitude of the screen-film combination, the inadequate compression of a sloped device results in relative underpenetration of the posterior aspect of the breast, and relative overpenetration of the anterior portion of the breast). The resultant more homogeneous film density produced by vigorous breast compression enables use of a lower kVp, and a more contrasty screen-film system, which then enables better calcium detection because of increased contrast (see figure 3).

f. More accurate assessment of the density of masses: The homogeneous degree of compression of the entire breast enables evaluation of the density of masses of variable diameter, in order to differentiate between benign low density objects such as cysts, versus higher density objects such as carcinomas. Cysts and normal glandular tissue are more easily compressed and flattened by vigorous compression, than are the more rigid less distensible carcinomas (thus accentuating the differences in density).

g. An added benefit of vigorous compression is the spreading apart of the islands of glandular tissue, so that the borders of suspicious lesions can be better seen.

(2) A. Soft x-ray beam: Calcium detection relies upon two factors: resolution and contrast. Specialized mammography units allow a soft beam to be utilized which is necessary in order to increase contrast, in order for calcifications to be better detected. Since the detector system resolution is less than that of direct film, a low kVp x-ray beam with a half value layer of .3 mm aluminum or less (95% of my mammograms are performed in the 25-26 kVp range), should be utilized in order to improve the contrast between the calcifications and surrounding tissue, to compensate for the diminished detector system resolution. The increased speed of the screen-film systems enables the lower kVp to be utilized without significant increases in time exposure. Attempts to perform screen-film mammography with harder beams (above 28 kVp), as is often utilized with direct film mammography, will result in impaired calcification detection (Fig. 6). The substitution of aluminum filtration for molybdenum filtration, in molybdenum target mammography, is detrimental for this reason, and should be reserved only for grid or magnification mammography.

B. New equipment modifications:

a. Increased focal spot to film distance - with mammography units utilizing larger focal spots, especially with shorter focal spot to film distances, geometric unsharpness can still be a problem, even with vigorous compression and utilization of a soft x-ray beam. An example of this is the original CGR unit, which has a nominal .6 mm focal spot, and a focal spot to film distance of only 35 cm. In this situation, the modification reported by Art Haus,[6] with use of a long cone, and adjustment of the focal spot to film distance from 35 cm to 66 cm will considerably reduce geometric unsharpness (this increased distance is permitted by the screen-film system speed, and has been adopted in the newer CGR model).

b. Grid use - A dramatic improvement in image quality has been obtained with the use of a grid developed by the Philips Company (see the chapter by Jost). When the grid is utilized with faster film-screen combinations (see Stanton's and Logan's chapters on the grid) the resulting improvement in images are dramatic, at no more average breast glandular dose than that utilized in non-grid studies with slower standard screen-film

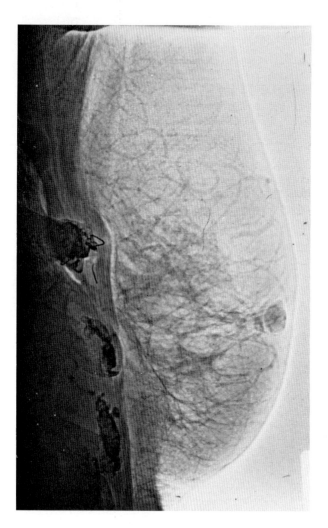

Figure 1A

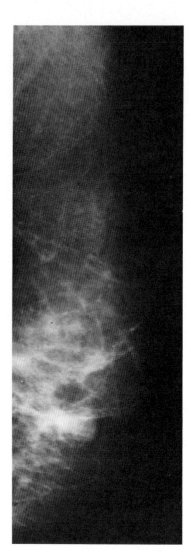

Figure 1B

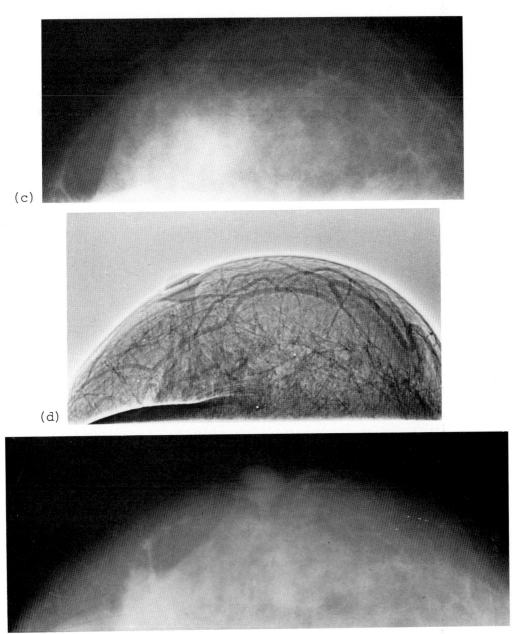

(c)

(d)

(e)

Figure 1: This patient's 20 pound weight gain over the past 5 years had resulted in breast enlargement and skin tightening. The lateral xeromammography
view (A), performed with balloon compression, as compared with a lateral
screen-film study (without ribs visualized, performed with a stiff compression
device - (B)), reveals an equal amount of glandular tissue. The original
cranio-caudad xeromammography view reveals glandular tissue extending from
the subareolar region posterolaterally (C). The original cranio-caudad
screen-film study (D), also reveals a considerable amount of glandular tissue
at the posterolateral aspect of the film. For this reason, an additional
slightly obliqued craniocaudad view was performed, with the patient rotated
slightly medially, in order to rotate the axillary tissue onto the film (E).
A large lobulated carcinoma with many small fine calcifications, now can be
visualized, which is not seen on the original 2 view study by either method.
Since 40% of all carcinomas occur in the axillary tail, this additional view
(which is necessary in only 5% of the patients), should be routinely performed
in all patients whose breast glandular tissue is difficult to pull away from
the ribs.

combinations. Scatter removal mechanisms are resulting in such significant improvement in mammography imaging, that it is inevitable that all dedicated mammography equipment will utilize them in the near future.

c. Small focal spots - The use of a small focal spot unit enables considerable versatility in situations where suspicious areas are visualized on contact mammograms (see Logan's chapter on grid versus magnification), since magnification spot views of these areas are then possible (a focal spot 300 microns or less in measured diameter is recommended).[7] Small calcifications can be magnified, while the background noise of the film remains unchanged (see figure 8).

SCREEN-FILM SYSTEMS

How does one decide which of the many available screen-film systems to use? In an attempt to further reduce breast glandular x-ray dose, some radiologists have advocated using screen-film combinations which have less detector system resolutions than the Kodak Min-R and DuPont Lo-dose II systems. This results in diminished detection of smaller calcifications, however, and for this reason their use is not recommended. The calculation of the average breast glandular tissue dose obtained with the soft x-ray beam utilized in screen-film studies, has been shown to be considerably less than that originally expected. Therefore, the possible carcinogenic effects are concomitantly considerably less (mid-plane breast dose is actually 5-10% of the breast entrance exposure, rather than the 25% originally assumed). Since the average glandular dose is therefore, much less than originally expected, strenuous efforts to resort to faster screen-film combinations are no longer necessary, (unless accompanied by improvements which will not impair detection of the smallest most easily treatable carcinomas). The recording film should have a single emulsion only, since image degradation results when films containing emulsion on both sides are used, due to angled spreading of the light produced by the screen phosphors. Double emulsion film should not be used unless this crossover can be eliminated. The use of the faster screen-film combinations with less resolution should be considered only when magnification studies are performed with the use of small focal spot mammography x-ray units, or with grids, or other scatter removal methods.

Once homogeneous breast thickness is accomplished by proper compression, the screen-film combination with the most contrast per given x-ray beam half value layer, may be used (or screen-film combinations of equal detector system resolution and speed). At this time I am presently utilizing Kodak NMB single emulsion automatic processed film (slightly more contrast and speed than the Kodak Min-R film) in contact with the Kodak Min-R rare-earth screen, placed in a Picker manufactured black, light-proof polyethylene bag, which is then vacuum sealed by a Picker vacuum sealer.[1] If this equipment is not available, I recommend placing the film in a screen enclosed cassette (both Agfa Gevaert and Kodak offer this option), rather than to enclose a screen-film system in an EZ-EM vacu-bag, because the EZ-EM vacu-bag absorbs and hardens the minimal $\pm$ 10 millirad x-ray beam exiting from the breast considerably more than do the cassette covers.* This attenuation is even less, when the Picker polyethylene bag is substituted, however, enabling both a slight decrease in patient x-ray exposure, and improved image contrast (as seen in figure 7). The screens are cleaned each day, with Kodak screen cleaning solution, followed by an application of Kodak antistatic solution. The Picker

*At this time the EZ-EM bag is being revised, using material which hardens the exit beam less.

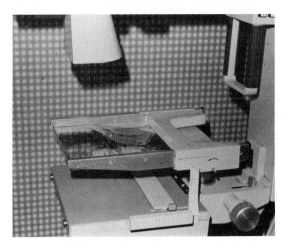

Figure 2: A posteriorly sloping compression device causes geometric unsharpness, and underpenetration of the posterior aspect of the breast tissue,
which is remedied by reversing the compression device. The GE unit with
the reversed compression device, is shown.

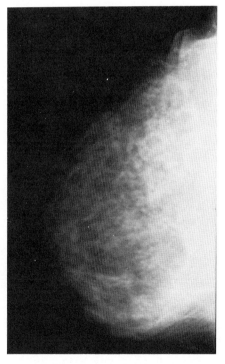

(a)

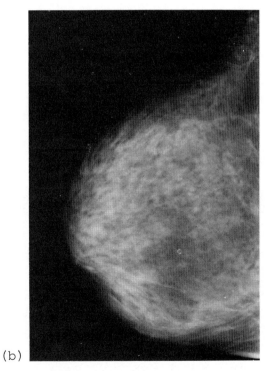

(b)

Figure 3: A lateral view mammogram (A), was performed with the original GE
sloping compression device, revealing underpenetration of the posterior aspect
of the breast. The study was performed on the GE unit, at 25 kVp at 1 second,
using Min-R single emulsion film in contact with a Min-R screen, packaged in
a Picker polyethylene bag. The repeat mammogram performed one year later at
which time the GE compression device had been reversed, shows much improved
compression of the posterior aspect of the breast (B). This study was performed at 25 kVp at .25 seconds, using Kodak NMB film in contact with the
Min-R screen, packaged in a Picker polyethylene bag. The proper posterior
compression of the breast, enables use of a slightly faster and more contrasty
film, which aids in dose reduction also.

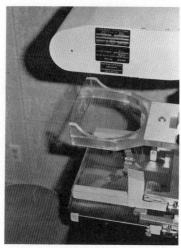

Figure 4: Compression device designed for use with the Radiologic Sciences Inc. mammography unit in my office. The plastic material is angled 90 degrees superiorly at the breast base, in order to push axillary fold and pectoral muscle tissue posteriorly so that it will not be superimposed over the glandular tissue. The sharp angle is preferable to a gently rounded angle for 2 reasons. The sharp angle enables the last few mm of glandular tissue, posteriorly, to be well penetrated with the x-ray beam. The sharp angle also grips the compressed breast tissue better, and does not enable the skin and tissue to slide posteriorly, as compression is performed.

(a)

(b)

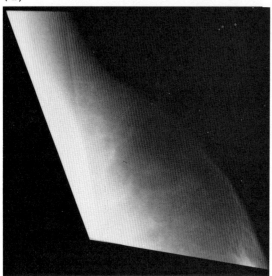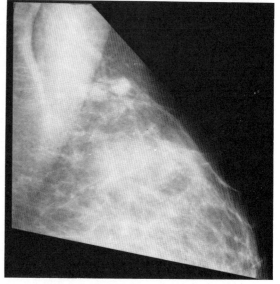

Figure 5: A mammogram was performed on this patient because of a palpable left breast upper outer quadrant density. The initial mammogram (A), utilizing Min-R film in a Kodak Min-R screen cassette, performed on a non-dedicated x-ray unit with a tungsten target, revealed poor contrast between soft tissue and fatty tissue. The second mammogram (B), performed 3 weeks later on a GE Mammex unit, at 25 kVp, utilizing the same Min-R screen-film combination, now reveals better contrast between the soft tissues and fatty tissues, with a 1 1/2 cm diameter lobulated soft tissue density now being readily visualized. The increased contrast is due to a combined effect of the soft x-ray beam available with a dedicated unit, plus the vigorous compression which can be obtained with dedicated mammography unit compression devices, which reduce scatter.

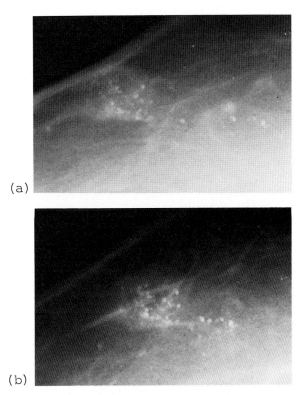

(a)

(b)

Figure 6: This patient has calcifications which have been followed with serial mammograms for a 5 year period. The first mammogram (A), was performed at 29 kVp, with the Min-R screen-film system, on the GE Mammex unit. Calcifications are visualized within a soft tissue density. The second mammogram (B), is performed on the same breast, with all other factors being equal, except that the exposure was performed at 25 kVp, at a slight increase in exposure time. The calcifications seen in A are more readily detected, and, more importantly, additional calcifications are now seen, because of the improved contrast.

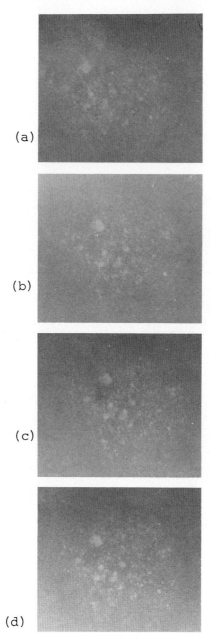

(a)

(b)

(c)

(d)

Figure 7: Radiographic images of the fine calcifications of the Kodak Pathe
Phantom (placed upon three 1 cm thick lucite blocks) were obtained. The
superior-most image (A) was obtained with Min-R film in contact with a Min-R
screen, esconced in a vacuum EZ-EM bag. The second image (B) was obtained
utilizing Min-R single emulsion film in a Kodak Min-R screen cassette. The
improved contrast occurs because the Kodak cassette cover attenuates the
beam less than the EZ-EM bag. The third image (C) was obtained utilizing the
Min-R film in contact with the Min-R screen, enclosed within a Picker polyethylene vacu-pack, rather than the Kodak cassette. The increased contrast
between the calcifications and surrounding lucite density occurred because the
Picker polyethylene cover attenuates the breast exit beam less than the Kodak
cassette cover. The fourth image (D), was obtained utilizing Kodak NMB single
emulsion film (slightly more contrasty and faster than the Min-R film), in
contact with the Min-R screen, enclosed in the Picker polyethylene bag. The
contrast between the calcification and surrounding lucite has been improved
further, because of the increased contrast of the film.

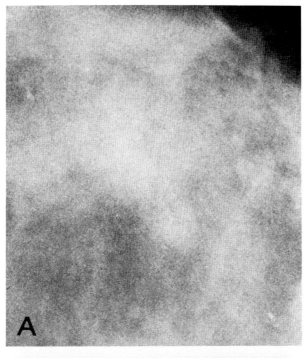

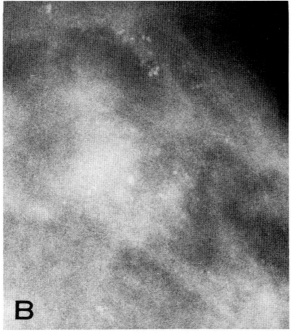

Figure 8: The contact film (A), reveals dense glandular tissue and several
small fine calcifications. For this reason a 1.5 magnification view was
performed with the RSI* unit with a measured 150 micron tungsten focal spot.
This magnification view (B), shows many more small fine calcifications. (The
image has been reduced in size to that of the original contact image, in order
to facilitate comparison).

---

*Radiologic Sciences Inc.

polyethylene bags can be re-used up to 5 times. The inside of each poly-ethylene bag is sprayed once with antistatic spray* before its first use, to prevent static marks on the film (screen and film should not be sprayed with this, as it leaves an elevated residue). As newer screen-film systems develop, they, of course, are continually being evaluated and compared with present methods.

Summary: Some of the technical problems encountered in conversion to screen-film systems for mammography use, have been described. When specialized mammography x-ray equipment, containing vigorous compression, and a soft x-ray beam to enable contrast, are utilized, the resultant images should be of superior quality. Under no circumstances, should screen-film mammography be attempted without these technical attributes. The many reasons for the most vigorous compression possible have been stated. Radiologists who perform mammography in this way will be rewarded by assisting in the re-emergence of mammography acceptance, even in the screening situation in young women. Inadequately performed mammography will only hinder this re-emergence.

*Price Driscoll Corporation, Farmingdale, New York.

1. Ostrum, B.J., Becker, W., Isard, H.: Low-dose mammography. Radiology 109: 323-326, Nov. 1973.

2. Chang, C.H., Sibala, J.L., Martin, N.L., Riley, R.C.: Film mammography: new low radiation technology. Radiology 121:121, Oct. 1976.

3. Skucas, J., Logan, W.W., Gorski, J., et al.: Improved mammography system. N.Y. State J.Med. 76:1992-1993, Nov. 1976.

4. Lundgren, B. and Jakobsson, S.: Single-view mammography screening. Radiology 130:109-112, Jan 1979.

5. Logan, W.W.: Overview of the radiologist's role in breast cancer detection. In, Breast Carcinoma: The Radiologist's Expanded Role, W.W. Logan, editor, Wiley and Sons, New York, 1977, pp 344-352.

6. Haus, A.G.: The effect of geometric unsharpness in mammography and xeroradiography. In, Breast Carcinoma: The Radiologist's Expanded Role, W.W. Logan, editor, Wiley and Sons, New York, 1977, pp 93-108.

7. Muntz, E.P., Logan, W.W.: Focal spot size and scatter suppression in magnification mammography. Amer. J. Roentgenol. 1979 (in press).

STATE OF THE ART PANEL
Art Haus, Moderator

Phillip Muntz: I would like to stress the slide I showed yesterday since
people seem to be forgetting this fact of life. If you are talking about low
half value layers, say .3 mm aluminum, then the ratio of the mid plane dose
to the average dose as you go through the breast varies significantly. We've
heard the mid plane dose treated as average, but it really isn't, it's a factor
of one half of the average glandular dose, for soft beams. For the harder
beam (as in xeroradiography) then the mid plane and the average are closer to
the same, say within 20%, but for the soft beams the average dose is a factor
of 2 times or more, higher than the mid plane. The thickness of the breast
matters considerably, in terms of what the average compared to mid plane or the
 entrance dose is (see my chapter). Therefore, neither breast entrance nor mid
plane doses are accurate representatives of the true average glandular dose.

Mary Ellen Masterson: If I might address Phil's point, the reason why the
data was originally presented back in '76-77 as mid plane doses, was because
that was what was being used for the risk-benefit analyses at that time. We
were apprehensive about that mid breast dose ourselves, and in our article
which has been submitted for publication, that point is made very strongly.

Phillip Muntz: I think the mid plane doses that have been circulated from
Northeast Center are for 6 cm breasts. I would like to point out that most
of the breasts we deal with in compression average about 4.7 or 4.8 cm. That
also makes a numerical factor difference in the numbers recorded. If you
aren't very careful you can generate factors of four difference, without trying
very hard, between a mid plane and say an actual average glandular dose. One
has to be quite careful.

Mary Ellen Masterson: We in the Northeast have realized for a long time that
the 6 cm thickness that was being employed nationally by the six centers for
Radiologic Physics was an overestimate and our survey of 276 patients at
Sloan-Kettering did indicate that we had a 5.1 cm average.

Wende Logan: I just want to plead to anybody reporting average glandular doses,
that if you don't have time to figure them out for your manuscripts at least if
you have an average breast thickness, breast entrance exposure, and a half
value layer we're all set. We must have a breast thickness if we really want
to know what the average glandular dose is going to be.

Attendee: Mr. Kaegi, when you were talking about the XERG system and the photon
energies used, you didn't say anything about filtration. Don't you see a
possibility to shift the beam energy to a certain point which might be optimal
for a XERG system? Don't you see that as a possibility?

Emil Kaegi: We used inherent filtration with the 50 mA units. Prior to that,
we used beryllium window tubes, so we added as much as 1.4 mm of aluminum. I
also recorded that one test condition, (44 kV) with the 50 mA unit; there we
added .5 mm of aluminum.

Attendee: And another question concerning the use of Xerox plates. You said
you were looking for possibilities to further reduce the dose. One of these
possibilities of course is to increase receptor sensitivity. This was said
several times, but I have never seen a receptor with increased sensitivity. Is

there a practice difficulty or are there some other reasons not to increase this sensitivity? You find some Russian papers for example where they tell you that they can go up to a mm of selenium thickness. They also claim they are able to get the whole charge out to the surface.

Dr. Rao: As far as I know, the receptor sensitivity in the case of xeroradiography depends on the nature of the material and the thickness of the material. Some years ago Boag published an article from England in which he established that in the case of selenium about 130 microns is the optimal thickness with which maximum sensitivity is obtained.

Dr. Fatouros: You cannot increase the thickness of the selenium. You cannot expect to halve the exposure by doubling the thickness, because of the field banding effect. The field banding effect inside the photoconductor causes degradation of the signal. In fact, the total calculations show that if you double the thickness in order to halve the exposure, we have a net loss of the signal output of about 25%. Similar results also are obtained with edges. So, increasing the sensitivity is not the way to proceed.

Dr. Rao: That gives an explanation of the findings that Boag projected years ago. Its a more accurate description of it.

Attendee: There still remains the question: is it in practice possible to increase the sensitivity or not?

Ellen Proctor: First let me address the thickness question. The 130 micron selenium plate is pretty well optimized for the mammography spectrum range. We have done work at double the plate thickness in which you have little or no improvement in radiation exposure for mammography. The sensitivity can be improved in looking at things beyond the photoreceptor.

Phillip Muntz: I would like to emphasize that the quantum efficiency or the absorption efficiency of the 130 micron plate of selenium for mammography is essentially better than any other systems around and the place to look is where Ellen said, in the processing. In other words in a xeroradiograph you discharge about 10% of the charge or something like that, Ellen? And so you double the sensitivity if you discharge 20%. That's the place to look.

Attendee: Then you degrade image quality.

Phillip Muntz: You change the edge effect, you do not degrade the image quality.

Attendee: Then you introduce granularity.

Phillip Muntz: Then you can change the toner characteristics.

Dr. Fatouros: You cannot overdevelop the image because, again, you degrade. At some point, the time of development is not optimal. At some point, the density of the signal stops growing. So you cannot do that. Both exposure and development are limited.

Attendee: We just received our XERG unit about 2 months ago and it produces rather good pictures. After we received the unit they told us that our machine would be down one full day for 5 working days, which means 20% of the time, and that it would cost 6-$10,000 per year to service the unit. This is a rather significant difference from what Dr. Saar Porrath has said, about this being the same service as the xeromammography unit. The cost of this service projected is as much as the rental was for the xerography unit. This is indeed a problem to clinicians and I hope that the people at Xonics will be working on that.

Dr. Hirschfeld: I just want to make a comment concerning the cost of the XERG system. We find in the Baltimore area, that supplies have averaged us between $1.10 and $1.20 an image. We decided not to take the contract that they offered at $260 a month, which is considerably less than what you are talking about, because for over the average 11 months that we had it, our service problems have not cost that. I don't know where you're getting your figures but our expenditures don't support that at all.

Attendee: They're doing something for 7 hours a week in the Cleveland area and its going to come between 6-$9,000 a year service.

Emil Kaegi: I think 7 hours a week is a little excessive. This can occur possibly during the first installation period of the unit. I spend approximately more time than an average service man with Dr. Porrath's unit because it is a test bed, in the sense that I am monitoring carefully the usage rates of consumables. In that line I would point out that the 50 mA unit there has been in operation 13 months and there has accumulated over 7,500 cycles on it. It can't be down too many days to accomplish that.

FALSE NEGATIVE AND HEROIC POSITIVE MAMMOGRAMS

Robert L. Egan, M.D.

Chief, Mammography Section

and

Professor of Radiology

Emory University

Atlanta, Georgia

The false negative mammogram is the bane of the mammographer. Lengthy delays in treatment of serious, perhaps only borderline clinically, breast disease or swaying the clinician not to act on definite breast changes cannot always be avoided. The knowledge that some breast cancers will still be found by clinical examination is slight comfort to those striving to bring early breast cancer to immediate therapy.

From the other side of the coin are non-palpable breast cancers to offset these embarrassing episodes. Clinical breast cancers not apparent on x-ray are often advanced, while those found solely by x-ray are most often free of axillary lymph node metastasis.

A challenging group of false negative mammograms are those with breast cancers developing after a non-cancer clinical and x-ray study. The realization upon review of the non-cancer mammograms that the cancer must be there and produces no overt x-ray signs is a great enigma. The philosophy of "fast growing" and "slow growing" tumors may soothe the conscience of the mammographer but does not eliminate the deficiencies of our screening methods. Too, these experiences loudly proclaim the necessity of maximal radiographic detail while maintaining a level of acceptable radiation exposure to the breast.

Supported in part by Grant R01 CA 14712 awarded by the National Cancer Institute, DHEW.

Acknowledgment: R. C. Mosteller, Ph.D., Assistant Professor of Radiology (Biostatistics), C. W. Stevens, Ph.D., Professor Biometry and K. L. Egan, Research Assistant, all of the Section of Mammography, prepared and tabulated the data.

MATERIALS AND METHODS

An ongoing prospective mammographic study has been in progress at Emory University for over 15 years designed to evaluate clinical examination of the breast and mammography while attempting to determine the contribution of history, physical and x-ray examination to risk profiles for breast cancer.[1] While over 1,200 breast cancers are in this data base, close follow-up on 7,127 women over age 30 years was available with 789 operable and treated breast cancer. Of these cancers 131 of them developed 6 to 137 months after a non-cancer clinical and x-ray examination.

Analysis of the 131 cancers, their relation to other cancers and non cancer studies was indicated to determine the reasons for being overlooked and possible better future patient care. Previous analyses of other data had revealed no single significant indicator of developing breast cancer but did show increased frequency of cancers in fatty breasts and in those with ductal hyperplasia.[2] As part of the evaluation we had included a simple classification of mammographic parenchymal patterns that had been reported as a highly successful risk indicator.[3] Such a workable scheme of ready classification of cancer risk would dramatically reduce radiation during mammography to the 94 per cent of the females destined never to get breast cancer.

Prerecorded categories of mammographic patterns contained four of breast consistency, six of parenchymal glandular patterns and three of major duct patterns. The 72 possible combinations were collapsed to the four patterns of increasing amount and density of fibroglandular tissue as illustrated and described by Wolfe as the standard: N1, P1, P2 and DY.

In this review the most recent non-cancer mammogram (based on the original interpretation) was always selected. Conventional mammography or xeroradiography, or both, once standardized did not vary throughout the period. In four classifications of the x-ray patterns of the breasts, two by each of two observers, there was minimal differences in placement into N1 as opposed to P1, or P2 as opposed to DY but no variation if N1 and P1 were combined and P2 and DY were combined.

RESULTS

Review of patient's charts included those with the 131 cancers developing under observation, many contemporary cancers and non-cancers revealed no specific characteristics that clearly separated these groups of patients. In no instance did the mammographer prospectively call attention to the site of a developing cancer and retrospectively no cancer could be identified despite knowledge of its location. In only 8 instances could any nonspecific change be noted in the site of the future cancer. This indicated to us a deficiency in our screening methods and that increased, not decreased, radiographic detail must be maintained despite publicized theoretical radiation harm.

The mammographic parenchymal patterns, the patients, the cancers and the developing cancers were distributed in the various age groups as follows:

	30-39 yrs.			40-49 yrs.			50-59 yrs.			60 and + yrs.			Total	
	Cases	Ca	% Dev. Ca	Cases	Ca	% Dev. Ca	Cases	Ca	% Dev. Ca	Cases	Ca	% Dev. Ca	% Ca	% Dev. Ca
N1	334	4	0%	490	15	.4%	642	44	.3%	997	141	7%	8.7%	.45%
P1	1,134	14	0	1,534	68	.2	927	55	1.0	531	67	2	4.7	.58
P2	1,278	12	0	1,336	50	1	739	61	3	583	75	2	5.0	1.2
DY	1,164	26	.3	1,638	80	1.3	550	48	3	266	32	5	5.1	1.4

From the table less glandular breasts (N1, P1) occur in older women with an increased number of proven cancers. The more glandular breasts (P2, DY) are more frequently studied, occur in younger women and have more cancers developing under observation. The number of developing cancers increased with the density of the breasts by a factor of 3 from N1 to DY. There was no pattern within the P2, DY groups that could predict which women would retain those patterns or would develop cancer. The rate of cancers in N1, P1 and P2, DY, the developing cancers and age groups are shown:

	% Cancer		% Developing Cancer	
Age, Yrs.	N1, P1	P2, DY	N1, P1	P2, DY
30-39	1.2%	1.5%	0%	4.1%
40-44	4.0	4.5	0	18.8
45-49	4.8	4.2	11.4	18.8
50-54	7.8	7.2	11.4	26
55-59	6.8	10.1	20.0	14.6
60-69	10.0	12.2	34.3	13.5
70-+	21.3	13.7	22.9	4.2

In both N1, P1 and P2, DY patterns the rate of cancer in all groups was identical as it gradually increased from 1 per cent in 30-34 year age group to about 10% in the 60-69 year age group. This smooth change was maintained despite heavy loading of P2, DY in the younger and N1, P1 in the older age groups. Yet 67.7 per cent of the developing cancers in P2, DY had been detected by age 55 years while only 22.8 per cent of cancers in N1, P1 had been diagnosed. As long as the detecting modality has a constant efficiency and with equal rates of cancers being found in N1, P1 and P2, DY, any shift from prevalence to incidence should be the same producing equal incidence in the two groups. The three fold increase in incidence in P2, DY merely represent retention of prevalent cancers under observation due to the increased delay of detection of breast cancer in dense breasts.

The stage of the disease was similar in the cancers (following non-cancer studies):

	Stage 0 No. Ca	Stage 1 No. Ca	Stage 3 No. Ca
N1	0	5	5
P1	5	11	5
P2	10	20	16
DY	13	21	16

Although non-palpable masses and areas of altered architecture that proved to be cancer were triumphs, our greatest heroic positives were in 204 cancer patients with borderline calcifications. These were demonstrated in 606 patients, with usually 4 to 10 calcific flecks in a cluster, coming to biopsy and specimen radiology. Of these cancers all were Stage 0 or Stage I (axillary lymph nodes histologically free of metastases). These were primarily intraductal carcinomas with an occasional cancer with minimal microscopic invasion and a few lobular carcinomas in-situ. None had a palpable mass even in the thinly sectioned biopsy specimen.

DISCUSSION

The application of clinical mammography required close cooperation between the radiologist, surgeon and pathologist. With radiography of the breast, biopsy specimens and whole organs, there was early recognition of changes of ductal epithelial hyperplasia, a process that was considered as non-obligate precursor of breast cancer. Cancer was 3 times as frequent in ductal hyperplasia by x-ray and 2 times as frequent in fatty breasts. Widefield mammography seemed ideal to select a parenchymal pattern to predict future cancer.

In some short-term studies there has been shown an increased number of developing cancers in denser breasts. With short follow-up after a non-cancer mammogram, our studies also showed this, but after follow-up well beyond 4 years the incidence of developing cancers were similar in all patterns. Of course with advancing age most of the P2, DY patterns had involuted into N1, P1. The unpredictable few remaining DY breasts after age 60 years had a larger percentage of developing cancers than P1 or P2 but less than N1. This suggests cancers are more readily masked in dense fibroglandular breasts and the normally prevalent cancers are detected in N1 while prevalent cancers become incident cancers in DY. If followed long enough the breast patterns become similarly involuted. This necessitates long follow-up periods for thorough evaluation.

Before mammography became a routine clinical procedure, most breast cancers presented with one or more inoperable grave signs of Haagensen. A most welcome respite from the frustration of oncologists attacking this advanced disease with extensive surgery and massive radiotherapy was a procedure to detect preclinical locally limited cancers. Surgeons insisted upon investigating fewer and fewer calcifications and less and less alterations in the fibroglandular patterns by x-ray. The mammographer was challenged to assure localization of these minimal changes, removal by biopsy and histologic study. Non-palpable masses and architectural changes became palpable after sharp dissection into the localized area by mammography. Every short-cut to study calcifications produced costly errors. We finally agreed that localization, tissue removal, radiography and precise localization of the calcification in that tissue for unhurried histopathologic study was mandatory in all cases despite the tedious and lengthy procedure. In such cases the mammographer was a hero.

Specimen radiography has done most to involve directly the surgeon and pathologist in early breast cancer and demonstrate to them unequivocally that 95% of patients with breast cancer can be cured. In these preclinical, and often preinvasive, cancers meticulous attention to mammographic technique cannot be sacrificed to undue concern about radiation carcinogenesis. A healthy and happy woman is far more important than arithematic legerdemain followed by the boast that .3 rad is infinitely superior to .5 rad.

CONCLUSIONS

Breast cancer is more frequent in older women with fatty breasts.

Cancers are harder to detect in glandular breasts than in fatty breasts by mammography.

Longer follow-up tends toward similar x-ray patterns and incidence of cancer.

There is no mammographic parenchymal pattern that indicates which women will maintain a glandular pattern or which women are at significantly higher risk of developing breast cancer.

Mammography has a prime role in detecting early breast changes or calcifications of preclinical and pre-invasive breast cancer. Meticulous radiographic detail is particularly required in this role of mammography.

REFERENCES

1. Egan, R. L., Mosteller, R. C.: High risk breast tumor patients. Acta Rad. Therapy Physics Biology 16: Fasc. 4:337-351 May, 1977.

2. Egan, R. L., Mosteller, R. C.: Breast cancer mammographic patterns. Cancer 40:2087-2090 November, 1977.

3. Wolfe, J. N.: Risk for breast cancer development determined by mammographic pattern. Cancer 37:2486-2492 May, 1976.

NEAR MISSES

Ruth E. Snyder, M.D.
Attending Radiologist
Memorial Sloan-Kettering Cancer Center
New York, New York

Good mammography depends not only on excellent technique and low absorbed dose but on an intelligent approach to the individual examination as well. The technologist must be able to establish rapport with her patient to obtain her cooperation, must know if there is a particular problem, must develop an appreciation of the type of breast with which she is dealing in order to establish optimal technique, and must be certain that all areas of concern have been demonstrated and localized. To illustrate how important all of this becomes, three cases are cited.

Case 1. A 60 year old patient had been followed by a breast surgeon for years for non-specific thickening in both breasts. A mammogram in 1967 using tungsten target and industrial film with no compression had shown no lesion, and a repeat study in 1971 with molybdenum target (fig. 1a) revealed no obvious change. However, in 1973 a mammogram done by a different technologist demonstrated an obvious 2 cm. cancer deep in the left breast against the chest wall (fig 1b,c). Comparing the 1971 and 1973 films, it was obvious that the 1971 films had not included the posterior portion of the breasts and a tumor could have been present on the earlier study. The technologist in 1971 used one film for two projections. We do not feel that this is a justifiable economy of film or effort except in patients with very small breasts. Positioning must be carefully planned and executed.

Case 2. A 56 year old patient had been under the care of a breast surgeon for years after an operation for a benign cyst of the left breast. On routine follow-up by another surgeon, a swelling was noted over the right chest anteriorly. The clinician could not determine if this was of rib or breast origin. Conventional mammograms by a good technologist were normal (fig. 2a,b). However, we try to examine all our patients, and after noting the fullness, obtained a coned lateral-medial view over the mass close to the chest wall. This clearly identified a breast primary (fig.2c). Patient underwent a radical mastectomy with chest wall resection for infiltrating duct carcinoma, grade II. Fortunately, all nodes were clear. A tumor not projected on to the film cannot be diagnosed.

Case 3. A very apprehensive 52 year old patient was admitted to Memorial Hospital because a routine xeroradiogram done elsewhere had demonstrated a small rounded nodule in the upper half of the breast, not located with certainty on the cranio-caudad view, and the report suggested that this might be an intramammary node (fig. 3a,b). However, it was not seen on a study two years previously. Her surgeon could palpate nothing

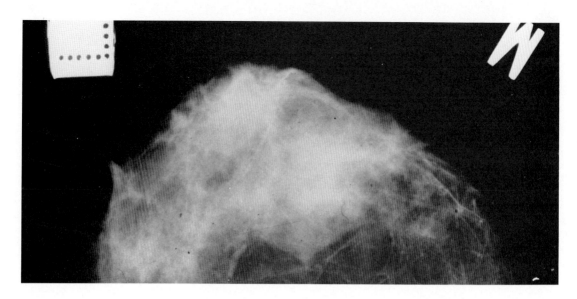

fig. 1a.   Case 1.   Cranio-caudad view in 1971 showing no tumor.
Lateral view was also uninformative.

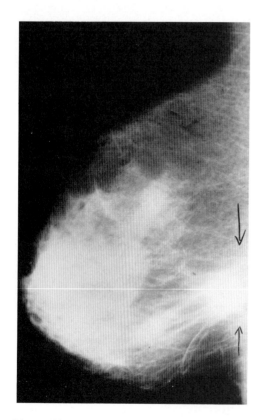
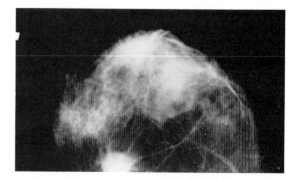

fig. 1b, c.   Same patient in 1973 with obvious carcinoma in
posterior breast.   Note this area was not
included in previous examination.

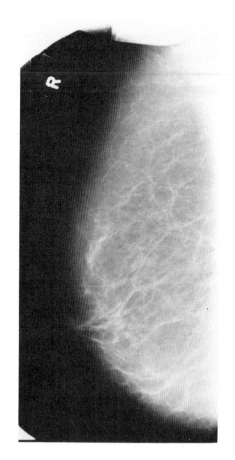
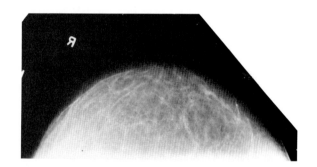

fig. 2a, b.   Routine views show no abnormality.

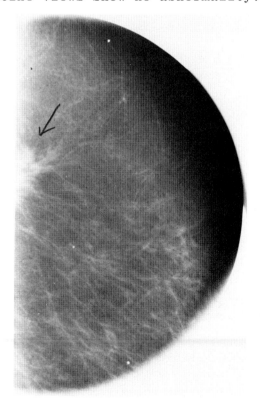

fig. 2c.   Cone view demonstrates cancer against chest wall.

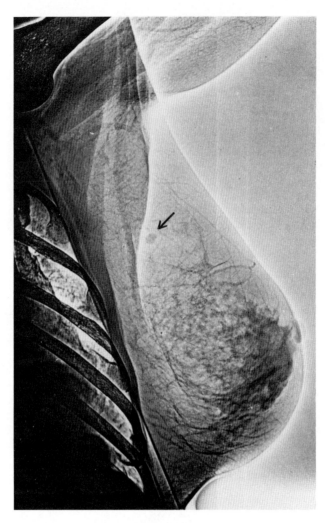

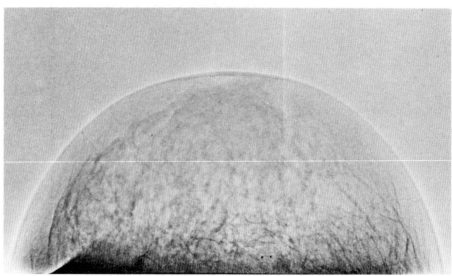

fig. 3a, b. Xeroradiograms demonstrate small nodule on lateral
view (arrow), not seen with certainty on
cranio-caudad projection.

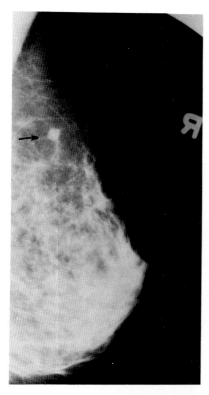
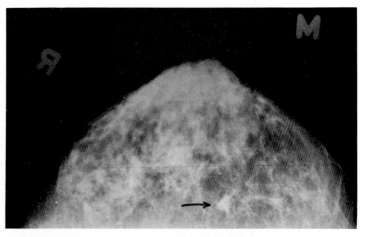
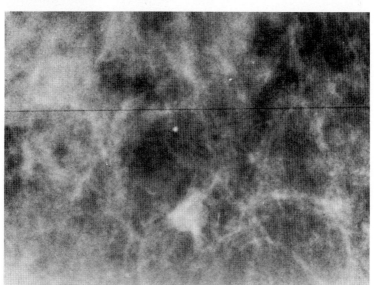

fig. 3c, d, e. Film-screen examination clearly demonstrates
malignant tumor, magnified in e.

443

and sent her for needle localization. Without knowing the exact location of the nodule, we felt it necessary to repeat the study with film-screen technique. A small irregular nodule was clearly located high in the breast in the 12 o'clock axis (fig. 3c,d,e) and could be diagnosed as a definite malignant tumor. It was easily localized for the surgeon and proved to be a 7 mm. infiltrating duct carcinoma with micrometastasis to 1 node at level I. Although the xeroradiograms were of good quality, the film-screen technique was definitely superior with better coverage than the xeromammograms.

SUMMARY: It is self-evident that good technique and low absorbed dose are not the only elements necessary for satisfactory mammography. A capable, conscientious technologist is a very necessary third ingredient. Film-screen mammography with molybdenum target has been more accurate with less absorbed dose than xeroradiography in our experience.

MAMMOGRAPHY: RISK, BENEFIT, DIAGNOSTIC PROBLEMS

Richard H. Gold, M.D.
Professor of Radiological Sciences
Chief, Diagnostic Division
Department of Radiological Sciences
UCLA Center for the Health Sciences
Los Angeles, California 90024

IS MAMMOGRAPHY WORTH THE RISK?

The main purpose of x-ray mammography is to detect cancer before it is palpable and when the disease is potentially curable. Through the use of mammography, moreover, it is possible to detect some cancers when they are still "minimal." So-called "minimal" breast cancer is defined as invasive or in situ carcinoma that forms a mass no greater than 0.5 cm. in diameter as measured pathologically. Women whose lesions are that small have a 10-year survival rate of 95%;[1] hence, early detection and treatment are of great importance.

In the past few years mammography has undergone a striking improvement in image detail along with a corresponding decrease in radiation exposure. The significance of this improvement can best be appreciated when the results of the ongoing Breast Cancer Detection Demonstration Project (BCDDP) are compared to those of the Health Insurance Plan (HIP) of New York Breast Cancer Detection Project of the 1960s: Both projects used a combination of physical examination and mammography. At the first annual screening in the BCDDP, mammography alone was responsible for the biopsy recommendation in 43.7% of the cancers, compared with 33.3% in the older HIP Study. When limited to the age group under 50, the corresponding figures were 43.5% in the BCDDP and 19.4% in the HIP Study.

Nevertheless, as promising as these comparisons seem, the efficacy of mammography in a screening program has yet to be validated in women under age 50. The lack of validation results from several factors. First, mortality was not lowered in the age group under 50 in the HIP screenees, perhaps because very few cancers 1 cm. or less were discovered among these screenees, whereas approximately one-third of the cancers detected among the BCDDP screenees were less than 1 cm. Second, the BCDDP is not a case-control study. Screenees lack a suitable control group against which breast cancer mortality may be measured. It is not possible, therefore, to accept the proposition that the high proportions of breast cancers detected in an early stage of disease among the BCDDP screenees provides evidence of benefit. We do not know when and at what stage of disease those cases would ordinarily have been detected without formal screening. Finally, we lack knowledge about the natural history of cases classified as non-infiltrating cancers, some of which might never have become clinically recognized.

(a)   (b)

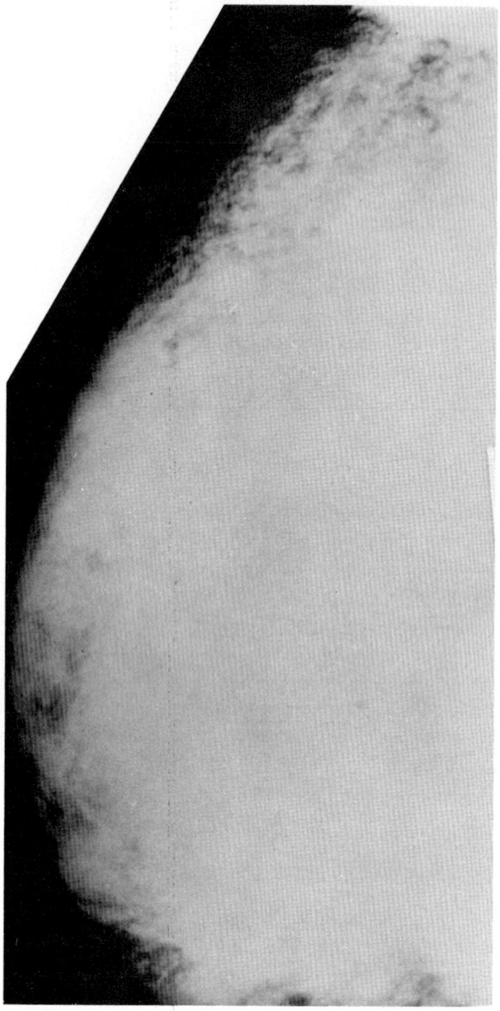

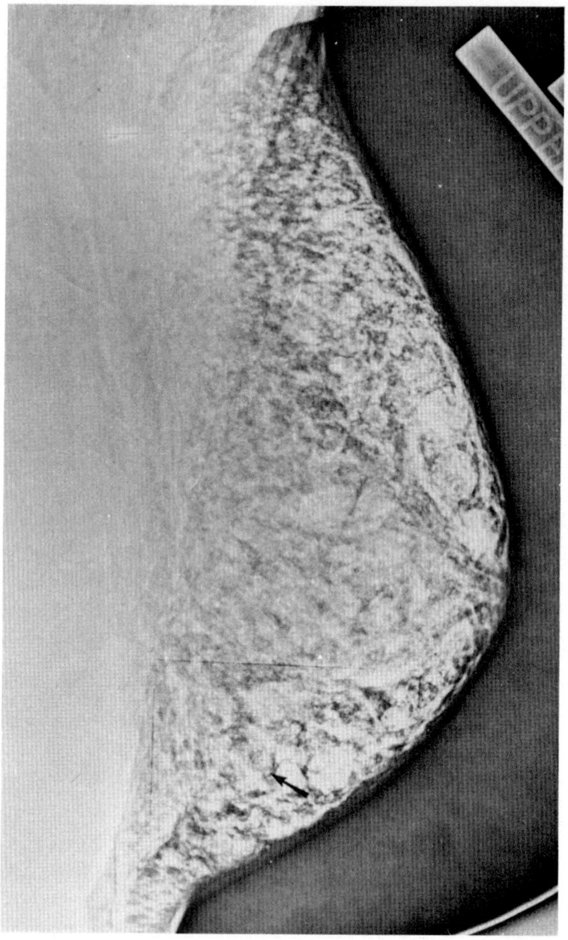

Figure 1. Injected silicone. A. Film mammography. B. Xeromammography
in the negative mode provides greater detail. The arrow points to a small
focus of fat necrosis represented by a lipid-filled cyst with a calcified
wall. This rather heroic observation was made in the face of almost
insurmountable odds. The chance of detecting any pathology, let alone
malignancy, in a breast of this tremendous density is small indeed.

WHAT IS THE RISK OF MAMMOGRAPHY?

The report of Dr. Arthur Upton[2] and his National Cancer Institute Working Group on the Risks Associated with Mammography in Mass Screening for the Detection of Breast Cancer, issued in February, 1977, noted that epidemiological studies revealed an excess of breast cancer in three groups: American women treated with x-radiation of the breast for postpartum mastitis; American and Canadian women subjected to multiple fluoroscopic examinations of the chest during artificial pneumothorax treatment of pulmonary tuberculosis; and Japanese women surviving atomic bomb irradiation who were more than 10 years old at the time of exposure.

From these observations, it was possible for Upton and his group to estimate the carcinogenic risk to the breast associated with the far lower doses of mammography, if the dose-response relationship was assumed to remain linear, irrespective of dose, dose rate, and age at irradiation. Based on this assumption, along with an adjustment for the effects of age difference and susceptibility, the risk was assumed to approximate 3.5 to 7.5 cases of breast cancer per million women of ages 35 or older at risk per year per rad to both breasts, from the tenth year after irradiation throughout the remainder of life.

According to this model, a single mammographic examination performed with a technique that involves an average dose to the breast of less than one rad should be expected to increase a woman's subsequent risk of developing breast cancer by much less than 1% of the natural risk of 7% at age 35 and by a progressively smaller percentage with increasing age at examination thereafter, i.e., from a risk of 7% (since one out of fifteen American women is struck by breast cancer) to a risk of 7.07%. Whether or not the risk is greater in women affected by other high-risk factors remains to be determined.

Through the BCDDP data, we know the least dose to the breast now attainable through mammography that is still consistent with maintenance of high diagnostic quality. In June, 1977, according to BCDDP data gathered by the regional Centers for Radiologic Physics and compiled by the American Association of Physicists in Medicine Coordination Office, Chevy Chase, Md., the average mid-breast dose for a complete film examination was 67 millirads and for a complete xeroradiographic examination, 0.61 rad. Assuming that the risk analysis of Upton and his Group is the best available, a total dose of 1 rad to the mid-breast would allow 13 annual mammographic examinations before the patient's risk is increased from the natural risk of 7% to a risk of 8%. A dose of 1/2 rad to the mid-breast would permit 26 annual mammograms to be performed before this 7% risk is increased to 8%; and a dose of 1/3 rad to the mid-breast would permit 39 annual mammograms to occur before the risk is increased to 8%.

At UCLA, using the Kodak Min R screen-film technique with a Senograph x-ray unit, the mid-breast dose is 40 millirads for a complete two-view examination. At this dose level, approximately 300 annual mammographic examinations are possible before risk is increased by 1%.

Xeromammography and film-screen mammography, while excellent methods of breast cancer detection, both have their advantages and drawbacks. Relative soft-tissue densities are sometimes more reliably evaluated in film-screen images, while calcifications are sometimes

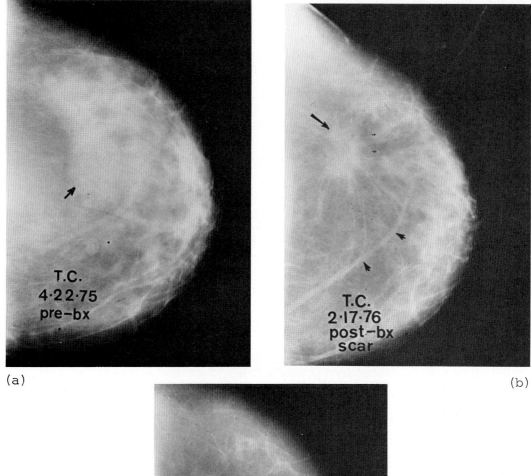

(a)

(b)

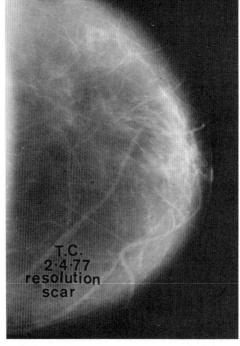

(c)

<u>Figure 2</u>. Biopsy scar mimicking carcinoma. <u>A</u>. Pre-biopsy.
<u>B</u>. Post-biopsy. The scar simulates the desmoplastic response to a
carcinoma. <u>C</u>. Complete resolution of the scar. A clue that the
connective tissue response results from a scar rather than a carcinoma
is that a scar is generally palpable only as a vague thickening, while
carcinoma generally feels two or three times larger than its mammographic
image and is usually rock hard.

more reliably evaluated in xeromammographic images. Film-screen
mammography tends to record fatty or fibrofatty breasts more reliably
than xeromammography, while the latter tends to record dense, dysplastic
breast tissue more reliably than the former.

At UCLA, we have at our disposal both film-screen and xeromammographic
techniques, enabling us to tailor our examination to obtain the greatest
information using the lowest dose of radiation possible. For women
under 35 who have strong indications for mammography, which usually means
signs or symptoms which could be those of breast cancer, two film-
screen images of each breast are obtained. For some women between 35 and
49, depending upon the contents of the film images, we may choose to
add a single negative-mode, highly filtered xeromammogram (150 mrad to
the mid-breast). For some women 50 and over, a single positive-mode,
highly filtered xeromammogram (200 mrad to the mid-breast) may be used
to complement the film-screen images. It is now possible for a radiologist
to perform a complete, high-quality mammographic examination using no
more than 500 millirads to the mid-breast. Referring physicians and
patients would do well to insist upon this (500 millirads to mid-breast)
as the highest dose they will accept. They need only to question the
radiologist regarding his dose. Most radiologists are extremely aware
of the sensitive nature of this problem and are willing to provide this
information.

DIAGNOSTIC PROBLEMS

The capability of mammography to record the shadow of a carcinoma
or of any lesion is largely dependent upon the presence in the breast of
sufficient fat to serve as a contrasting radiolucent background. An
atrophied breast in which all glandular tissue has been replaced by fat
may be shown by mammography to contain an obvious carcinoma only a few
millimeters in diameter, while a breast packed with radiographically
dense glandular or mammary dysplastic tissue may contain a large carcinoma
that is completely masked by the tissue which surrounds it. Therefore,
mammography must be supplemented with clinical examination. Just as
mammography cannot replace a thorough physical examination, the physical
examination cannot replace mammography. Moreover, a negative mammogram
or a negative physical examination should never deter the performance
of a biopsy with histologic examination of a suspicious lesion that has
been detected by either method.

The breast must be compressed during each x-ray exposure. Compression
not only reduces the possibility of breast motion during the exposure,
but it diminishes the thickness of tissue being radiographed, thus
decreasing scattered radiation and diminishing the superimposition of
both anatomic and pathologic structures. The fraction of scattered
radiation decreases as the volume of irradiated tissue decreases. Thus,
the thinner the part and the smaller the area being radiographed, the
smaller will be the fraction of scattered radiation. It is important
to restrict the x-ray beam to the smallest area that will include the
selected anatomic region. But an even more important factor in diminishing
scattered radiation is compression of the breast. The effect of compression in limiting scattered radiation is considerable; however, once
compression and coning have been achieved, the effect of further coning
is relatively insignificant.

449

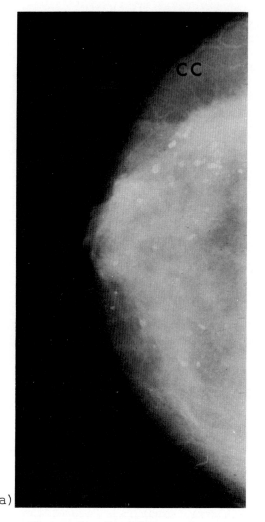
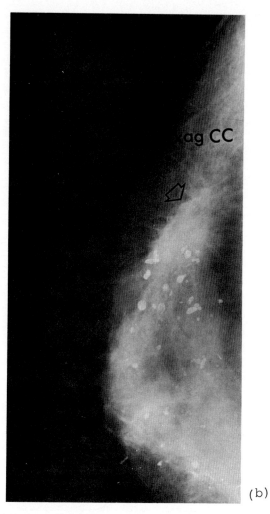

(a)

(b)

Figure 3. Usefulness of an exaggerated cephalocaudal view.
A. Routine cephalocaudal view. The carcinoma in the upper part of the
illustration is difficult to appreciate because its posterior margin is
cut off by the edge of the film. B. When the cephalocaudal view is
performed with the film beneath the outer (axillary) portion of the
breast, the full extent of the carcinoma is revealed, making diagnosis
easier. The coarse, ring-shaped calcifications represent benign
secretory disease, while some of the smaller calcifications may result
from the carcinoma.

450

Just as mammary dysplasia may completely mask an underlying carcinoma, the increased density of the breast that results from pregnancy, lactation, or injected silicone may also prevent detection of underlying cancer. When faced with any of these conditions, the mammographer should alert the referring physician to the difficulty in detecting cancer in breasts of such increased density.

Retromammary implants within the breast prohibit adequate compression during the x-ray exposure, making visualization of the anteriorly displaced breast tissue less than optimal. In the face of retromammary silicone implants or intramammary silicone injections, the best commonly available technique for visualization of the breast is xeroradiography utilizing the negative mode.

A mole or a senile keratosis on the skin of the breast may simulate an intramammary lesion in the mammogram. Similarly, a biopsy scar, particularly of relatively recent origin, may simulate the desmoplastic reaction of a carcinoma. A suggestion: After performing the physical examination, the mammographer should record on a line-drawing of the front of the breasts the location of all moles, scars, and masses. It is convenient to outline each breast as representing the face of a clock; but remember, the lateral aspect of the right breast is 9 o'clock while that of the left is 3 o'clock.

To localize a lesion for the surgeon, it must be visible in two views at 90-degree angles. If the standard views show the lesion only in the mediolateral view, it will usually be found at the base of the axillary tail of the breast. An exaggerated cephalocaudal view, with the film beneath the axillary portion of the breast, will usually disclose the lesion.

One last admonition: While breast carcinoma in some cases yields characteristic radiographic findings, there are no pathognomonic signs. Two lesions in particular that may be difficult to distinguish from carcinoma are sclerosing adenosis and traumatic fat necrosis. Both of these lesions may result in calcifications and spiculations that mimic those of carcinoma. Remember that the most common cause of traumatic fat necrosis is the trauma of surgery.

REFERENCES

1. Wanebo JH, Huvos AG, Urvan JA: Treatment of minimal breast cancer. Cancer 33:349, 1974

2. Final Reports of National Cancer Institute Ad Hoc Working Groups on Mammography Screening for Breast Cancer and A Summary Report of Their Joint Recommendations. Washington, U.S. Dept of Health, Education and Welfare, National Institutes of Health, DHEW Publication No. (NIH) 77-1400, March 1977

HEROIC POSITIVES AND FALSE NEGATIVES PANEL FOR REDUCED DOSE MAMMOGRAPHY

Myron Moskowitz, M.D.

University of Cincinnati, College of Medicine

In Cincinnati we believe that a heroic positive is the detection and treatment of highly curable carcinoma of the breast. We believe minimal breast cancer (0.5 cm invasive carcinoma without evidence of axillary metastases, or tumor which is wholly in situ lobular or intraductal) fits this criteria. We don't care whether the detection was by physical examination or mammography. We consider any case to be a tragic negative when the disease is not found until invasive and well established.

By periodically reviewing our efforts in this direction, hopefully we can learn from past mistakes and successes and expand our future horizons.

We are aware that there is some skepticism concerning the significance of the minimal breast cancers detected to date. Suffice it to say that during the first 2½ years of annual incidence screening, including the count of all cancers incident and interval, if we were to eliminate the minimal breast cancers from consideration, we would have found less than half of the expected incidence of carcinomas. This data includes all interval as well as incident cancers. When the minimal breast cancers are included, the total number of cancers during this period matches the number one would have expected. This would lead us to believe that the minimal breast cancers are in fact real cancers, and the likelihood is that at least 90% of them would have presented as invasive cancer, not only within the projected lifetime of the patients, but included within the projected time frame of the screen.

Furthermore, as a result of continued followup of the 6,000 women under the age of 50 who have not been offered full screening since April, 1977, we are able to state with confidence that the clinical lead time gained by aggressive full sensitive screening including mammography is two years.

Based on our prior screening experience, we would have expected in these 6,000 younger women that 14 cancers would develop through the month of October. As of October 24 we are aware of 12 such cancers which have developed. Allowing for some lag time in reporting we believe that this is well within expected range. Had the patients been fully screened we would have expected 6.5 of these cancers to have been minimal. In fact only 2 of the cancers were minimal and these were found in the 1,000 women who did receive screening because they fit the appropriate criteria. The remaining 10 cancers were invasive, 5 were Stage I, and 5 were Stage II.

Thus, the predicted effect of not screening is simply delay in time to diagnosis. Since there are data now indicating over 93% 20 year relative survival rates for minimal cancer (1), and since our experience suggests that the lead time gained to clinical detection is two years, we believe the clinical imperative to detect these minimal lesions is quite clear.

Recently, the accuracy of the histopathologic diagnoses of minimal breast cancers has been called into question. In fact, certain self proclaimed patient advocates have risen in pious indignation and proclaimed a pox on the medical profession for the "mutilation" of innocent women. The facts of the matter are quite different.

There were 506 cases of minimal breast cancer reviewed by an independent team of pathologists. The diagnosis of minimal breast cancer was not confirmed in only 48 cases.

We have unequivocal evidence that this review team did not see the correct slides on four of our own patients. Two of these patients had invasive carcinomas with either lymph node involvement, or frank lymphatic permeation. In no way were these cases minimal. They have been re-examined and are unquestionably malignant.

In the two additional cases of intraductal carcinoma, three pathologists have concurred in the diagnosis in one case, and two pathologists in the other.

Doctors Robert McDivitt, and Peter Paul Rosen have just recently completed review of additional material submitted on all four of these cases. They concur completely in the diagnosis of invasive carcinoma in two, and intraductal carcinoma (carcinoma in situ of duct origin) in one. In the fourth case they feel that the primary diagnosis of sclerosing adenosis with severe lobular atypia, not quite carcinoma in situ is more appropriate. Thus, no significant divergence of pathological opinion is thought to be present in any of these instances.

If this degree of error exists for 4 of the 48, how many more must exist in the reviewed group?

Let us assume for the moment that all 48 cases were not, in fact, cancer. This represents an area of disagreement of less than 10%! Not only is this an acceptable concordance of medical opinion, it is absolutely remarkable. For example, Wallgren (2) has reported that of 91 breast cancers, pathologic concurrence was found in 75, or 82%. The overwhelming majority of these cancers were invasive, well established, not minimal breast cancers. Gordon, et al (3), found pathologic agreement in the diagnosis of endometrial cancer in 66/89 cases or 74%.

Pathologists, like all medical specialists will disagree. This disagreement will occur even when great care is taken to ensure that all observers have access to the same material.

Prior to mass screening for breast cancer, the rate of detection of minimal breast cancer was less than 5% nationwide.

In our screening center the rate of detection of minimal breast cancer for younger women is 54%. If it is necessary to accept a false positive pathology diagnosis rate of 10-20% to increase the yield of highly curable cancers by over ten times, then that is what must be done.

We have found that one of the most frequently overlooked signs of minimal breast cancer is the sign of asymmetry. In Figure 1 the increased density in the upper outer quadrant of the left breast as compared to the right is quite apparent. In the absence of a palpable mass or any palpable thickening or minimal abnormality whatsoever, the yield for cancer under these circumstances is very small, I would judge less than 5%. If there is any palpable thickening or resistance whatsoever, the likelihood of finding an underlying carcinoma rises dramatically. In fact, when the latter situation pertains we increase the strength of our likelihood of finding carcinoma, on a scale of 0 to 10 with 10 being the highest, from 1 to approximately 8 or 9. Figure 2 is the same patient one year later. There is both clinical and radiographic evidence of classical inflammatory carcinoma.

The question of when to biopsy small calcifications has often been raised. Radiologists, generally, are aware of the classical criteria for calcifications which are very strongly associated with carcinoma. Unfortunately many of the very early carcinomas are not associated with such obvious well defined calcifications. We try to recommend biopsy for small punctate calcifications numbering 3 or more, clustered in a circle whose circumference is less than a centimeter, as well as those which are linearly arranged. We do so even though our degree of confidence in a diagnosis of malignant on a scale of 0 to 10 with 10 being the highest is probably on the order of 1. Figure 3 demonstrates an array of calcifications which were not biopsied. One year later, Figure 4 demonstrates where there had been 3 there are now perhaps 3,000 calcifications. The cancer was a 5 mm lobular carcinoma with microinvasion.

That these lesions progress and develop is further attested to in the next image, Figure 5. You will note a single punctum of calcification. However one year later there are now three little calcifications in the same area and there is a little tiny density of nonspecific nature. This was a 5 mm microinvasive carcinoma of the breast (Figure 6).

Figure 7 demonstrates the reason for doing mammography in a clinically palpable lesion. The lesion at the equator which was small and readily palpated was a benign fibroadenoma. The larger deeper seated lesion not clinically palpable was the malignancy. Although this was a detecting triumph for mammography I'm not certain that it significantly affects the patient's long term survival.

Martin and Gallaher first drew our attention to the significance of the neodensity sign. They stressed that any new density occurring in the breast, no matter what its radiographic appearance, was highly likely to be neoplastic (Figure 8-9). Although, in our experience, the frequency of neoplasm has not been as high as reported in their experience, we do believe that neodensities should be biopsied. In Figure 10 we see a nonspecific new density forming deep in the substance of this patient's breast. Biopsy was performed and the pathologic diagnosis was severe atypical epithelial hyperplasia. Thus, while not true malignancy was found here, a high risk marker was discovered which indicates this woman, who was under the age of 40, deserves annual lifetime screening with mammography and careful physical examination. She has no other known risk factors for carcinoma of the breast.

The next four images demonstrate why we believe it is extremely important that we biopsy benign masses. All of these lesions are fibroadenomas which contain minimal breast cancer either within the lesion or immediately adjacent to it. In our experience these minimal lesions have virtually all been intraductal lesions. Ten percent of 63 fibroadenomas in women in this age group have, in our experience, been associated with minimal breast cancer. We believe that fibroadenomas are not premalignant in and of themselves, but represent a hallmark of the proliferative stimulus to the breast epithelium. In younger women with developing breasts these are essentially normal, frequent findings. In premenopausal and postmenopausal women, we believe the presence of an active fibroadenoma is not a normal finding, but rather it

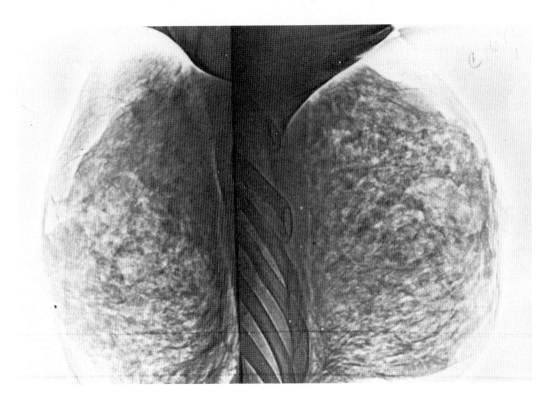

Figure 1:   Asymmetrical density, left breast.

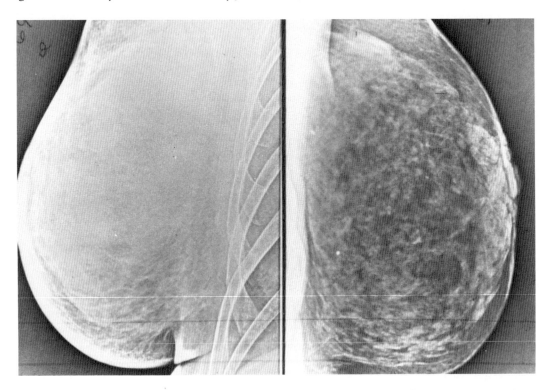

Figure 2:   Same patient as Figure 1, one year later; inflammatory carcinoma, left breast.

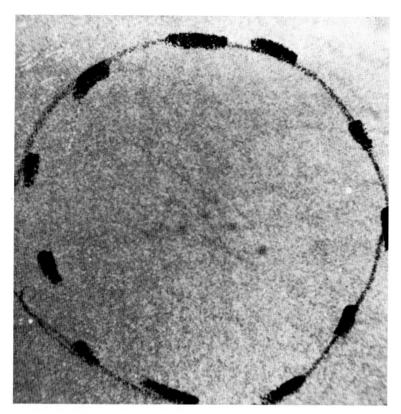

Figure 3:   Few calcifications clustered.

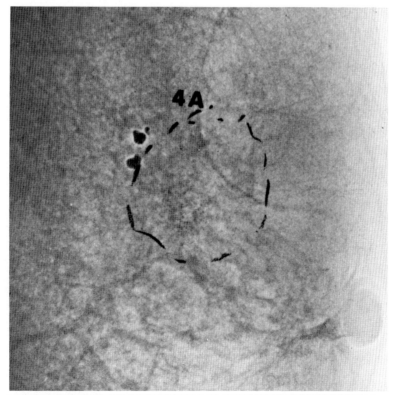

Figure 4:   Same patient one year later; innumerable calcifications have
              developed.

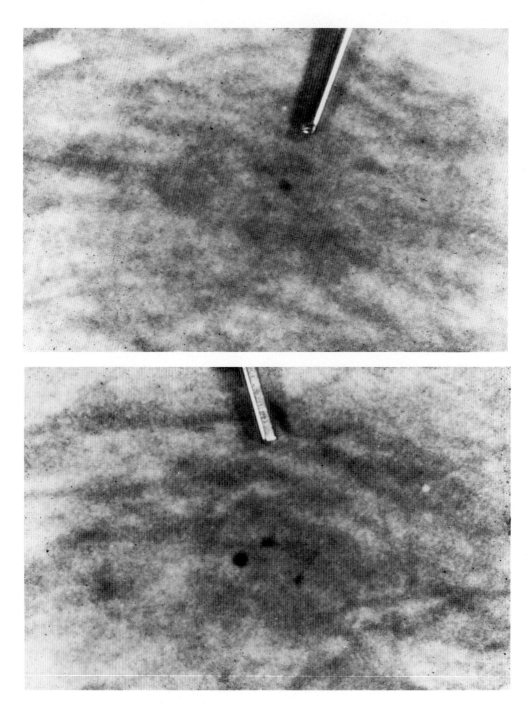

Figure 5 & 6:One calcification progressing to three associated with tiny, nonspecific density.

indicates a group of women at very high risk. We believe that excisional
biopsy should be undertaken for definitive diagnosis, and a reasonable cuff
of tissue should be obtained so that careful pathologic evaluation of the
surrounding tissue and the fibroadenoma itself can be made for the presence
or absence of microcarcinoma.

Our detecting methods at this point in time are crude. Nevertheless
by aggressive use of them we have the opportunity to detect a significant
number of suspicious abnormalities, many of which will turn out to be highly
curable small breast cancers. Until a more sensitive/specific diagnostic
tool comes about, we must rely on the methods which are available.

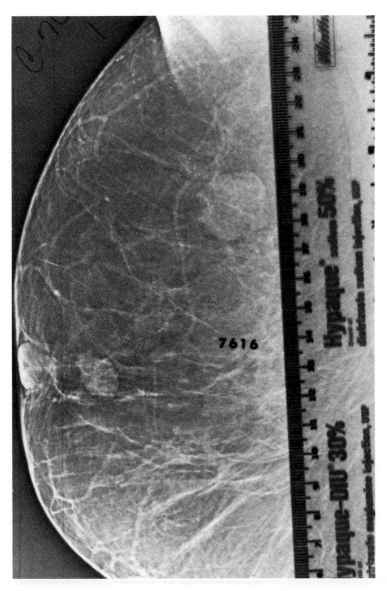

Figure 7:   Smaller palpable lesion was fibroadenoma. Larger lesion, which
              looks not dissimilar was not palpable. It was cancer.

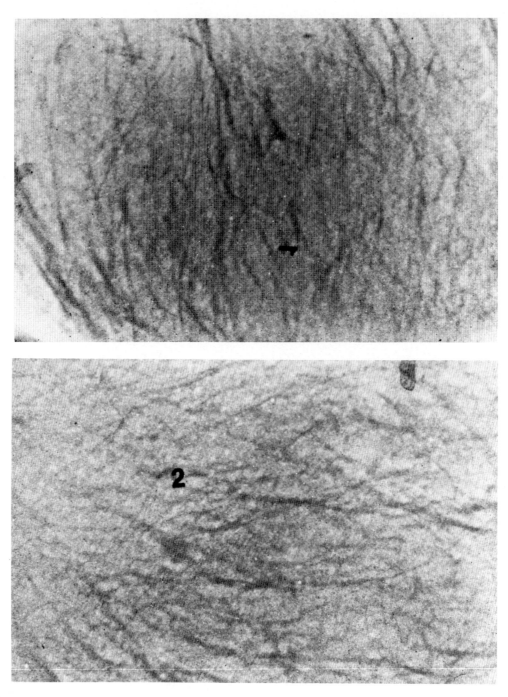

Figure 8 & 9: Neodensity sign. This was cancer.

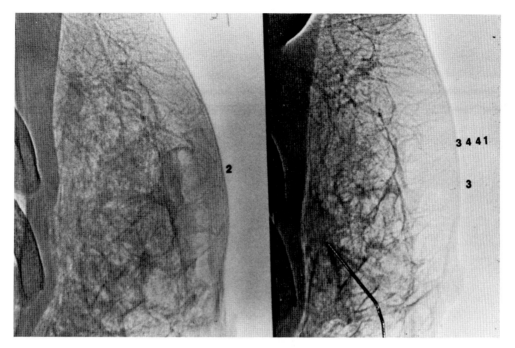

Figure 10:   Neodensity sign.   This was atypical epithelial hyperplasia.

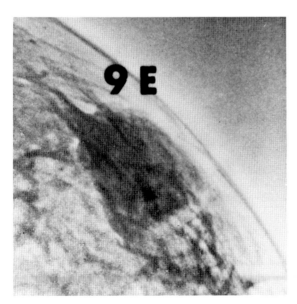

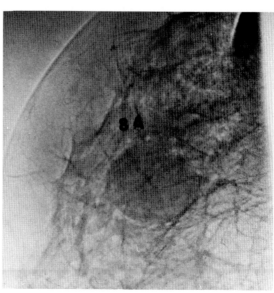

Figure 11   Figure 12

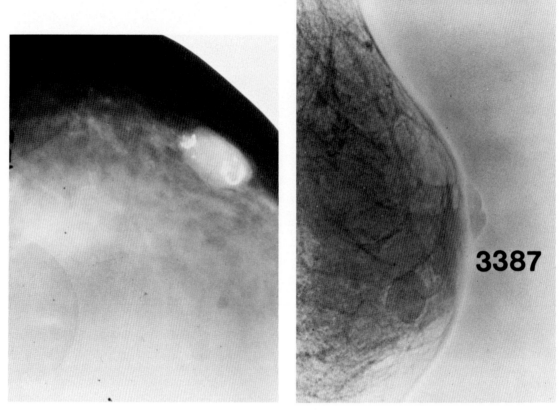

Figure 11-14:Fibroadenomas proven to be associated with small microinvasive cancer or foci of intraductal cancer.

REFERENCES

1. Frazier, T.G., Copeland, E.M., Gallager, H.S., Paulus, D.D., and White, E.C.: Pronosis and treatment in minimal breast cancer, American Journal of Surgery: 133 (6): 697-701, 1977.

2. Wallgren, A., Silfversward, C., Hultborn, A.: Carcinoma of the breast in women under 30 years of age, Cancer 40: 916-923, 1977.

3. Gordon, J., Reagan, J.W., Finkle, W.D., Ziel, H.K.: Estrogen and endometrial carcinoma: Pathological support of original risk estimates, New England Journal of Medicine, 297: 570-571, 1977.

MALIGNANCIES MISSED BY MAMMOGRAPHY

John J. Gisvold, M.D.
Consultant, Department of Diagnostic Radiology
Mayo Clinic and Mayo Foundation

At the Mayo Clinic, mammography is done by using either the Min-R screen-film method or xeroradiography. Overhead tubes are used, with the craniocaudad view done in a sitting position and the oblique view performed with the patient recumbent. Long cones, measuring 22 inches, are used with a target-film distance of approximately 33 inches. Balloon compression is used for all mammography.

Three examining rooms are devoted to mammography. Two rooms have molybdenum target tubes, and one room has a tungsten target tube. Only xeromammography is done with the tungsten target tube; 1.5-mm Al filtration is added. One molybdenum target tube is used only for film mammography. The second molybdenum target tube is used for either film or xeroradiographic studies; when xeromammograms are done with this latter tube, 1.75-mm Al filtration is added. All three tubes have dual focal-spot sizes, and the larger focal spots are used. The nominal focal-spot sizes used are 1.2 mm for the molybdenum target tubes and 1.0 mm for the tungsten tube.

Table 1 show the exposure factors used for mammography. Table 2 shows the measured half-value layers for each tube. Table 3 shows the radiation exposures measured at skin level without backscatter. Values given are for techniques used for the craniocaudad views of a breast 7 to 8 cm thick. Measured exposures are shown for all techniques used with each tube.

Table 1--Exposure Factors

Factor	Film mammography	Xero-mammography
mA	300	300
Time (s)	0.2-0.4	1-1.25 (positive mode) 0.7-0.8 (negative mode)
kVp	27-44	47-60

Only one method of examination is used for each patient, except for occasional instances in which it is considered desirable to check questionable findings by using both techniques. The selection of method is made randomly by the technicians, depending on availability of examining rooms. An attempt is made to do an approximately equal number of examinations with each technique.

Table 2--Half-Value Layers (HVL) in mm Al

Tube	kVp	HVL
Moly I	30	0.40
Moly II	30	0.48
Moly II + 1.75 mm Al	50	1.12
Tungsten + 1.5 mm Al	50	1.74

Table 3--Radiation Exposure (Craniocaudad Views)

Tube	Method	Technique s	kVp	Exposure, R
Moly I	Film	0.3	31	0.133
Moly II	Film	0.2	28	0.121
	Xeromammogram, negative mode	0.7	53	0.527
	Xeromammogram, positive mode	1.0	51	0.679
Tungsten	Xeromammogram, negative mode	0.8	52	0.463
	Xeromammogram, positive mode	1.25	50	0.723

Rather than deal mainly with so-called heroic positive results, this discussion will be concerned primarily with missed lesions. Many reports concerning accuracy of mammography have appeared in the literature in the recent past. Some of these results, which are listed in Table 4,[1-8] range as high as 98% for xeromammography and 95.3% for film mammography.

Table 4--Accuracy Rates

Film mammography	% Accuracy
Block & Reynolds	66
Karsell	85
Brebner & Judelman	95.3

Xeromammography	
Wolfe	95.3
Kalisher & Schaffer	95
Cramer	96.2
Frankl	98
Feig	78

A series of 429 patients who had surgery for breast malignancies at the Mayo Clinic was reviewed. Eleven patients had a preliminary biopsy at a home hospital, 20 had only mammograms at the local institution, and 44 had no mammograms. Subtracting these patients, 354 are left who had a Mayo Clinic mammogram. Eleven of these had simultaneous bilateral lesions, and so a total of 365 malignancies were available for review on these mammograms. One hundred fifty-one malignancies were removed from patients who had xeromammograms and 214 from patients who had film mammograms.

The accuracy rate for xeromammography was 81% and for film mammography, 82%. The studies were interpreted by any 1 of 14 radiologists involved in this work. A retrospective review of all missed lesions was carried out by the author, and the conclusion of the review was that of 29 lesions missed on initial xeromammography interpretation, 31% could have been diagnosed. Similarly, for film mammography, it was thought that of 39 lesions initially missed, 36% could have been diagnosed. Overall, it was believed that 66% of the missed lesions were not visible, even in retrospect.

No lesions were missed in patients who were more than 80 years old. Otherwise, with both techniques, the misses were fairly evenly distributed over all age groups, probably because women of all ages can have dense parenchymal patterns that obscure malignancies. This does not agree with the oft-stated opinion that mammography is much more accurate at older ages than in women less than 50 years old.

Calcification was visible in 33% of malignancies on xeromammograms and in 35% of those on film mammograms.

Table 5 shows the breakdown of parenchymal patterns for patients in this series. Ten lesions were missed in breasts with an N pattern, 10 in P1 type breast, and 9 in patients with a P2 pattern. The remaining 39 misses, or 57% of total misses, were in breasts with a Dy pattern. It was surprising to note that 10 lesions were missed in fatty, N type breasts. Review of these 10 lesions showed that 5 of them could be seen in retrospect. The other five lesions were all small, 1 cm or less in size. Two of these were infiltrating lobular carcinomas. Two of the lesions were infiltrating duct cell carcinomas, both 6 mm in size, and one of them was located in the nipple. The fifth lesion missed, and not visible in retrospect, was a 1-mm focus of carcinoma found in a small area of adenosis.

Table 5--Parenchymal Pattern*

Type	Xeromammogram No.	Xeromammogram %	Film mammogram No.	Film mammogram %	Total No.	Total %	Avg age (yr)
N	43	29	55	28	98	28	65
P1	39	26	37	19	76	22	65
P2	17	12	21	10	38	11	62
Dy	48	33	86	43	134	39	55
Total	147	100	199	100	346	100	

*Only 346 cases available for review.

The largest percentage of malignancies overlooked were missed because they were obscured by dense parenchyma and were not associated with visible calcification (Fig. 1 and 2). When carcinomas are calcified, they can be seen even

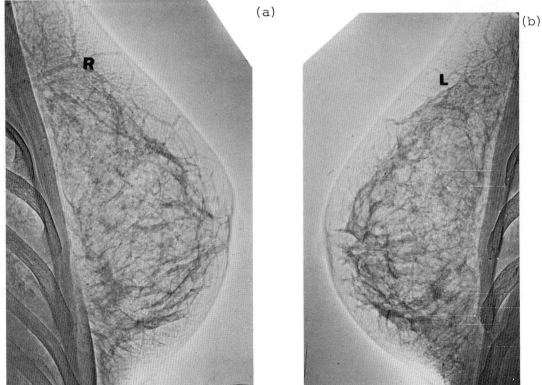

Fig. 1. A, Right oblique view. B, Left oblique view. These oblique views are from the xeromammogram of a 45-year-old woman who had a palpable mass in the 10 o'clock position of the right breast. A 2.5-cm grade 3 adeno-carcinoma was removed from the upper outer quadrant of the right breast. This is an example of a case in which there is some fibrocystic disease and the lesion is not imaged well enough to allow a mammographic diagnosis. No calcification is evident in the area where cancer was located.

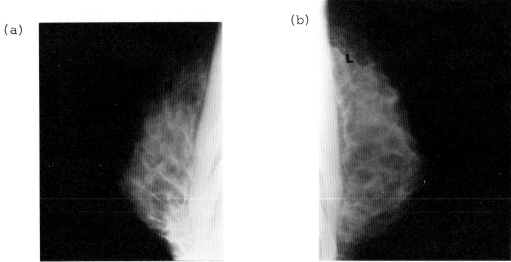

Fig. 2. A, Right oblique view. B, Left oblique view. A 46-year-old woman had two palpable masses in the left breast, one at 6 o'clock and one at 9 o'clock. At surgery, a 2-cm cancer was removed from the 6 o'clock position and a 3-cm carcinoma from the 9 o'clock position. Review of the oblique views from the film mammogram shows that neither of the carcinomas in the left breast can be separated visually from the marked dysplastic changes in the breast. There is a similar degree of mammary dysplasia in both breast.

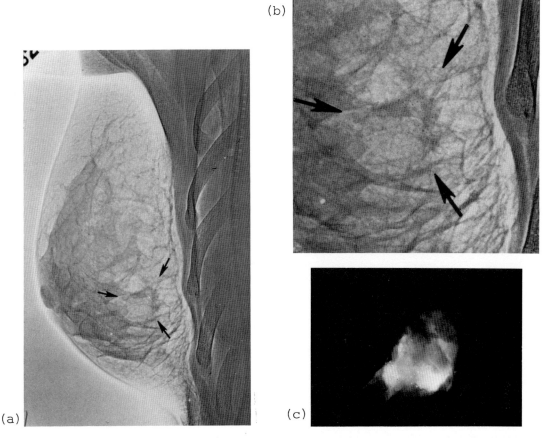

Fig. 3. A, Left oblique view. B, Enlargment of the involved area of the left breast. C, Specimen radiograph. This is a 28-year-old woman who came for an evaluation primarily because of a palpable mass in the right breast. No mass was palpable in the left breast. The xeromammogram shows an area of calcification and slightly increased density in the lower portion of the left breast, deep within the breast. This clinically occult lesion was removed and proved to be a small grade 3 adenocarcinoma. (The lesion in the right breast was a benign fibroadenoma.) This malignant lesion is discernible in the midst of dense fibrocystic changes because of the presence of calcification and a slight distortion of architecture. Despite the fact that this was a clinically occult lesion, the patient had two positive axillary nodes.

in the midst of dense parenchyma. Even if carcinomas are not calcified, they can be recognized in the midst of dense parenchyma if they create enough architectural distortion (Fig. 3 and 4).

Table 6 shows the frequency of localized disease for several reported series of cases[9-13]. Sixty-six percent of the patients in this series had negative axillary nodes and no evidence of other spread. By comparison, 82% of patients with clinically occult lesions had negative nodes. This series consisted of a large percentage of symptomatic patients or those with suspicious physical findings rather than of a basically screening population. Only 10% of the malignancies were clinically occult. It is interesting to note that 81% of the radiographically missed lesions were associated with negative nodes. This points up the fact that the clinicians examining these patients were skillful in finding even fairly small lesions when they could not be seen on mammograms. The favorable lymph node status for missed lesions also raises a question of whether this group of malignancies was less aggressive and thus created less architectural distortion even though pathologically they appeared no different.

Table 6--Localized Breast Malignancies

Study	No. of Patients	% with localized disease
Fischer	2,578	49
HEW Cancer		
Pt survival	33,619 white pt	49
Report #5	3,045 black pt	32
Egan	53	72
Feig	138	71
		88 (occult group)
Frankl &	133	61
Rosenfeld		78 (occult group)
Malone, Frankl,	185	56
et al.		68 (occult group)

One important finding of this review is that teamwork among clinicians, surgeons, and radiologists is important--certainly not a new point but one worth emphasizing. The best prognostic indicator for breast cancer patients today is the presence or absence of known spread beyond the breast, and this is best indicated by the status of the axillary lymph nodes at surgery. Overall, the patients in this series had a better than average lymph node status. The frequency rate of uninvolved nodes is similar to that in some reports in which mammographic accuracy rates were approximately equal to or slightly better than those in this series. The lymph node status is somewhat better than that in some series in which the mammographic accuracy was significantly better. Although mammographic accuracy is very important, the overall result for the patient is a much more important factor than the accuracy rate alone.

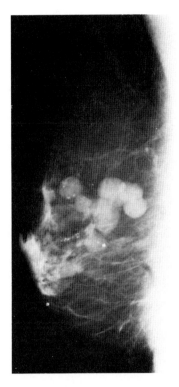

Fig. 4. This 80-year-old woman had some nodularity in this breast on
physical examination but showed no signs that suggested malignancy. The film
mammogram shows a spiculated density in the midst of multiple benign-appearing
masses and an area of calcification extending from the spiculated density
toward the nipple. This clinically occult lesion was a grade 4 comedo carcinoma, 0.8 cm in diameter. A simple mastectomy was done with a low axillary
dissection, and no involvement was found in the low axillary nodes. This
carcinoma is also evident because of a combination of calcification and a
mass with characteristics different from those of most of the benign-appearing
masses in the breast.

REFERENCES

1. Block MA, and Reynold W: How vital is mammography in the diagnosis and management of breast carcinoma? Arch Surg 108:588-590, 1974.

2. Karsell PR: Mammography at the Mayo Clinic: A year's experience. Mayo Clin Proc 49:954-957, 1974.

3. Brebner DM, Judelman E: Comparison of xeromammography and film mammography in the diagnosis of breast lesions. S Afr Med J 49:1380-1382, 1975.

4. Wolfe JN: Analysis of 462 breast carcinomas. Am J Roentgenol 121:846-852, 1974.

5. Kalisher L and Schaffer DL: Xeromammography in early detection of breast cancer. JAMA 234:60-63, 1975.

6. Cramer GG: Xeromammography. IN: Najarian JS, and Delaney JP: Advances in cancer surgery. New York, Stratton Intercontinental Medical Book Corporation, 1976, pp.419-420.

7. Frankl G, Ackerman M: Xeromammography: Five years and 559 carcinomas. Am J Obstet Gynecol 129:61-64, 1977.

8. Feig SA, Shaber GS, Patchefsky A, Schwartz GF, Edeiken J, Libshitz HI, Nerlinger R, Curley RF, Wallace JD: Analysis of clinically occult and mammographically occult breast tumors. Am J Roentgenol 128:403-408, 1977.

9. Fisher B, Slack, NH, Bross IDJ, and Cooperating Investigators: Cancer of the breast: Size of neoplasm and prognosis. Cancer 24:1071-1080, 1969.

10. Asire AJ, Shambaugh EM: Cancer of the breast. IN: Axtell LM, Asire AJ, Myers MH: Cancer patient survival: Report number 5. DHEW publication No. 77-992. US Government Printing Office, Washington, D.C., 1976.

11. Egan RL, Goldstein GT, McSweeney M: Conventional mammography, physical examination, thermography and xeroradiography in the detection of breast cancer. Cancer 39:1984-1992, 1977.

12. Frankl G, Rosenfeld, DD: Breast xeroradiography: An analysis of our first 17 months. Ann Surg 178:676-679, 1973.

13. Malone LJ, Frankl G, Dorazio RA, Winkley JH: Occult breast carcinomas detected by xeroradiography: Clinical considerations. Ann Surg 181: 133-136, 1975.

DOUBT AND CERTAINTY IN XERORADIOGRAPHY - THE FALSE NEGATIVE

Lester Kalisher, M.D.

Saint Barnabas Medical Center
Department of Radiology
Livingston, New Jersey 07039

Mammography, whether photochemical (film) or photoconductive (Xerox), has been accepted as a highly accurate means of discovering breast cancer and is usually included in the evaluation of symptomatic or high-risk women with breast problems. Xeromammography has been utilized clinically for the past six years and has demonstrated that like its film counterpart there appears to be a fairly constant, although comparatively low, error rate inherent in the technique. The purpose of this paper is to evaluate specific Xerographic false negatives in a large series of breast cancers in order to ascertain the reason for the errors and to see if they might be reduced. False positives are inconvenient and increase the cost of medical care as well as decrease the confidence in mammography as a diagnostic tool. There usually is little long term harm to the patient. On the other hand, the false negative is a far more serious situation. Not only is the patient given a false sense of security and confidence in mammography undermined, but the delay in diagnosis may be the difference between cure and death. Keeping the error rate low is especially important since the risk and efficacy of mammography has recently been under strong attack.

This paper analyzes and attempts to define the causes of the false negative group in order to decrease the error rate in this important population. Although this paper specifically addresses the Xerographic false negative, stressing some of the technical pitfalls, most of the causes of the false negatives also pertain to film mammography.

MATERIALS AND METHODS

The Xeromammographic case load at Massachusetts General Hospital from January 1, 1973 to October 1, 1977 was searched and 52 cases of misdiagnosis were found in a total series of 1,214 proven breast cancer cases. In retrospect, 27 of these cancers still were not seen.

DISCUSSION

It became quickly evident that mammographic errors could be divided into certain reproducible groups.

Past experience suggests they should be divided as follows:

A. Not Visualized

    1. Obscured by Surrounding Breast Parenchyma
    2. Location Outside the Breast
    3. Obscured by Thick Skin
    4. Poor Technique

B. Misinterpretation

    1. Lesion Demonstrates No Malignant Criteria
    2. Palpating One Lesion, Imaging a Different Lesion
    3. Lesion Not Recognized by Observer
    4. Non-Belief

NONVISUALIZATION

SURROUNDING BREAST DENSITY

Over 50% of missed breast carcinomas fall into the first group. (Table I) The most difficult breast to evaluate radiographically is the small, dense breast usually found in the young, nulliparous woman.

Since 80% of carcinomas manifest themselves as masses and only 30-40% demonstrate radiographically visible microcalcifications (1) it is easy to see why a certain percentage of non-calcified carcinomas cannot be imaged. Without a fatty background to image margins and no microcalcifications to act as a guide, the radiologist must rely on differential assymetrical density. Unfortunately, Xeroradiography is limited in grey scale and subtle differences in density may be more difficult to appreciate. This is further complicated since this parenchymal pattern is usually found in women under 35 years of age, and the incidence of breast cancer in this group is quite low. (Table II). 21 of the 52 errors fell into this category and in an earlier series Wolfe stated that 50% of errors fell into this category (2). It appears that the error rate in this group must be considered irreducible and that careful reassessment of these mammograms will fail to demonstrate the carcinoma. Obviously, the same limitations apply to any woman with extremely dense, dysplastic breasts, regardless of age. This type of breast pattern has also demonstrated a greater risk for the development of mammary cancer. (3) Recent work with C.T. Breast Scanning (Chang) (4), Ultrasound (Teixidor) (5), and Thermography (Barash) (6) may have further impact on reducing the errors in this group.

LOCATION

The second group is those not imaged due to location of the lesion. Certain areas of the breast may not be imaged, especially if a fixed, dedicated mammographic unit is utilized. Approximately 6% of all breast cancers lie against the chest wall and could be easily missed with certain types of equipment. It is imperative that the entire breast is imaged to the chest wall level. Lesions high on the chest wall are usually difficult to image with any system.

Occasionally, a lesion is too medial or lateral to be imaged on a routine cranio-caudal view and can only be imaged on the medio-lateral projection. Clinical correlation of all women undergoing mammography is imperative in order to ascertain that the lesion in question is properly positioned and imaged. It is also helpful in proving that the palpable lesion is the same one that is imaged. If a lesion is palpable, but not imaged on either one or two routine views, the examination should be tailored to the specific location of the lesion. Exaggerated views, contact views, obliques, axial and axillary views have all proven helpful and should be utilized whenever necessary. If the clinically palpable lesion still cannot be imaged the radiographic report should mention this in the discussion so that the referring physician is not lulled into a false sense of security.

SKIN PROBLEM

A third cause of carcinoma non-imaging is skin thickening from an extraneous process. Classically, burn victims develop small contracted breasts with thick skin in which carcinomas cannot be imaged. Thickened skin and soft tissues secondary to congestive heart failure, anasarca, acromegaly, psoriasis, dermatomyositis and other diffuse skin disorders have the capability of obscuring carcinoma. (7) Obviously inflammatory carcinoma, cellulitis, and diffuse metastatic carcinoma from one breast to the other also obscures an underlying carcinoma. Often subtle skin thickening is the only sign of metastatic carcinoma of the breast to the opposite breast. (8) Missing a new primary breast lesion in these cases would probably be of less importance to the patient's prognosis.

TECHNIQUE

Proper technical factors are extremely important in both film and Xeromammography. The latter demonstrates several unusual characteristics which must be specifically considered when critiquing image quality as errors in technique may obscure an otherwise obvious lesion.

Toner rob is a characteristic of the edge enhancement properties inherent in Xeroradiography. Toner is attracted from one side of a discontinuity and deposited on the other side. If the charge attraction is too great an area of toner depletion will result in which a small lesion would not be imaged. In order to prevent this phenomenon skin folds, calcific densities, and implants must be noted and technical adjustments made.

Under or overexposure is a common error which may obscure lesions. Numerous technical treatises explain how to differentiate exposure errors. Underexposure, though aesthetically pleasing, must be condemned because of the ease with which obvious lesions can be overlooked. Careful attention to halo width can solve this problem.

Image smear is a plate charging defect which has numerous causes. Definition is underenhanced and detail is destroyed. A lesion could be easily missed especially near the skin surface. Other artifacts (pressure, spatter, plate crystallization, etc.) should be immediately corrected and the images repeated.

Motion is an obvious problem usually caused by a small generator with a slow time. Modern three phase generators have almost completely solved this problem. Small microcalcifications, abnormal ducts, and small cancers will be obliterated by motion artifact.

Likewise, poor geometry will also fail to image small lesions. A small focal spot, long target/object distance and short object film distance with good compression is vital for excellent detail. Presently, high resolution magnification units are available which have proven very useful in selected cases. (9)

Errors in the first three categories discussed above are almost impossible to reduce and are probably defensible until new techniques such as C.T. and Ultrasound become universally available and efficacious. The last category can be corrected if technicians and radiologists adhere to careful radiological technique and clinically evaluate each patient.

MISINTERPRETATION

This category should decrease as the radiologist obtains experience in interpretation. Radiographic criteria are well established for benignancy and malignancy. Unfortunately, these signs may occasionally fail even the most astute, experienced mammographer.

LESIONS DEMONSTRATING NO MALIGNANT CRITERIA

A well demarcated mass with a thin radiolucent halo, no architectural distortion, and no microcalcifications usually represents a benign lesion. However, certain malignancies can mimic a benign lesion. Notorious amongst these is the medullary carcinoma, a solid, well differentiated, slow growing, adeno-carcinoma with concomitant lymphoid stroma. Intracystic carcinomas also have a benign appearance. (10) They are quite rare, representing only 0.4% of all carcinomas, and consist of a cystic cavity filled with bloody fluid and a small papillary mass. They are usually found in older women near the chest wall. Colloid carcinomas often have a lobulated border, but are smooth and demonstrate well defined margins. (11) They can be easily misinterpreted. Occasionally, a "garden variety" well differentiated adenocarcinomas can mimic an adenoma or cyst with peri-cystic fibrosis. Ultrasound and C.T. may be helpful in differentiating cystic from solid masses, but a non-cavalier attitude in which any dominant mass is aspirated and/or biopsied is the safest course. Fortunately all of these rare carcinomas have excellent prognoses.

PALPATING ONE LESION, IMAGING A DIFFERENT LESION

Numerous cases of a palpable lesion growing over a non-palpable carcinoma have been reported. Several carcinomas have been obscured by cysts and fibroadenomas. As discussed earlier in this paper, it is imperative that the radiologist examine the patient before interpreting the images. Often the palpable lesion and the carcinoma are in different areas of the same breast or in the opposite breast. Therefore, in order to avoid this type of error, continue searching the breast after the palpable lesion has been located and always try to radiograph the opposite side.

LESION NOT RECOGNIZED BY OBSERVER

Fatigue, inattention, and inexperience may enter into many diagnostic errors. If the mammograms are read by an inexperienced, non-interested observer at the end of a long, hard day the error rate will increase sharply.

Numerous refresher and training courses are available to radiologists to keep their degree of expertise at a proper level. If possible, mammograms should be interpreted when they are completed rather than at the end of the day so that the case is fresh in the examiner's eye. If this is not feasible, good notes and clinical drawings are extremely helpful.

NON-BELIEF

This last category is difficult and fortunately not too common. It usually occurs in a very young woman with dense breasts who may demonstrate a few microcalcifications or minimal architectural distortion. In view of her age, perhaps her appeal or apparent innocence, the subtle warning signs are suppressed by the radiologist with such statements as "she is too young to have cancer, it is only a little adenosis or a scar," etc. Psychologically, the radiologist does not want this woman to have carcinoma and unconsciously ignores the minimal radiographic findings resulting in a missed diagnosis. Obviously, this last situation is rare, but it has occurred.

CONCLUSION

There are numerous reasons why Xeromammographic false negatives occur. They can be divided into two broad categories: Nonvisualization and Misinterpretation.

About half of the Xeromammographic errors occur because of surrounding parenchymal density which obscures the lesion. The rest are evenly distributed amongst the other causes for error. This study suggests that a certain percentage of false negatives is irreducible with present techniques, but other errors can be sharply reduced by paying particular attention to technique, carefully examining the woman clinically, making certain that radiologists assigned to interpreting mammograms are interested and well trained, and lastly, that the images must be painstakingly evaluated with magnification for any subtle changes and that the radiologist must have sufficient confidence to comment on these findings.

If these criteria are followed the number of false negatives should be substantially reduced.

TABLE I

FALSE NEGATIVES

CAUSE	#	%
A. NOT VISUALIZED	27	51.9
1. Obscured by Surrounding Dense Breast Parenchyma	12	23.1
2. Location Outside Breast	8	15.4
3. Obscured by Thick Skin	3	5.8
4. Poor Technique	4	7.7
B. MISINTERPRETATION	25	48.1
1. Lesion Has No Malignant Criteria	15	28.8
2. Palpating One Lesion, Imaging a Different Lesion	4	7.7
3. Lesion Not Recognized by Observer	5	9.6
4. Non-Belief	1	1.9

TABLE II

AGE - SPECIFIC BREAST CANCER INCIDENCE RATES

AGE	35	35-44	45-54	55-64	65-74	75
New Cases per 100,000 per year	3	87.5	162.1	197.7	237.8	311.3

OVERALL INCIDENCE   71.5/100,000

Connecticut Tumor Registry, State of Connecticut, 1968.

BIBLIOGRAPHY

1. Wolfe, John N. : Analysis of 462 Breast Carcinomas.
   Am. J. Roent. Vol. 121, #4, 846-853, August, 1974.

2. Wolfe, John N. : Mammography: Errors in Diagnosis.
   Radiology 87: 214-9, August, 1966.

3. Wolfe, John N. : Risk for Breast Carcinoma Development
   Detected by Mammographic Parenchymal Patterns.
   Cancer 37: 2486-2492, 1976.

4. Chang, C.H.; Sibala, Justo L.; Fritz, Steven L.;
   Gallagher, Joe H.; Dwyer, III, Samuel J.; Templeton, Arch W.;
   Computed Tomographic Evaluation of the Breast.
   Am. J. Roent. 131: 459, 1978.

5. Teixidor, H.S. and Kazam, E.: Combined Mammographic-Sonographic
   Evaluation of Breast Masses.
   Am. J. Roent. 128: 409-417, March, 1977.

6. Barash, I.M.; and Pasternack, B.S. : Quantitative Thermography
   as a Predictor of Breast Cancer.
   Cancer Vol. 31, 769-776, April, 1973.

7. Hall, D.; and Kalisher, L.: The Breast as a Mirror of
   Systemic Disease.
   Journal of Interamerican College of Radiology,
   Vol. II, pp. 211-217, October, 1977.

8. Toombs, B.D.; and Kalisher, L.: Metastatic Disease to the
   Breast: Clinical, Pathologic and Radiographic Features.
   Am. J. Roent. 129:673, April, 1977.

9. Sickles, Edward A.; Doi, Kunio; Genant, Harry K.: Magnification
   Film Mammography: Image Quality and Clinical Studies.
   Radiology 125:69, 1977.

10. Kadir, S. and Kalisher, L.: Colloid Carcinoma of the Breast.
    Breast, Vol. 3, pp. 42-45, April-July, 1977.

11. Kalisher, L.: Intracystic Carcinoma of the Breast Presenting
    as a Benign-Appearing Mass.
    Breast 3(1):32-33, January-March, 1977.

MAMMOGRAPHIC INTERPRETATION: FALSE NEGATIVES AND HEROIC POSITIVES

Edward A. Sickles, M.D.
Department of Radiology
University of California School of Medicine
San Francisco, CA 94143

Mammography is both a sensitive and a specific indicator of the presence of breast cancer, and often will delineate a carcinoma well before it is large enough to be palpable. On the other hand, some palpable breast cancers, occasionally even large ones, will not be found by mammography. This paper deals with these two extremes of mammographic capability: 1) false negative interpretations, in which existing breast carcinomas are missed by mammography but detected by other means, and 2) "heroic" positive interpretations, which I define as those cases where mammography is the only examination that demonstrates a carcinoma thereby permitting timely therapeutic intervention that results in cure. The fact that heroic positives occur more frequently than false negatives is the basis for the current widespread acceptance of mammography as the most accurate non-invasive technique for the detection and diagnosis of breast cancer.

FALSE NEGATIVE INTERPRETATIONS

NON-REMEDIABLE

Of the many causes of false negative mammography interpretations, some are due to limitations in image quality resulting from deficiencies in currently available radiographic equipment.

Breast carcinoma is usually detected on mammograms by the demonstration of clustered microcalcifications having characteristic shape and distribution (1,2) or by delineation of a mass with spiculated or knobby margins (3,4). Conventional mammography techniques indicate the presence of microcalcifications in only 30-50% of breast cancers (5-7), while 60-80% of these cancers can be shown to have calcifications by subsequent histological examination (8,9). Clearly, many breast cancers contain microcalcifications that are smaller than the limits of resolution of conventional mammography. One possible approach to minimize such missed diagnoses is the more widespread use of microfocal spot x-ray tubes adapted for mammography. The small focal spot results in decreased geometric unsharpness, thereby improving resolution (10) and facilitating microcalcification detectability. Microfocal spot mammography, with either a contact or magnification technique, has indeed been shown to permit superior microcalcification detection compared to conventional contact techniques (11).

The radiographic visibility of a non-calcified breast carcinoma depends primarily on demonstration of the tumor mass itself. This is accomplished without difficulty if the mass is surrounded by fatty tissue, but in the densely glandular breast conventional mammography often provides insufficient contrast to allow the cancer to be distinguished from the adjacent benign fibroglandular tissue. Several newly developed techniques promise to improve detectability of non-calcified masses, by increasing the contrast of the mammographic image. These techniques include scatter-reduction mammography with moving grids (12) or scanning multiple slit assemblies (13), use of very high-contrast (currently experimental) screen-film combinations (14), contrast-enhanced CT scanning (15), and heavy-particle mammography (16). The clinical value and feasibility of these techniques has not yet been determined.

REMEDIABLE

The remainder of false negative mammography interpretations can be attributed to improper radiographic technique or observer error. These types of missed diagnosis are avoidable and merit more detailed discussion.

Observer error occurs in the interpretation of all radiographic examinations, including mammography. Inexperience can be corrected by appropriate training, observer fatigue by double reading (two radiologists) or repeat reading all cases one day later. In addition, it is very important to obtain clinical follow-up on as many completed examinations as possible; this is perhaps the best way to refine interpretive skills and to adjust personal criteria to decide which specific radiographic features are necessary to make the diagnosis of benignity or malignancy.

Improper radiographic technique results in a false negative interpretation when the mammograms do not adequately image a carcinoma to permit its detection and diagnosis. This can occur not only if the films are too unsharp to portray the important features of the lesion but also if the lesion is not included on any of the available films. The best way to avoid either of these situations is to have the radiologist who will read the mammograms check all the films before the patient leaves, so that appropriate extra exposures are taken. I do not believe that this responsibility should be delegated to a technologist, no matter how skilled she might be, because she cannot be expected to read the mind of the radiologist to know whether additional films will be requested. I am not arguing against allowing technologists to take as many exposures as they consider necessary to complete the examination; I am simply suggesting that since it is the radiologist who must interpret the study, it should be the radiologist who makes the final decision as to whether additional films are needed. If, under specific circumstances, it proves impossible for the radiologist to monitor the mammography examination, there must never be any hesitation in recalling the patient for additional films, even though such a recall results in both inconvenience and emotional strain to the patient.

In order to avoid missing breast cancers because they are not included on available films, the radiologist must know the precise location of all palpable masses, especially the ones for which the mammography examination is requested. Since this information is often not supplied by the referring physician, the radiologist (or a properly trained technologist) must take an appropriate medical history and perform the necessary physical examination, noting the locations that all palpable masses occupy as the breast is compressed for both craniocaudal and lateral projection mammograms. Lesions high in the upper outer quadrant of the breast are frequently not included on either craniocaudal or lateral projection mammograms. Under these circumstances, additional exposures using oblique or axillary projections are necessary. Lesions at 3 o'clock and 9 o'clock positions close to the chest wall may be missed on standard craniocaudal projection. These can be imaged successfully on an "exaggerated" craniocaudal view, with the patient turned either medially or laterally, as needed. Finally, a lesion at 12 o'clock position close to the chest wall may also be left out on the craniocaudal projection, especially in a woman with small breasts; if this occurs, the lesion may well be included in the craniocaudal projection image if only the upper part of the breast (that portion above the nipple) is radiographed.

There are slight but definite differences in the amount of breast tissue that can be included on mammograms taken with screen-film vs. xeroradiographic recording systems. However, no controlled studies have been done to determine whether these differences significantly affect the false negative cancer detection rate.

Many radiologists contend that among lateral projection images, only the standard mediolateral xeromammogram includes all the breast tissue close to the chest wall, since it images structures back to and including the pectoral muscles and ribs (17,18). My experience with standard contact lateral screen-film mammograms confirms this observation. However, if the technologist pays special attention to pulling the breast away from the chest wall at the moment compression is applied, the entire volume of breast tissue can indeed be included, even though the ribs are not seen (Fig. 1). Therefore, when proper patient positioning is achieved, the same amount of breast tissue is included on lateral projection screen-film mammograms as is included routinely on standard mediolateral xeromammograms.

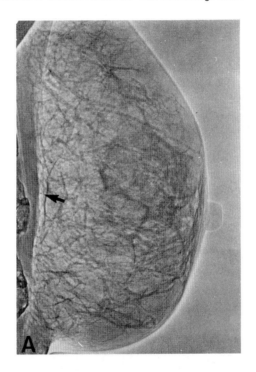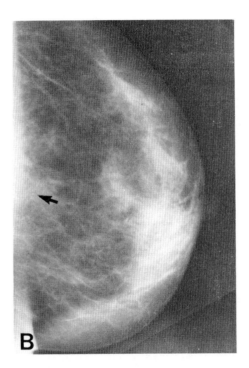

Fig. 1. Lateral projection mammograms of a breast that contains a single microcalcification close to the chest wall, at nipple level (arrows).
   A. The standard mediolateral projection xeromammogram includes all the breast tissue back to the chest wall.
   B. A properly positioned contact lateral projection screen-film mammogram includes the same amount of breast tissue, even though the ribs are not included in the image.

The situation is quite different for the craniocaudal projection, in which screen-film images usually include more breast tissue than xeromammograms. Two reasons help to explain this finding. First of all, the dead space between the outer margin of the xeroradiographic cassette and the edge of the selenium-coated plate is 5/16", compared to a dead space of less than 1/16" for screen-film mammography done with vacuum-sealed plastic envelopes. This permits the screen-film images to include tissue at least 1/4" closer to the chest wall than xeroradiographic images. Secondly, the rigid flat compression devices used mostly for screen-film mammography (to produce uniform-thickness breast compression) allow the breast to be pulled much further away from the chest wall than do the gently contoured compression devices used primarily for xeromammography (balloon compression, Xerox Corp. "independent" mammographic positioner), again permitting more breast tissue to be included in the screen-film images.

Improper radiographic technique can also result in a false negative interpretation if the cancer is not portrayed with sufficient clarity to allow for its detection. Artifacts can mask the presence of an underlying carcinoma, as can either markedly overexposed or underexposed images. However, these errors in technique are usually recognized by the technologist, and are frequently corrected by a repeat exposure before the radiologist even sees the films. Motion unsharpness can also interfere with detection of a subtle carcinoma, especially if a long-duration exposure is required or if there is inadequate breast compression. Geometric unsharpness is more difficult to recognize, but is best corrected by a repeat exposure in a projection that places the lesion closer to the film (e.g., a contact lateromedial or medio-lateral xeromammogram as opposed to a standard mediolateral projection image). This problem is encountered less frequently with techniques employing long focus-film distances; it is almost never the cause of a missed diagnosis when a microfocal spot x-ray tube is used.

The edge enhancement property of xeroradiography can produce relatively large areas of deletion (toner robbing) immediately adjacent to an abrupt interface between dense and less dense tissue. This situation often occurs on standard mediolateral projection xeromammograms of small-breasted women, in whom the axillary skin fold can cause a substantial deletion of the image in the superficial portions of the axillary tail of the breast. A single exposure in the negative mode should be obtained whenever such areas of deletion occur, to avoid missing lesions in the deleted portion of the image.

Finally, the slight differences in image quality between xeroradiographic and screen-film recording systems can occasionally account for a false negative interpretation, in that under certain circumstances a carcinoma may be missed with one technique when it could have been detected with the other. It must be emphasized, however, that this occurs only when the radiographic features of malignancy are subtle indeed. Xeromammography demonstrates superiority in the detection of breast microcalcifications, probably because of its edge enhancement capability; this has been shown most convincingly in controlled studies of whole, fresh (unfixed) breast specimens obtained at autopsy, in which xeroradiographic recording systems consistently permit detection of smaller "microcalcifications" (aluminum oxide specks) than do screen-film systems (11). On the other hand, poorly defined breast masses are more readily detected on screen-film mammograms (Fig. 2), probably due to the relatively poor broad-area contrast of xeroradiography. All in all, there is no clear-cut advantage to one technique over the other, since mammography demonstrates calcifications in only about half the breast cancers (xeromammography favored), and since the other half are diagnosed primarily by visualization of a poorly defined mass (screen-film mammography favored). Furthermore, based on my own experience involving cancers radiographed with both types of recording system, one will be more helpful than the other in the differentiation of benign from malignant lesions approximately 25% of the time, but the detection of a cancer with one technique alone occurs very infrequently (certainly less than 5%, possibly less than 1% of cases).

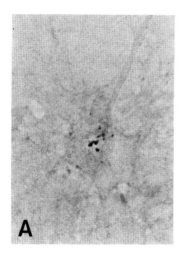 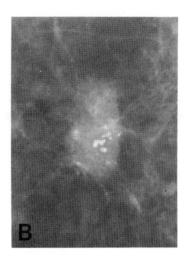

Fig. 2. Xeromammogram (A) and screen-film
mammogram (B) of a 9 mm infiltrating
ductal carcinoma that was not palpable.
Microcalcifications characteristic of
malignancy are highlighted by the edge
enhancement property of the xeroradiographic
process, but the poorly defined mass of the
tumor itself is seen well only in the
relatively high-contrast screen-film image.

HEROIC POSITIVE INTERPRETATIONS

At the other end of the spectrum of mammographic capability we find the
so-called heroic positive cases, in which mammography is the only examination
that indicates the presence of a carcinoma. The great majority of these cases
involve cancers with a highly favorable prognosis, since they tend to be both
small in size and limited in extent (few give evidence of hematogenous
metastasis or spread to regional lymph nodes).

Heroic positive interpretations will be made by every mammographer,
regardless of the radiographic equipment used or of the degree of attention that
is paid to proper radiographic technique. However, the frequency of heroic
positive cases can be expected to increase as the quality of the mammographic
images improves. By tailoring the mammography examination to each individual
patient, ordering additional exposures whenever helpful (as described above),
high quality images can indeed be obtained. The second step to maximize the
yield of heroic positive cases is to use the best possible radiographic
equipment. I have had the greatest success with a microfocal spot x-ray unit
specially adapted for mammography, with a built-in uniform-thickness compression
device included. This system not only produces standard contact (1X) mammograms
of quality equal to or better than that of any other available equipment, but it
also has the capability to produce magnification (1.5-2X) mammograms, which are
of even higher quality (19). I have not used the magnification mode for my
routine examinations since it results in an increased radiation dose, but among
patients specially selected because their contact mammograms are difficult to
interpret, an additional magnification exposure substantially increases the
ability to detect heroic positive cases (10). Figure 3 illustrates an example;
such diagnoses are truly "heroic", for these cancers are detectable neither by
physical examination nor by conventional mammography.

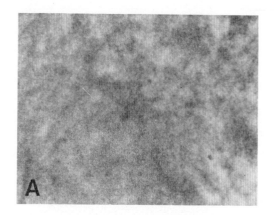 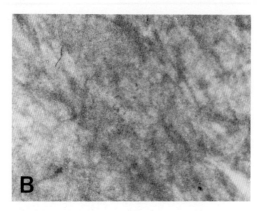

Fig. 3. Craniocaudal projection xeromammograms of a small area in the right breast of a woman who had no abnormality palpable in that location.
   A. Contact (1X) exposure made with a conventional overhead x-ray tube, showing no evidence of malignancy.
   B. Microfocal spot magnification (1.5X) exposure, of considerably superior image quality, demonstrating numerous clustered micro-calcifications highly suspicious of carcinoma (biopsy-proved intraductal carcinoma). Note that the two images have been made equal in size photographically to facilitate comparison of image quality.

Another method that has proved successful in increasing the yield of heroic positive interpretations is the adjustment of diagnostic criteria to consider as malignant all lesions which demonstrate any radiographic features even remotely suspicious of carcinoma (20). The disadvantage of such an approach is the concomitant increase in false positive diagnoses, resulting in the biopsy of as many as 10 benign lesions for every cancer found. Nevertheless, for screening asymptomatic patients, it is probably the best available method with standard mammography equipment to detect early breast cancer. However, the use of microfocal spot mammography, with selective additional magnification exposures when necessary, appears to be the optimal technique currently available, since it not only maximizes heroic positive diagnoses while decreasing the false negative rate, but it also results in a substantial reduction in false positive interpretations, saving many women from the physical and emotional morbidity of biopsy for benign lesions (10).

CONCLUSIONS

False negative mammography interpretations can be minimized by rigorous adherence to optimal radiographic technique, in particular by careful monitoring of all examinations by the radiologist, to ensure that any palpable masses are included on available films, and to be certain that any areas of radiographic abnormality are imaged with maximum clarity. This involves an aggressive approach to obtaining additional films whenever there is any doubt about the possibility of carcinoma. This same method also facilitates detection of heroic positive cases, but the best results can be expected only with use of state-of-the-art radiographic equipment.

REFERENCES

1. Wolfe JN: Xeroradiography: Breast Calcifications. Springfield, Thomas, 1977, pp 3-43.
2. Martin JE: Benign vs. malignant calcifications. In Margulis AR, Gooding CA, eds: Diagnostic Radiology 1977. San Francisco, University of California Press, 1977, pp 831-836.
3. Wolfe JN: Xeroradiography: Uncalcified Breast Masses. Springfield, Thomas, 1977, pp 3-41.
4. Martin JE: Correlations of mammography and histology of the breast, benign and malignant. In Margulis AR, Gooding CA, eds: Diagnostic Radiology 1977. San Francisco, University of California Press, 1977, pp 807-821.
5. Black JW, Young B: A radiological and pathological study of the incidence of calcifications in diseases of the breast and neoplasms of other tissues. Brit J Radiol 38:596-598, Aug 1964.
6. Gershon-Cohen J, Berger SM, Delpino L: Mammography: some remarks on techniques. Radiol Clin N Amer 3:384-401, Dec 1965.
7. Wolfe JN: Analysis of 462 breast carcinomas. Am J Roentgenol 121:846-853, Aug 1974.
8. Fisher ER, Gregorio RM, Fisher B, et al: The pathology of invasive breast cancer. A syllabus derived from findings of the National Surgical Adjuvant Breast Project (Protocol No. 4). Cancer 36:1-85, Jul 1975.
9. Millis RR, Davis R, Stacey AJ: The detection and significance of calcifications in the breast, a radiological and pathological study. Brit J Radiol 49:12-26, Jun 1975.
10. Sickles EA: Microfocal spot magnification mammography using xeroradiographic and screen-film recording systems. Radiology, in press.
11. Nguyen MT, Sickles EA: Radiographic detectability of breast microcalcifications: in vitro studies using a wide variety of mammography techniques. In Application of Optical Instrumentation in Medicine VII. Bellingham, WA, Society of Photo-Optical Instrumentation Engineers, 1979, Vol 173, in press.
12. Jost G: Evaluation of grid technique in mammography. In Logan WW, Muntz EP, eds: Reduced Dose Mammography. New York, Masson, 1979.
13. Barnes G: Characteristics of scatter. In Logan WW, Muntz EP, eds: Reduced Dose Mammography. New York, Masson, 1979.
14. Sickles EA: Controlled evaluations of image quality and diagnostic accuracy of low-dose mammography screen-film systems. In Logan WW, Muntz EP, eds: Reduced Dose Mammography. New York, Masson, 1979.
15. Chang CHJ: Computed tomographic mammography (CT-M): experiences with 1000 patients. In Logan WW, Muntz EP, eds: Reduced Dose Mammography. New York, Masson, 1979.
16. Sickles EA, Benton EV, Tobias CA, et al: Mammography using Bevalac-accelerated heavy particles: a novel approach to dose reduction. In Logan WW, Muntz EP, eds: Reduced Dose Mammography. New York, Masson, 1979.
17. Libshitz HI, Fetouh S, Isley J, et al: One-view mammographic screening? Radiology 120:719-722, Sept 1976.
18. Buchanan JB, Jager RM: Single view negative mode xeromammography: an approach to reduce radiation exposure in breast cancer screening. Radiology 123:63-68, Apr 1977.
19. Sickles EA, Doi K, Genant HK: Magnification film mammography: image quality and clinical studies. Radiology 125:69-76, Oct 1977.
20. Moskowitz M, Gartside PS, Gardella L, et al: The breast cancer screening controversy: a perspective. In Logan WW, ed: Breast Carcinoma. The Radiologist's Expanded Role. New York, Wiley, 1977, pp 35-52.

MAMMOGRAPHY MISS PANEL

Wende Logan, Moderator

Cameron: I notice that the negative mode is seldom used, even though it uses less radiation. I have seen some pretty samples where a negative mode really helps. I wondered if one of the reasons is that the PDS spots show up the same way that calcifications do? Why isn't negative mode used more often?

Gisvold: We are using negative mode routinely right now. I didn't show any cases because these were old but I am becoming more and more bothered by PDS spots. I have occasion to compare with the positive mode from a year or two ago. I really think we are seeing a lot of little tiny powder deficiency spots so I think it is a concern of mine, currently.

Cameron: On these powder deficiency spots - if you go around in our own department we find often, that a lot of the xerox plates should have been pulled much sooner. I wonder if this is a lack of quality control that we are seeing, and if you have any suggestions to improve that.

Kalisher: I think in part you're right. Quality control is very important. I've seen completely crystallized plates that have been used in some institutions where you're no longer dealing with vitreous selenium, you're dealing with crystal selenium, and get multiple PDSs to the point of a snowstorm. Yet those plates have not been pulled. I use negative mode only in selected cases because even with dropping the back bias there is some flattening of the image and I still like to use a fairly soft beam. Negative mode I find more useful in a very dense breast, such as a younger patient, or the patient with some type of implant. I think it's a matter of choosing what you want to use. My technologists will switch in the middle of an exam: if they do a craniocaudal view and find the breast to be too dense to see adequately, they'll go into a negative mode.

Moskowitz: We routinely use negative mode, and have been for about a year and a half now. But since I do my own photography I haven't gotten off my duff to photograph too many slides recently and so those come from our prior experience.

Sickles: I have one comment on the negative mode. Could I see my last slide? We have recently started doing a lot of work with breast specimens that I removed at autopsy (whole breast specimens) and we have been radiographing them in the fresh nonfixed state and putting calcifications on and in them (simulated calcifications) the size of which we can measure. We've compared screen-film techniques to xerox positive and xerox negative mode techniques with varying x-ray tubes, and with both magnification and nonmagnification techniques I have found that you can detect smaller calcifications in the positive mode than you can in the negative mode.

Moskowitz: I agree.

Sickles: That's one facet. The other facet is, and this is very subjective - I don't know that anyone can prove it with any hard data - I find it very difficult to read negative mode images and to see masses.

Gold: We have kind of a funny system at U.C.L.A. If a woman is under 35 and she really needs a mammogram we just perform screen-film mammograms. If she's between 35 and 50, in some women we augment those film mammograms with a mediolateral xeromammogram in the negative mode because of the lower dose. If she's over 50 we use the positive mode, with the augmenting mediolateral xero-mammogram. I don't feel as comfortable interpreting the negative mode as I do the positive mode. I too feel that calcifications are easier identified on the positive mode, than the negative mode.

Egan: I think you should individualize. You make a mistake if you stick with one entirely.

Cameron: Could I make a comment also about quality control? I noticed that enough of the xeromammogram images did have artifacts on them. I'm sure all of the practitioners here are aware of those, but there are many other people who might not be. At the University of Wisconsin at the Midwest Center for Radiological Physics, Larry Dewerd has prepared a booklet on artifacts in xeroradiography. If you want copies of it you can order them from the University of Wisconsin for $2.50. If you want to save money you can order one from the AAPM Coordination Office in Washington but I won't give you the address for it.

Dr. Alcorn: In the situations where you see a mass in one view and not on the other there has been something written recently (I think it's in the Sept. A.J.R.*) by a gentleman from Boston, to the effect that if you do an oblique view which would be upper-inner to lower-outer, that it dispels this doubt.

Robert Wagner: I'm getting more and more convinced that the human eye really is limiting us and that there is a lot of information on the films that the eye has trouble to fill out. Would you comment on the possibility of using more of the industrial film idea of routinely overexposing, especially the denser breasts. Are there good enough hot lights available? Do any of you use them routinely and would you all just reemphasize your use of magnifying glasses for those who don't use them?

Egan: There is no way to properly or adequately project mammograms, to compare to xeromammograms, which have very little range of density in them - about 15 or 18, whereas the film may have 256. Now there is an old saying: the worse the mammogram the better it projects. There is a lot of truth to that. It is a very good trick to put a xeromammogram beside a mammogram and any fool can see how much worse it is, but the reason is the inability to project the mammogram.

Snyder: May I say also that if you overexpose a film-screen mammogram, you lose all your soft tissue detail, and your calcifications. We need the magnifying glass.

Moskowitz: We routinely use the magnifying glass on all our evaluation of all the mammogram screening or consults, symptomatic or asymptomatic. I happen to agree with you that the limiting factor at this point is the human eye, and brain. There may well be a pattern of recognition assist that can be achieved by computer reconstruction and we are involved in that now, at least in the evaluation of calcifications, specifically. We hope ultimately to expand it. An intriguing idea is what information we can reconstruct from an underexposed film.

---

* Hall, FM, Berenberg, AL, "Selective use of the oblique projection in mammography". A.J.R. 131:465-468, Sept 1978.

Kalisher: There have been recent articles (and it's an interesting idea that the Swedes have been doing for a long time) about a single oblique view. Some people I know who have specialized units are trying it and we'll see what their experience is. As far as the other question you had asked, Bob: in xeroradiography, one of the first questions that we asked three years ago was, why use toner as a means of transferring information since it is really one of the clumsiest methods. You have 5 micron particles that you are attracting by a magnetic field. You have basically a charged field on that plate and if you can read it by use of scanning it by somehow collecting the charges and putting them through a computer you should be able to get a tremendous amount of information. I know that there are several groups that are working on scanning or otherwise collecting the charges on the plates and then processing this information; I don't think there is much of a secret in that. It would be a slow scan, not the 525 of television, or something of this type but I think this is really the direction that we would have to go rather than using liquid toners and solid toners and so on.

Moskowitz: I do think its important to realize that the Swede's view that they're doing is not the same view that we do as a routine lateral-medial here and shouldn't be interpreted as that. I sent Skip Libshitz all the minimal cancer cases that we had at that time and mixed them with our normals (just lateral views) and asked him to evaluate them. He was able to pick up 80% of the carcinomas on the lateral view only, which I think was remarkable because often, as you all know, you see something on one view and then you go back and say "oh I see it on the other view". The 20% diagnostic loss that we would have picked up was perhaps not worth it in terms of the possible cancer induction.

Sickles: I would like to make just one comment on this paper about oblique views. We have been using them for several years. I don't really think there's anything magic about the particular positions that they describe in the paper. When you think you see something on only one projection and you're trying to convince yourself that it's real and not superimposition of structures you just have to vary the patients position in almost any way. I don't think you have to use that particular scheme, you can just try another view that's very similar and frequently you will be able to show just with subtle patient positioning differences that you're not seeing a real mass.

Snyder: As far as oblique views go, that's our routine. We don't do a straight 90° lateral, it's always been a 30°-60° oblique, as necessary.

Logan: I would like to disagree with Ed Sickles. The oblique view actually allows maximum visualization of the posterior breast tissue. Ruth's "30° to 60°" touches upon a key point, and that is that it is best if you individualize each patient. In my office, after the craniocaudad view, we examine the patient to determine the direction of the pectoral muscle. Our routine second view is performed with the breast pulled forward from the ribs at that same angle, because it is possible to pull the breast further away from the ribs when you aren't fighting the direction of the pectoral muscle when you compress (see chapter on Screen-Film Technique: Compression and Other Factors). This method has enabled us to see much more axillary tail tissue than the usual lateral view does. If we find a lesion on the oblique view, we perform a lateral view for the surgeon, because surgeons have difficulties understanding where the lesion is, when they see it on an oblique view.

Robert Jennings: A couple of people have said you have to have a molybdenum target to do film-screen imaging. I hope that I can convince some of you that perhaps you can do the same job with K edge filters and a tungsten target. You can then do xeromammography and film-screen mammography with the same tube. K edge filtered spectra don't harden in the same way that the molybdenum spectra harden. That means that you not only get better contrast in the uniform sections of the breast you also get better latitude because you don't have the extreme darkening at the edges of the film. Finally, for Dr. Gisvold, the BHR handbook discussing mammographic spectra indicates that your physicist's half value measurements are correct. The apparent discrepancy is born out in our data in almost the same numbers.

Dr. Muntz: I would just like to ask Dr. Gisvold if he has ever done film mammograms with lower half values. Your numbers are rather high for some techniques and your doses are correspondingly low and I suspect your calcification detection rate is directly connected with the difference between that and other techniques is directly connected to the half value layer you are using.

Gisvold: Which was .4. The other tube was a little higher than .4.

Muntz: I think .3 is the typical number from Sloan-Kettering Memorial.

Gisvold: I was surprised when I heard our half value layers were that high.

Muntz: Your exposure image doses are very low, and I think that probably would explain the calcification detection differences.

Gisvold: You know a lot of people have reported 30-35%. Now people are reporting more. Series are going to vary.

Logan: 50-60% of lesions have calcium on specimen radiography.

Gisvold: We know that with specimen mammography we see a lot more than with the regular mammogram. There is no way that we are going to match that but its certainly food for thought.

Cameron: Do you do specimen radiography afterwards to look for the calcium in the biopsy?

Gisvold: No one I know does routine specimen radiography of every obvious cancer. It would be extremely time consuming.

Kalisher: The Japanese pathology literature mentions 80-85% microcalcifications in their specimen work, with careful analysis of specimens. The best figures I have seen on a mammographic study, is generally around 50%. We used to say 40 was great so we're missing some.

Sickles: Just as an additional statement to this, we have found when we use our magnification mammography (direct magnification, not using a magnifying glass) that we can see calcium in upwards of 60% of cases, and it's probably just because of the better quality image.

Snyder: 80% is too high actually for specimen radiography. We found that about 55% of our cancer specimens have calcification. Dr. Rosen says some of the things that are called calcifications are not.

Gisvold: Can I poll the panel for my own interest to see what your percentages are? I know John Wolfe and Gloria Frankel both say 50%. What do you find? What percentage of your mammographically diagnosed cancers have you seen calcium in, on the radiograph?

Snyder: Not more than 45%.

Egan: I would say 80%, in stage 0 or stage I. On routine mammograms I would say about 40%. We ran a series where we used a coned down view, and ran it up maybe to 45 or 50. I think, on the specimens that we had, it went up to maybe 60.

Gold: I don't think it's unusual to go back retrospectively and look at a cancer and find 2 or 3 calcifications. We do that all the time. If you do that then I think you are going to find a lot of calcifications. But if you use a prospective view on what percentage of calcifications did you observe before the biopsy was made, then I think its going to be more like a third.

Moskowitz: In our younger women, something like 78% of the cancers that were found on mammography alone, were found on the basis of occult cancer with calcification. In a dense breast, that often is the only thing that leads me to biopsy, is the calcifications. In older women, however, we see more small tiny masses, and the percentage of cancers with calcium is probably less.

Dr. Seidband: The lack of dynamic range capability of the film-screen systems is pretty obvious from the range of densities in some of the films. Has anyone done any work or does anyone know of any work going on with the use of, say, aluminum wedge filters or fluid filled field flattening devices for mammography which would permit us a more uniform film density such that the contrast range could be extended by technique?

Egan: In the mid 50's when I was working on this technique we used parafin plastic shaped wedge, but we didn't get it up to aluminum. Aluminum is too dense to have any thickness at all. Anything you put in this soft x-ray beam flattens out extremely rapidly. As far as we can determine we could never find the magic material to put in there.

Kalisher: I think the problem is that different patients have different sized breasts. Therefore, to set up a reverse wedge filter with the thin part next to the chest wall the thick part under the nipple is very very difficult to do. We have toyed with this idea on a moly tube, with moly wedge filter with 10 micron at one end and 50 micron in the other, and 30 in the center, to see what would happen. We could never get the central beam right where we wanted it to be.

Egan: Also, if you place the central beam right at the base of the breast chest wall, with good collimation your energy falls off about the same speed at which the slope of the breast falls off. Therefore, even though we thought we might need this wedge filter we never actually did. Now on the Senographe, you'll notice the heel effect is much more apparent because you're using such a short target-film distance. But when you get back to 30-36 inches, with good collimation, you are only using the central beam and it works out pretty well if you aim it at the base of the breast. The normal skin often times, par- ticularly in a dense small breast may well be burned out, but if it's diseased, and thickened, you'll see it.

Jennings: All the measurements we made at the Bureau have been made with glass window tubes. At 30 kVp with a moly tube, whether it has a filter or not, we can't get below about .48 mm of aluminum half value layer. It's .48 without a filter, .49 with a filter, so those numbers are correct. Since all those experiments comparing K edge filters with moly tubes were done with glass window tubes, I suggest that if you are going to experiment with that and you have a beryllium window tube to compare to, you may find that the results are a little bit different. I would suggest a little bit of caution if you want to start out on that route.

Attendee: Doesn't the Senographe have a beryllium window?

Jennings: Yes, it has a beryllium window and a much lower half value layer. A .3 mm half value layer corresponds to about 15 KEV photons. You have a large exposure fraction below the molybdenum characteristic lines with those beryllium window tubes.

PART IV

LOOKING AHEAD

COMPUTED TOMOGRAPHIC MAMMOGRAPHY (CT/M): EXPERIENCES WITH 1000 PATIENTS

C.H. Joseph Chang, M.D.
Department of Diagnostic Radiology
University of Kansas Medical Center
Kansas City, Kansas 66103

Computed tomography is a revolutionary new method of studying breast disease. We have been evaluating the General Electric CT/M system since October 1976. Earlier experiences with this technique have been reported by this author and his co-investigators (1,2) and we now wish to present our clinical experiences in 1000 patients.

THE GENERAL ELECTRIC CT/M SYSTEM

The General Electric CT/M system is a CT fan-beam scanner which is specially designed for breast scanning. The system includes a three-phase x-ray generator, GE Maxtray 75 tube with a focal spot measuring 0.6 x 0.6 mm., an array of 127 high - pressure Xenon-gas detectors, Data General S/200 Eclipse computer with magnetic tape drive, Control Data Corp. (CDC) disc, RAMTEC display console, Versatec printer and Dunn Camera. The scanning is done at 120 Kvp, 20 mA (HVL - 3.4 mm. Al) and 10 sec per 360° rotation. The scanning field is 20 cm. in diameter. Resolution volume for each picture point is 1.56 x 1.56 x 10 mm. Reconstruction time per slice is 90 sec. Images from a 127 x 127 matrix are displayed on a scale of -127 to +128 CT numbers according to calibration with water at zero. The exposure dose to the patient's skin is 240 mR per breast.

MATERIALS

From October 1976 through August 1978 1000 patients were studied. All patients had a physical examination, film mammography and thermography. Two general groups of cases were selected. One group had physical, mammographic and/or thermographic abnormalities. The other group consisted of asymptomatic patients in the high risk group and asymptomatic dense breasts. In addition 5 cases were studied to check the status of their breast cancer after cobalt therapy or lumpectomy and chemotherapy. Two cases with silicone mammoplasty were also studied to appraise the postoperative status of their breasts.

METHOD

The patient lies prone on a canvas table with an opening for the dependent breast. Scans were performed from the chest wall to the nipple in horizontal position to permit the breast to be completely immersed in a water bucket. The required CT slices are determined by looking through a mirror system viewer and CT scans are obtained before and after rapid intravenous drip infusion of 300 ml diatrizoate meglumine (RENO-M-DIP). The patient received a drip infusion in a comfortable sitting position within 10 minutes. For every lesion, the highest CT number is identified on the display. All final CT values are obtained on hard-copy print.

FINDINGS

BREAST CARCINOMAS

There were 44 histologically proven cancers detected in 41 patients. The range of CT number for cancer is -19 to +39 (mean 21) on initial scans and +10 to +96 (mean 57) on postinjection scans. The range of contrast medium enhancement (Δ CT number) in proven carcinomas is 26 (5.2% increase in density) to 64 (12.8% increase in density) with the mean of 36 (7.2% increase in density). All malignant lesions showed an increase of at least 26 CT numbers after contrast medium enhancement.

Breast cancer in a fatty breast can be identified as an irregular mass on a breast scan. In moderate to markedly dense fibrocystic breasts, a tumor mass cannot be distinguished from the surrounding tissues on a preinjection scan. The mass, however, becomes obvious on a postinjection scan because of preferential high iodide uptake by the tumor (Fig. 2). Malignant microcalcifications without an associated mass cannot be identified on an initial scan but can be identified as a tiny area of marked contrast enhancement on a postinjection scan.

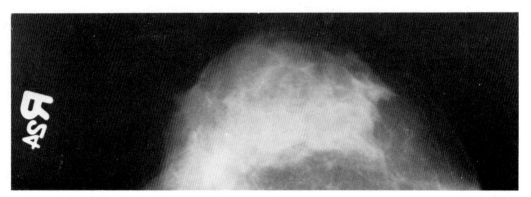

Fig. 1 Film mammogram of the right breast failed to identify a discrete mass in moderate fibrocystic disease.

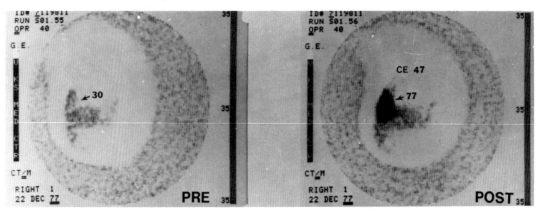

Fig. 2 CT/M scans of the same patient. Preinjection scan (PRE) failed to identify a discrete mass. Postinjection scan (POST) now clearly shows a

cancer mass (arrow). Contrast medium enhancement (CE) was 47 CT numbers (9.4% increase in density) indicating cancer.

The size of cancers in this series ranged from 2mm. to 9cm. in the maximum diameter. Twelve were less than 1cm., twelve were 1-2cm., ten were 2-3cm., six were 3-5cm. and four were over 5cm.

The sensitivity of CT/M for 44 cancers compared to film mammography and thermography is summerized in Table 1. All carcinomas but three were diagnosed by CT/M. One cancer was situated in the lower, most posterior aspect of the breast and could not technically be included in the scan field. The second cancer missed was a tiny focal lobular in-situ carcinoma with maximum diameter of 1mm. This in-situ cancer was discovered accidently by breast biopsy for suspicious calcification in the same quandrant but different location of the breast. The microcalcifications were benign lesions. The third cancer with a diameter of 1cm. was missed due to a registration problem. The lesion was not included on the same pre and postinjection slice. The CT/M detected two totally unsuspected very small breast cancers which were unable to identify by conventional mammography or physical examination. One lesion measuring 2x2mm in size, was in a dense fibrocystic breast and another lesion measuring 3x4mm in size was in a fatty breast. Mammography missed 9 of 44 cancers, all in dense dysplastic breasts; thermography correctly identified 24 cancers.

Biopsy-proven recurrent cancer in a post-cobalt therapy patient for advanced breast cancer also showed high contrast enhancement of 30 CT numbers. However, patients with benign post-irradiation fibrosis failed to show any significant contrast enhancement.

TABLE I

Sensitivity Analysis
(44 Cancers)

	Benign	Suspicious	Malignant
Film Mammography	9	15	20 (80%)
Thermography	20 (normal)	13	11 (55%)
CT/M	3	–	41 (93%)
Mammography + CT/M	–	1	43 100%)

BENIGN LESIONS

There were 70 biopsy-proven benign lesions in 66 patients. These included 49 fibrocystic diseases, 3 fatty necrosis, 2 focal duct ectasia, 2 intraductal papillomas, 1 gynecomastia, 8 fibroadenoma, 3 abscess and 2 normal breast tissues.

The initial CT number of fibrocystic disease is similar to cancer ranging from -16 to +40 (mean 20). However, the degree of contrast medium enhancement (Δ CT number) is less than that of malignant lesions ranging from 4 to 47 (mean 17). The scan of diffuse fibrocystic disease shows increased density and obliteration of the normal mammary architecture by duct dilations, fibrotic reactions and multiple masses. Fat necrosis can mimic a cancer on the mammogram but the CT/M study reveals minimal contrast medium enhancement (mean 6).

High contrast enhancement, over 25 CT numbers, was identified in non-calcified fibroadenomas. However, their initial CT reading is lower than carcinoma (mean 12). Additionally fibroadenomas appear as well defined smooth, homogenous oval mass. A densely calcified fibroadenoma showed a high initial CT number but displayed only minimal contrast enhancement (3 CT numbers). There were 3 cases of breast abscesses in this series. Even though these lesions showed high contrast medium enhancement, ranging from 26 to 45 (mean 33), their initial CT numbers were lower than would have been expected for a malignant lesion of such sizes. The abscesses are also located close to a skin. If a skin is involved, the skin may also display high contrast enhancement (over 25 CT numbers).

Table 2 compares the diagnostic accuracy of CT/M for benign lesions with that of film mammography and physical examination. There were 11 false positive cases in younger patients with markedly fibrocystic breasts (mean age of 44). Our clinical observations suggested that there is a definite relationship between increased iodide concentration in mammary tissue and high progesterone level. Hence the CT/M study should not be performed 1 week before to the immediate end of menstruation. 2 cases of this group had hyperprolactinemia.

TABLE 2

Specificity Analysis
(70 Benign Lesions)

	Benign	Suspicious	Malignant
Film Mammography	38 (54%)	31	1
Physical Examination	39 (56%)	31	-
CT/M	59 (84%)	7	4

SEVERE TERMINAL DUCT HYPERPLASIA

In proliferative mammary dysplasia severe terminal duct epithelial hyperplasia and atypia has been considered a potential precancerous lesion by many knowledgeable investigators (3-8). Subsequent development of in-situ carcinoma in these areas of abnormal ductal hyperplasia has been reported (6&9). A five-fold increased risk of developing breast cancer in women with this condition was reported by Black and his co-workers (3). CT/M has preoperatively demonstrated and biopsy has proven 41 such areas of cellular abnormality in 34 patients.

The preinjection CT number in this group ranged from -17 to +39 (mean 22) and increased by 24-49 CT numbers (mean 33) after contrast medium enhance-ment. The scan characteristically showed more than one tiny area, usually 2-4mm in size, of high contrast enhancement. Majority of the patients had diffuse fibrocystic disease. Mammography, thermography and physical examinations were otherwise negative. Biopsies were performed mainly on the basis of the CT/M findings.

The age of these patients ranged from 35 to 76 years (mean 46.6 years). Seventeen of 34 women had a positive family history of breast cancer. One patient had a family history of breast cancer in her father and brother. Four patients had had a previous mastectomy. Two patients had concomitant cancers in other parts of the breast. There were 31 whites, 3 blacks and 1 oriental.

DISCUSSION

Increased iodine and iodide concentration in the tissue of normal and diseased breasts in human and animals is well documented in the literature (10-12). Our results showing contrast medium enhancement in various mammary lesions support these previous findings.

Marked contrast medium enhancement (CT number), over 25 CT numbers (5% increase in density) was noted in cancers, severe terminal duct epithelial hyperplasia (potential precancerous lesions), fibroadenomas ans abscesses. However, only minimal (less than 10 CT numbers) contrast enhancement was demonstrated in the predominantly fibrotic and cystic lesions. This suggests that increased contrast medium enhancement may not only be due to increased vascularity but also may be due to the status of epithelial cells.

Our clinical experiences indicate that there is a definite relationship between higher iodide concentration in mammary tissue and high level of progestrone and prolactin. Estrogen and other hormones may also effect the iodide concentration in breast tissue. We need further investigations in this matter. This may result in possible elimination or reduction of false positive in CT/M but may also open a way to understand a complicated relationship between hormones and mammary diseases.

Since CT/M is now able to discover totally unsuspected very small cancers and tiny potentially precancerous lesions, extraordinary cooperation from the surgeon and pathologist is required to find these lesions in the specimen.

Present table design of CT/M unit is such that it is very difficult to accommodate women with a large protuberant abdomen for lower posterior aspect of the breast and with a severe kyphosis of thoracic spine for upper posterior portion. The CT/M is capable to identify lesions in diameter of 2mm or larger with contrast medium enhancement technique but it failed to demonstrate a lesion with a diameter of 1mm. This is smaller than one pixel size (1.56x1.56mm) and probably beyond the resolution capability of CT/M system. Other problems which we have experienced with CT/M was a registration of lesions, especially of 1cm or less in diameter, on the same slice of pre and postinjection scans.

The question of dose reduction for CT/M can be considered in three ways: (1) improving sensitivity of detectors; (2) Omitting water path. Recent CT technology is capable to omit a water bath for scanning but a new fixation device for breast is needed; (3) Using filtration, possibly Cerium, to match the energy of the K-edge absorption peak of Iodine (33 KeV). The recent works on iodine imaging using K-edge energies in CT offer an encouragement for CT/M-iodine contrast agent system.

SUMMARY

CT/M examination using our contrast medium enhancement technique identifies both the morphological changes in the breast and any altered iodide concentration in mammary tissue. This unique capability of CT/M provides many advantages as compared to film mammography for diagnosing both benign and malignant breast disease especially in dense breasts. CT/M can also detect totally unsuspected very small breast cancers which were unable to identify by conventional mammography or physical examination. CT/M system also has the capability of differentiating potentially precancerous lesions from benign fibrocystic disease. The CT/M is a significantly improved diagnostic tool for evaluating breast diseases.

ACKNOWLEDGEMENTS

The author expresses his sincere thanks to co-investigators, Drs. Justo L. Sibala, Steven L. Fritz, Samuel J. Dwyer III and Arch W. Templeton for their contribution and assistance in this study.

REFERENCES

1. Chang CHJ, Sibala JL, Gallagher JH, Riley RC, Templeton AW, Beasley PV, Porte PV: Computed tomography of the breast: A preliminary report. Radiology 124:827-829, 1977.

2. ChangCHJ, Sibala JL, Gallagher JH, Dwyer SJ III, Templeton AW: Computed tomographic evaluation of the breast. Am J Roentgenol 131:459-464, 1978

3. Black MM, Barclay TH, Cutler SJ, Hankey BJ, Asive AJ: Association of atypical characteristics of benign lesions with subsequent risk of breast cancer. Cancer 29:339-343, 1972.

4. Cheatle GL: Desquamative and dysgenetic epithelial hyperplasia in breast: Their situation and characteristic, their likeness to lesions induced by tar. Br J Surg 13:509-532, 1926.

5. Dawson EK: Carcinoma in mammary lobule and its origin. Edinburgh Med J 40:57-82, 1933.

6. Foote FW, Stewart FW: Comparative studies of cancerous versus noncancerous breasts. Ann Surg 121:6-53, 1945

7. Kern WH, Brooks RN: Atypical epithelial hyperplasia associated with breast cancer and fibrocystic disease. Cancer 24:668-675, 1969

8. Willings SR, Jensen HM: An atlas of subgross pathology of the human breast with special reference to possible precancerous lesions. J Natl Cancer Inst 55:231-273, 1975

9. Moskowitz M, Wirman J: Proliferative mammary dysplasia with subsequent development of in-situ cancer. Breast 2:34-35, 1976

10. Eskin BA, Parker JA, Bassett JG, George DL: Human breast uptake of radioactive iodine. Obstet Gynecol 44:398-402, 1974

11. Freinkel N, Ingbar SH: The metabolism of ^{131}I by surviving slices of rat mammary tissue. Endocrinology 58:41-45, 1956

12. Miller JK, Swanson EW, Lyke WA: Iodine concentration in nonthyroid tissues of cow. J Dairy Sci 56:1344-1346, 1973

MAMMOGRAPHY USING BEVALAC-ACCELERATED HEAVY PARTICLES: A NOVEL APPROACH TO DOSE REDUCTION

Edward A. Sickles, M.D., Eugene V. Benton, Ph.D.,
Cornelius A. Tobias, Ph.D., and Kay H. Woodruff, M.D.
Lawrence Berkeley Laboratory, Berkeley, CA 94720
and
University of San Francisco, San Francisco, CA 94117

Heavy-particle radiography is an experimental imaging technique that produces superior density resolution at low radiation dose (1-4). _In vitro_ studies using whole, fresh (unfixed) mastectomy specimens have demonstrated increased detectability of malignant breast tumors with heavy-particle radiography as compared to conventional screen-film mammography (5,6). This experience, as well as the relative ease with which the breast can be examined radiographically, led us to initiate a pilot _in vivo_ study of heavy-particle mammography in an attempt to evaluate its potential for detecting breast cancer at a low radiation dose.

HEAVY-PARTICLE IMAGING PROCEDURE

The Bevalac accelerator at the Lawrence Berkeley Laboratory is used to produce the heavy-particle beams. Atoms of carbon are stripped of all their electrons and then accelerated to energies of approximately 250 MeV/nucleon (3 GeV/particle), resulting in an essentially monoenergetic beam of particles. The monoenergetic nature of the heavy-particle beam and the known beam stopping power of given thicknesses of breast tissue permit precise modification of the beam before it enters the breast, so that the vast majority of particles are made to stop immediately downstream from the breast, within a stack of 25 thin plastic detector sheets. The detector sheets are then developed in 6.25 N NaOH, to etch the tracks of stopped particles so that they become visible. The composite patterns of visible particle tracks in each of the detector sheets constitute the multiple heavy-particle images produced for each exposure.

The slightly higher density of breast cancer as compared to surrounding benign tissues causes areas of malignancy to decrease the kinetic energy of the heavy-particle beam to a slightly greater extent, so that particles passing through such tumor stop and are recorded in detector sheets further upstream than particles traversing benign breast tissue. Therefore, by examining the developed detector sheets in sequence, those portions of the breast containing cancer (e.g., those with the highest density) will be imaged first. The superb density resolution of heavy-particle radiography is to a great extent due to the ability of the plastic stack recording system to image heavy particles only at their stopping points; indeed, very subtle differences in tissue density (stopping power differences of only 0.005) can be readily detected by heavy-particle radiography (5).

The low radiation dose of heavy-particle imaging is in part due to the concentration of energy deposition (the so-called "Bragg peak") within the recording system itself, in contrast to conventional x-ray mammography, in which deposition of energy decreases exponentially and only a very small portion of the incident beam reaches the recording system. Furthermore, the quantum efficiency for detection of heavy particles is 100%, whereas a much smaller proportion (usually less than 50%) of conventional x-rays that pass through the breast are in fact recorded.

PILOT CLINICAL STUDIES

Our pilot clinical studies with heavy-particle mammography involve patients with clinical suspicion of breast cancer either by physical examination or conventional mammography. The patient lies prone on a canvas sheet containing an 8-inch circular hole into which one breast is placed, suspended in a water bath directly beneath the hole. Compression is applied to achieve uniform breast thickness by moving one wall of the water bath in or out. The detector stack of plastic sheets is placed immediately downstream from the water bath, and the exposure is made. Measurement of absorbed radiation dose (mid-breast dose) is made simultaneously with the exposure by measuring the entrance dose with previously calibrated ionization chambers. Current heavy-particle mammography techniques impart 20-80 mrad per exposure. The relative biological effectiveness (RBE) of the heavy-particle carbon beams used for in vivo mammography is not known precisely; the RBE of similar Bevalac-produced beams on mouse skin is reported to be 1.0-1.2 with reference to 230 kVp x-rays (7).

The heavy-particle mammography examination involves a craniocaudal and lateral projection exposure of each breast. Each exposure produces a series of images, which are viewed in sequence along with the images of the corresponding projection of the opposite breast, in search for asymmetric areas of increased tissue density (Fig. 1). In our study, each heavy-particle examination is interpreted independently from the conventional mammograms, and the accuracy of interpretation is determined by correlation with the pathological diagnosis at subsequent biopsy.

To date we have studied 25 patients. Results show that heavy-particle mammography accurately delineates tumor masses, including some very small non-palpable masses, with much greater contrast than corresponding conventional mammography. On the other hand, spatial resolution is inferior to conventional mammography, such that clustered malignant microcalcifications are not portrayed as discrete radiopaque objects. However, these cancers are detectable in heavy-particle images as asymmetric "masses" of increased beam stopping power (density), even though mass lesions cannot be seen on the corresponding conventional mammograms. Among the 25 patients studied, overall diagnostic interpretation of the heavy-particle examination differed from that of the conventional mammograms in only one woman. She had abundant (water-density) fibroglandular tissue distributed symmetrically in both breasts, seen on both conventional and heavy-particle examinations, but only the heavy-particle study visualized a mass of slightly greater density than surrounding tissue, biopsy of which showed infiltrating lobular carcinoma. It is in such women, in whom conventional mammography shows diffusely "dense" breasts, that heavy-particle mammography seems most advantageous, by virtue of its exquisite density resolution.

We have recently developed the ability to generate a single composite image of beam stopping power (density) values for the entire set of images produced by each heavy-particle exposure. The developed images on the individual detector sheets are scanned with a Vidicon television camera and then digitized, using a Quantimet 720 digitizer interfaced to a PDP 1110 computer. A computer-assisted composite of absolute beam stopping power is then provided, either in the form of a print out or displayed on a cathode ray tube (CRT), from which a permanent photographic record can be made. Computer-generated composite CRT

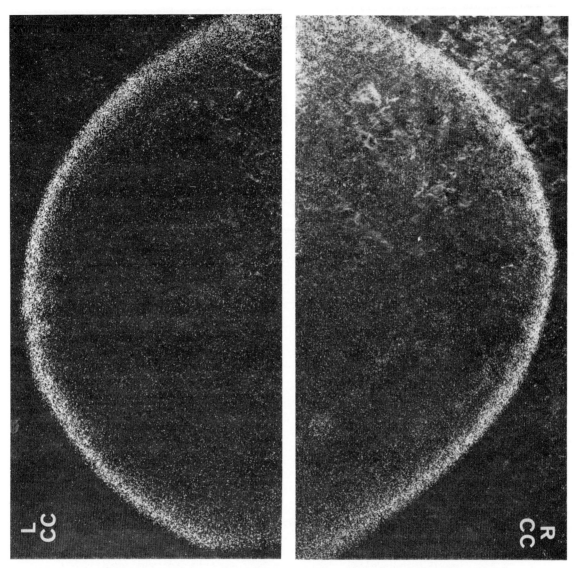

Fig. 1. Craniocaudal projection heavy-particle mammograms of an elderly woman
with fatty breasts, showing a small area of increased stopping power
(density) in the outer aspect of the right breast. Subsequent biopsy proved
this to be an 8 mm infiltrating ductal carcinoma. The wavy cloud-like white
markings overlying the water bath and inner portions of both breasts are
artifacts of photographic reproduction and were not seen on the original
images.

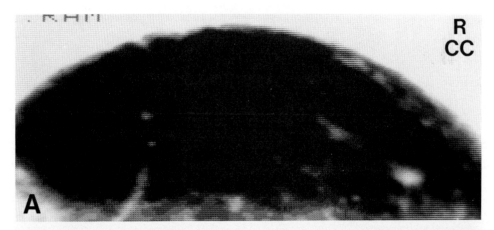

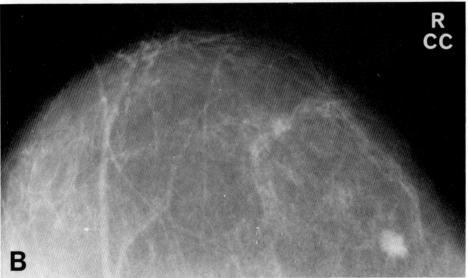

Fig. 2. Craniocaudal projection mammograms of the same right
breast shown in Fig. 1, containing an 8 mm infiltrating ductal
carcinoma.
   A. Computer-generated composite heavy-particle mammogram
displayed on a CRT. Note the dramatic improvement in image
quality (increased contrast, reduced noise) afforded by computer
processing. The carcinoma demonstrates far greater stopping
power (density) than adjacent areas of benign (water-density)
breast tissue or than the large vein in the inner portion of
the breast.
   B. Conventional screen-film mammogram (DuPont Lo-dose-2)
showing superior spatial resolution but substantially less
contrast than the composite heavy-particle mammogram.

images not only require less time and effort to interpret, but also provide the capability for independent adjustment of contrast (window width) and absolute density level (window height), after the exposure is completed, similar to the capability of present-day CT scanners (8). An additional advantage to composite imaging is a marked reduction in background noise level, since the random distribution of quantum mottle is for the most part cancelled out in composites of the 25 individual images (Fig. 2). This ability to overcome noise limitations promises to permit a substantial decrease in radiation dose for heavy-particle mammography, perhaps down to or even below the millirad level.

Current heavy-particle mammography techniques are far from optimized. Anticipated future developments involve the use of: 1) heavier atomic particles, including oxygen and neon, which are capable of better spatial and density resolution than carbon; 2) three-dimensional image reconstruction techniques; and 3) imaging following administration of contrast material specially formulated to enhance the beam stopping power of malignant tissue.

CONCLUSIONS

Heavy-particle mammography is one of the lowest-dose systems employing ionizing radiation that has been designed to image the breast. Heavy-particle mammograms have poorer spatial resolution than conventional x-ray film images, but they compensate for this deficiency by providing exquisite density resolution, permitting accurate detection of breast cancer, including clinically occult carcinomas at least as small as 6 mm in size. In the "dense" breasts of younger women, the superb density resolution of heavy-particle mammography may provide even greater diagnostic accuracy than conventional mammography. Recent development of computer-generated composite heavy-particle mammograms allows for improved image quality and also promises to permit substantial further reduction in radiation dose.

REFERENCES

1. Benton EV, Henke RP, Tobias CA: Heavy-particle radiography. Science 182: 474-476, 2 Nov 1973.
2. Tobias CA, Benton EV, Capp MP: Heavy-ion radiography. In Biological and Medical Research with Accelerated Heavy Ions at the Bevalac. Berkeley, CA, Lawrence Berkeley Laboratory, 1977, Publication # 5610, pp 164-186.
3. Tobias CA, Benton EV, Capp MP, et al: Particle radiography and auto-activation. Int J Radiat Oncol Biol Phys 3:35-44, 1977.
4. Tobias CA, Benton EV, Capp MP: Heavy-ion radiography. In Lawrence JH, Budinger PF, eds: Recent Advances in Nuclear Medicine. New York, Grune & Stratton, 1978, Vol 5, pp 71-102.
5. Sommer FG, Capp MP, Tobias CA, et al: Heavy-ion radiography: density resolution and specimen radiography. Invest Radiol 13:163-170, Mar-Apr 1978.
6. Sickles EA: Heavy-particle mammography. In Logan WW, ed: Breast Carcinoma. The Radiologist's Expanded Role. New York, Wiley, 1977, pp 239-241.
7. Alpen E: Tissue radiobiology: acute and chronic effects. In Biological and Medical Research with Accelerated Heavy Ions at the Bevalac. Berkeley, CA, Lawrence Berkeley Laboratory, 1977, Publication # 5610, pp 111-126.
8. Kreel L: A general view of computed tomography. In Norman D, Korobkin M, Newton TH, eds: Computed Tomography 1977. San Francisco, University of California Press, 1977, pp 1-20.

OPTIMAL XEROMAMMOGRAPHIC IMAGES AT REDUCED DOSES

Panos P. Fatouros, Ph.D. and Gopala U.V. Rao, Sc.D.
Medical College of Virginia
Radiation Physics Division, Box 72, Richmond, VA 23298

I. INTRODUCTION

The value of mammography in diagnosing breast cancer prior to signs and symptoms is well-established. The early detection of non-invasive carcinoma leads to prolonged survival or improved surgical procedures. Nevertheless, the application of mammographic examinations in large scale screening has raised many concerns over the possibility of radiation-induced cancers. The result has been a continous decrease in exposure levels deriving mainly from faster recording systems (e.g., Dupont Lodose, Kodak Min-R etc). In addition to dosage, however, the diagnostic quality of the image must be carefully maintained if fine details and subtle changes are to be visualized.

This paper will examine the optimization of the xeromammographic image through a systems-based approach. Ways to reduce the incident exposure will also be suggested.

II. THE XERORADIOGRAPHIC PROCESS

Xeroradiography is an electrostatic imaging process which exhibits very limited macro response and relies principally on border exaggeration for detail detection. The subdued response leads to a wide recording latitude which permits the simultaneous display of skin, vessels, ducts, tumor masses and microcalcifications. The edge enhancement which is primarily responsible for the visualization of soft-tissue details arises whenever there is an abrupt difference in the radiation transmitted through adjacent anatomical structures. Such sudden variations in the transmitted x-ray intensity cause "steps" or edges of discontinuities in the originally uniform charge distribution on the selenium layer. This gives rise to strong, rapidly varying, fringe electrostatic fields. During development the amount of toner deposited depends on the normal electric field component (E) which acts as the driving force for the charged particles. If E is unidirectional across the entire image, as is the case with low-contrast inputs, then it is linearly related to the density D (or toner mass). However, when a high contrast edge is imaged (e.g., a bone-tissue interface) a depletion zone (or white gap) appears where no toner accumulates. This is due to a change in sign of E adjacent to the edge. In xeromammography with its inherently low-contrast details, edge enhancement is manifested as a continous density profile and small or no white gaps are present. The process is then ideally suited for analysis by the standard Fourier methods.

There are three steps in the xeroradiographic process which are independently controlled:

(a) The plate is sensitized by corona charging to an initial uniform potential V_0.

(b) Exposure: an object is irradiated creating an electrostatic image on the plate. Radiological contrasts $C = \Delta R/R$ are converted into potential steps ΔV. R is the exposure in roentgens.

(c) Development: a stream of charged pigmented particles is delivered to the plate with the help of a bias potential V_B and it is sorted out at the Se surface by the strong fringe fields. Potential steps are converted into density profiles or white gaps.

In the entire process the operator has control over V_0, R (and hence ΔV), V_B and t, the development time. In the following we will examine separately steps b and c above.

III. The Exposure Step

Following the corona charging, the photoconducting plate is exposed to the x-rays emerging from the object being imaged. The absorbed x-rays in the Se layer produce charge pairs which are separated by the strong internal electric field and drift towards the charged surface or the aluminum substrate depending on their sign. The surface charge is thus neutralized according to the amount of radiation incident in different areas of the plate and the radiological image is converted into an electrostatic one. This process faithfully reproduces the image during the initial period of exposure. However, as the exposure continues, the electric field lines inside the photoconductor bend due to the developing, uneven surface charge distribution. Newly generated charges are displaced on their way to the surface leading to a blurring of surface details (1-3). In fact, as it will shortly be shown, there exists an optimal exposure which maximizes the signal. Two separate cases will now be considered: broad area and detail irradiation.

(a) When an extended area on the Se layer is "uniformly" irradiated, the surface voltage (or charge) neutralization rate, dV/dR, is proportional to the electric field, E_i, in the bulk (4). This finding leads immediately to a simple exponential law for the voltage discharge curve:

$$V = V_0 \, e^{-R/Ro}$$

(1)

where V is the surface potential remaining following an exposure R. R_0 is a constant related to the sensitivity S of the selenium layer. We will define S as the reciprocal of the exposure R required to reduce the voltage to 1/e of its initial value:

$$S = \frac{1}{R_0}$$

(2)

R_0 is inversely proportional to the energy absorbed by the selenium, and depends on the Se thickness and the incident x-ray spectrum. Measured R_0 values are shown in Figure 1. These measurements were performed using a Siemens Mammomat x-ray machine (Mo target with 0.5 mm Al filtration operated at 49 kVp). The beam quality was changed with lucite blocks of different thickness.

The speed increase as function of HVL reflects the increasing energy fluence per roentgen. This trend continues for higher HVL over the mammographic range and points into a possible direction for dosage savings.

(b)   Consider now the irradiation of some detail represented by an edge in Figure 2:   a uniform x-ray beam is modulated by the edge, producing a potential discontinuity $\Delta V = V_1 - V_2$. Using equation 1 we can express ΔV in terms of the exposure R

$$\Delta V = V_0 \, e^{-R/R_0} \, (e^{CR/R_0} - 1) \qquad (3)$$

where C is the subject contrast $(R-R^1)/R$. ΔV can be viewed as a function of exposure R for a given edge and x-ray beam quality The optimal exposure R_{opt} is given by:

$$dV/dR \;=\; 0$$

or $$R_{opt} = \frac{-R_0}{C} \ln(1-C) \qquad (4)$$

For the small C the above expression reduces to

$$R_{opt} = R_0 \qquad (5)$$

Notice that R_{opt} is independent of C and hence a single exposure will simultaneously optimize all soft-tissue details as they are mapped onto the Se layer. The existence of an optimal exposure results from the field-bending effect mentioned earlier. The signal ΔV is initially growing in size with increasing exposure while the uniform charge background is exponentially decaying. As the exposure continues the field-bending effect becomes more serious leading to a signal erosion for $R > R_{opt}$.

Because this effect is more pronounced in thick Se layers, the use of thicker plates for dose reduction is limited.   For example, for a sinusoidal signal (3) a reduction of 25% in the amplitude of the charge signal is caused at 2 cycles per mm, when the exposure is halved and the thickness is doubled.   For a step discontinuity (1-2) the amplitude is proportional to 1/L which leads to a 50% reduction in the density profile.

It should be emphasized, that the formation of the latent electrostatic image during the exposure step, is governed by the internal electric field E_i.

IV. The Development Process

During development the plate is exposed to a stream of charged toner particles in the presence of a bias potential V_B (Fig. 3). V_B is necessary for improving toner delivery to extended, uniformly charged areas where the fields are weak (the electrostatic fringe fields are largely confined in the vicinity of the discontinuities). It may also be used to control the magnitude of the white gap appearing near edges. We will first consider broad-area development, i.e., development in regions away from charge discontinuities. This will be followed by an analysis of edge development.

(a) Broad-Area Densitometry: During development the charged toner particles will be deposited in a given area on the plate at a rate proportional to the local normal electric field. Detailed analysis (2) shows that

$$D_B \simeq 0.43 \ a \ n \ \mu \ t \ E_B \ (0) \qquad (6)$$

where D_B is the optical density, E_B (0) the initial bias field, a the toner mean area, n the cloud number density, μ the mobility and t the time of development. By introducing D_0 and D_∞, the densities under a given set of development conditions for zero and for infinite exposures, equation 6 becomes:

$$D_B = D_\infty + (D_0 - D_\infty) \ e^{-R/R_0} \qquad (7)$$

This equation describes the characteristic curve for broad area densitometry. Figure 4 shows measured image densities for both positive and negative mode xeroradiography. The solid lines are predictions from equation 7 using the experimentally determined values of D_0 and D_∞.

(b) Edge Development: The electrostatic image contains now a step charge discontinuity $\Delta V = V_1 - V_2$ superimposed on an average background $V = V_B + (V_1 + V_2)/2$ (positive development). Toner deposition is controlled by the total normal electric component.

$$E(x,y,t) = E_B \ (t) + E_y \ (x,y,t) \qquad (8)$$

E_B is the average dc field V/d, and E_y is the fringe electrostatic field arising from ΔV. In Figure 5, E (x,y,0) corresponding to ΔV = 100 volts and V = 2500 volts is plotted against x. Note that the field is enhanced for x < 0 while for x > 0 it changes from negative to positive again at $X = X_R$. For points far away from the edge the total field approaches asymptotically the bias field E_B. If now the plate undergoes powder cloud development, the negative toner particles (which are preferentially arriving at the plate due to the applied bias potential) will deposited in the region $x < 0$ and $x > x_R$ where E is attractive and repelled in the segment $(0, x_R)$. The point x_R will then mark the right-hand edge of the white gap, and can be found by solving the equation $E(x,0,0) = 0$. This forbidden zone where no toner can land, is better illustrated by plotting the lines of force near the edge (Figure 6). It is seen that the "maximal" field line which determines the white gap, extends partially into the step, intersecting the plate at the point x_L.

In general, determining the white gap $\delta = x_R - x_L$ requires numerical calculations. An analytical expression for δ, which is essentially equal to the exact solution for δ greater than about 2 mm, is (2)

$$\delta \simeq \frac{1.28 \ d}{\pi} \ \frac{\Delta V}{V + V_B} \tag{9}$$

i.e., the white gap is directly proportional to the electrostatic contrast $C_E = \Delta V / (V + V_B)$.

The white gap δ can be determined as outlined above provided that E crosses the x - axis for $x > 0$. However, this is not always the case as shown in Figure 7: E can remain positive for all x's. The situation depicted in Figure 7 will arise whenever (E_y) max $< E_B$, or equivalently (2), whenever

$$C_E < \frac{2L \ (1 + \kappa)}{\kappa \ d} = 0.003 \tag{10}$$

where $d = 10$ cm (Figure 3), $\kappa = 6.3$ for selenium and $L = 130\mu$. According to relation 10, the appearance of a white gap requires a minimum electrostatic contrast $\Delta V / (V + V_B)$ of about 0.003 for present day Se plates and development chamber. In the way of illustration we calculated the white gap for the case of $C = 0.25$ $V_B = 2000$ volts and $V_0 = 1600$ volts. In Figure 8, δ is plotted versus C_E. It is zero for $C_E < 0.003$ and rises monotonically with increasing C_E. For $C_E >_\sim 0.01$, δ is proportional to C_E as given in equation 9. In xeromammography, low-contrast details are predominantly present leading to small electrostatic contrasts C_E. For a given edge, depending on the exact value of C_E, either a continous density profile $D(x)$ will be observed across the edge or a small white gap. $D(x)$ is given by

$$D(x) = 0.43 \ a \ n\mu t \ E \ (x,y,0) \tag{11}$$

An optimal $D(x)$ corresponds to an optimal ΔV, obtained with $R = R_{opt}$ (See earlier discussion). When $C_E \gtrsim 0.003$, the quantity to be maximized is the white gap or equivalently (See Figure 8) C_E. This operation yields in the limit of low C (2,5).

$$(R_{opt}/R_0 - 1) \, e^{-R_{opt}/R_0} = V_0/V_B \qquad (12)$$

The optimal exposure R_{opt} is again independent of C for low-contrast objects and for a given ratio V_0/V_B depends only on the beam quality (through R_0). The solution of equation 12 for $V_0/V_B = 1600/2000 = 0.80$ is

$$R_{opt} = 1.2 \, R_0 \qquad (13)$$

The above value of R_{opt} required to yield maximal low-contrast white gaps, is close to $R_{opt} = R_0$ required to optimize density profiles. The implication of xeromammography is that a single exposure $R = R_{opt}$ will simultaneously optimize <u>all</u> low-contrast edges in a given breast.

During development, in contrast to the exposure step, the electric fields above the Se layer control the process.

V. Factors Degrading The Density Profiles

In Figure 9, optimal edge profiles are shown for a charged circle (radius = 50 microns) representing a microcalcification, a long narrow strip (halfwidth = 50 microns) and a uniformly charged infinite half-plane. In all cases the step was assumed to be 6 volts with $V_B = 2000$ volts and $V_0 = 1600$ volts. Edge profiles can be degraded by several factors:

(a) Incorrect Exposure: Figure 10 shows the effect of under and over exposures for an extended edge with $C = 0.01$. When $R = R_{opt} = R_0$ the density profile is maximized.

(b) Beam Quality: The main effect of beam hardening is the reduction of the subject contrasts C which leads to a proportional reduction in $D(x)$. One way to compensate for the lost contrast is to introduce a white gap. This may be done by reducing the bias potential V_B and hence make the electrostatic contrast C_E larger than 0.003. This procedure will also enhance already existing white gaps.

(c) Scattered Radiation: The effect of scatter on density profiles is similar to (a) and (b). It turns out (2) that the density profile is degraded exponentially:

$$D_S(x) = D + e^{-S/R_0} \{ D(x) - D_\infty \} \quad (14)$$

where D_S is the profile in the presence of scattered radiation S.

(d)   Thick Se Layers: This effect has been mentioned before. It leads similarly to loss of edge contrast.

(e)   Diffuse Borders: Edge unsharpness leads to profiles which are reduced in height and extended in width (1).

(f)   Time of Development: In the present discussion we have assumed that the step potential ΔV is not degraded during development. For long development times, however, we must consider the exponential time decay (2) of ΔV:

$$\Delta V(t) = \Delta V(0) \, e^{-t/\tau} \quad (15)$$

This leads to a further reduction of $D(x)$ by a factor τ/t.

(g)   Initial Potential V_0: Detailed analysis (2) shows that the density profile $D(x)$ is directly proportional to V_0 and hence the highest possible value (~ 1600 volts) should be used.

The factors listed above cause similar degradation of any white gaps present.

VI.   Effect of Lower Bias Potential

One of the parameters affecting the white gap during development is the bias potential V_B (See Equation 12). The higher the V_B the smaller the electrostatic contrast and hence the smaller the δ. We can understand this effect by referring to Figure 11 a. Negative toner particles are driven into the shaded areas in amounts dependent on the local $E(x)$. The region OA represents the white gap. The average bias field E_B is $V/d \simeq 0.026$ V/μ while Δ^+, the maximum edge difference, is $E_B + (E_y)$ max. Reducing E_B means decreasing Δ^+ but in the process the white gap O A is increased. The increased visibility afforded by a greater δ apparently more than compensates for the reduction in Δ^+, as it was found clinically by Van de Riet and Wolfe (6). These authors achieved significant dose reductions with increased filtration and were able to restore some lost edge contrast by a lower bias potential.

Negative mode development is illustrated in Figure 11 b. The bias potential is ~ 2000 volts in positive mode. Maximizing the white gap O B leads to an equation similar to equation 12 with solution

$$R_{opt} = 0.8 \, R_0$$

i.e., the use of the negative mode will result in additional dose savings of the order of 40% (1.2 R_0 vs 0.8 R_0). This is due to the higher bias potential which lowers the optimal C_E. In fact, it is easy to show with the potentials and R_{opt} values quoted that C_E (opt) = 0.9 C_E^+ (opt) for a given subject detail C.

VII. Discussion

Some features of the xeromammographic process were discussed and their role in optimizing the image was analyzed. Proper choices of the parameters involved in the different stages may lead not only to optimal images but also to reduced exposure levels. In particular, it was indicated that increased beam filtration is desirable from the point of view of dosage reduction especially when coupled with lower bias potential.

The optimal exposures corresponding to a maximal low-contrast white gap were found to be 1.20 R_0 and 0.8 R_0 for positive and . negative development respectively. Optimizing the density profiles leads to an optimal value of 1.0 R_0. The appropriate choice for the exposures is presently unclear. Some physicians prefer a slightly under-exposed image (R = R_0) and some insist on the 1 mm rule (R = 1.2 R_0).

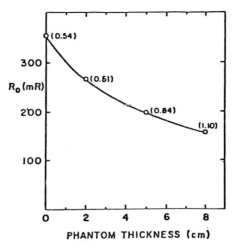

1. Receptor optimal exposures as a function of beam quality.

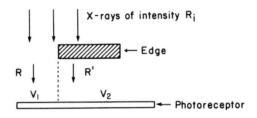

2. The radiological problem: incident x-rays are modulated by an edge, creating a potential step ΔV on the plate.

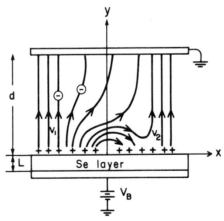

3. Schematic of the development process in the Xerox processor unit. A bias potential is applied between the back of the plate and the chamber (positive development).

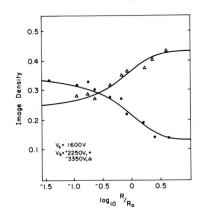

4. Measured image densities for both positive and negative mode xero-radiography. The solid lines are theoretical predictions as discussed in the text.

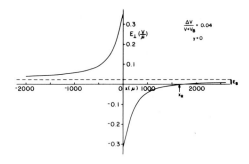

5. The total normal electric field plotted at y = 0 against distance. The application of a bias field E_B, causes the field to change sign at the point X_R which marks the right hand edge of the white gap.

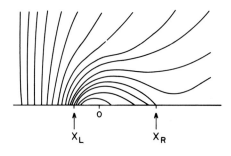

6. Lines of force indicating the extent of the white gap. No toner particles can land in the region (X_L, X_R) where the field lines are arching back to the plate.

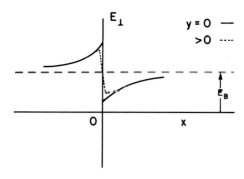

7. For small electrostatic contrasts, E can remain positive for all X's. In the case no white gap is possible. Instead, a continous density variation across the edge is seen.

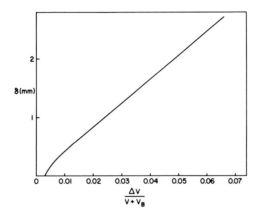

8. Calculated white gap versus electrostatic contrast C_E. Note the existence of a threshold value in C_E below which no white gap is present.

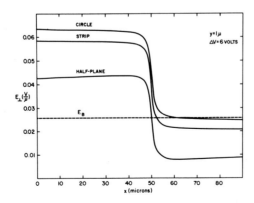

9. Optimal edge profiles across a circle (R = 50 microns), a strip (width = 100 microns) an infinite half-plane.

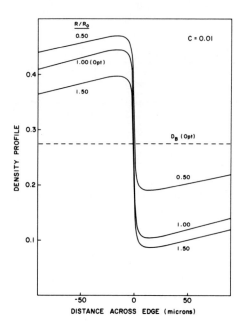

10. Density profiles across a low-contrast edge for different values of R/R_0. The profiles corresponding to $R/R_0 = 1.0$ yields the greatest density variation across the edge. The dashed line represents the solid-area density away from the edge for $R = R_{opt}$ ($y = 1$ μ).

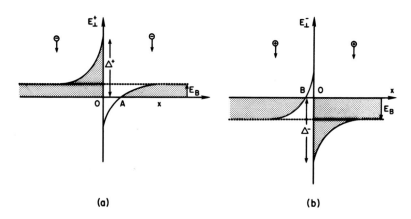

11. Schematic representation of the positive (a) and negative (b) development process.

ACKNOWLEDGMENTS

This work was supported in part by Grant 7 R01 FDO 1004-01 from HEW. We would like to thank Dr. G. Zeman for permission to use the data in Figures 1 and 4.

We would also like to thank Miss Inez Wasicki for her secretarial assistance.

REFERENCES

1. Fatouros, P.P. and Rao, G.U.V.: Detail Visibility In Xeromammography (To be published).

2. Fatouros, P.P. and Rao, G.U.V.: On Optimizing the Xeromammographic Image. Medical Physics (In Press).

3. Kao, C.C. and Lewis, R.B.: Dynamic Latent-Image Formation in Xeroradiography. J. Opt. Soc. Am. 65, 1189 (1975).

4. Fender, W.D.: Quantification of the Xeroradiographic Discharge Curve. SPIE 70, 364 (1975).

5. Zeman, G.H., Rao, G.U.V. and Osterman, F.A.: Evaluation of Xeroradiographic Image Quality. Radiology 119, 689 (1976).

6. Van de Riet, W.G. and Wolfe, J.N.: Dose Reduction in Xeroradiography of the Breast. Am. J. Roentgenal. 128, 821 (1977).

FUNDAMENTAL ASPECTS OF MAMMOGRAPHIC RECEPTORS

FILM PROCESS

R. E. Wayrynen, Ph.D.
E. I. du Pont de Nemours & Co., Inc.

HISTORICAL

A low dose film-screen system for mammography was introduced by Du Pont in 1972. Since then, other film manufacturers have introduced other film-screen systems for mammography. Before considering further system speed increases to further reduce patient exposure, we should review the steps which have led us to where we are today.

Radiographic imaging of the breast is a difficult task because of the need to image both soft tissue tumors and cysts, and small microcalcifications down to about 0.1mm. Films and screens designed for general purpose radiography had been tried by many radiologists and considered unacceptable in image quality. The chief deficiencies of these film-screen combinations were excessive noise, unsatisfactory sharpness, and inadequate recording range. Radiologists evaluating techniques at that time were convinced that significantly better image quality was required.

As a result, prior to 1972, most film mammography was done using industrial type radiographic films. These films are designed for use without intensifying screens to image very fine detail in metal castings and parts. The mammography techniques required with such films were characterized by relatively high patient dosage, long exposure times, and the corresponding risk of unsharpness due to patient motion. The sensitometric curve shape of these industrial films when used in mammography was typical of that for non-screen film imaging. The contrast is low at low densities and gradually increases continually as exposure is increased. The low contrast at low density made images of small calcifications in the thick portion of the breast difficult to see, and the continually increasing contrast at higher densities limited the exposure range. As a result, many radiologists found it necessary to simultaneously expose a pair of industrial films of different speed in order to extend the exposure range so the entire breast could be imaged.

Working with Drs. Isard and Ostrum at the Albert Einstein Medical Center in Philadelphia, goals for a film-screen imaging system were established. The basic goal was to obtain maximum patient exposure reduction consistent with maintaining the image quality required for diagnostic accuracy.

But, the image quality required for satisfactory mammography was not readily defined. Radiographic image quality, in general, is determined by three characteristics--contrast, sharpness and noise. Each was considered in establishing the goals.

High contrast improves image perceptibility but reduces exposure range or latitude. High contrast also increases the visibility of quantum noise which interferes with the perceptibility of detail at low density. Based on experience with industrial films, the exposure range required to image from the chest wall to the nipple had to be at least 25 to 1 (log exposure scale at least 1.4). To avoid bright-light film reading, which was characteristic of industrial films, it was desirable to limit the breast image to densities less than 3.0. The film contrast should be the maximum possible within these limits for good imaging of small calcifications.

Sharpness in film-screen receptors is determined by the screen sharpness. For mammography, the screen sharpness should be sufficient to image calcifications as small as 0.1mm. Although the sharpness of intensifying screens is significantly less than that of film alone, film sharpness far exceeds that required for mammography as was later shown by Haus et al.

Noise due to random distribution of X-ray photons limits visibility of low contrast images at low density. Therefore, in mammography, this quantum noise can interfere with visibility of both calcifications and soft tissue tumor edges which appear at relatively low film density. The noise observed by the radiologist is also dependent on screen sharpness, and it is quite possible for these noise-limited images to be less perceptible if the screen is too sharp. To avoid image degradation by noise, it was desired to achieve as much speed increase as possible through improved absorption over industrial films.

The Du Pont Lo-dose Mammography Film-Screen System announced in 1972 reduced patient exposure by a factor of 7, compared with high-speed industrial film, and by a factor of 15, compared with the slower industrial film also being used at that time. The system consisted of a single-emulsion film and a single intensifying screen held together in intimate contact in a flexible vacuum cassette. Calcium tungstate was chosen as the intensifying screen because it is a very good absorber below 30 keV. Most of the speed increase was due to improved X-ray absorption as shown in Table I.

TABLE I. Comparison of nominal exposure, fraction of X-ray beam absorbed, and effective exposure for the film-screen system and nonscreen film. Data were obtained at 30 kVp.

	Exposure	Absorption	Exposure X Absorption*
Mammography Film-Screen System	25 mAs	80%	20.0
NDT 75 - Nonscreen Film	175 mAs	10%	17.5

*Approximately proportional to the number of X-ray quanta absorbed.

Compared with film alone, the intensifying screen provided an unusual opportunity to increase speed through improved absorption. Table I shows that the film-screen combination absorbs about 80% of the X-ray beam, compared with only about 10% for film alone. It is also clear that similar increases in absorption are no longer possible.

The sharpness of the film-screen combination, as illustrated by modulation transfer curves, is compared with that of film alone and with a conventional film-screen combination in Figure 1. Although the sharpness of the mammography film-screen combination is obviously much better than that of the film-screen combination for general diagnostic work, the system's capability of imaging small calcifications was not established until clinical films showing calcifications were obtained.

The sensitometric curve of the film-screen combination is compared with that of industrial film in Figure 2. Note that the film-screen combination provides higher contrast at low densities which is helpful in imaging small calcifications. The contrast does not continue to increase with increasing exposure as it does with industrial film so that the exposure range can be extended. Assuming the lower exposure limit is the point at which the gradient is 0.4, the exposure range for industrial film is about 1.2, while that of the film-screen combination is 1.5 to 1.8, depending on whether densities over 3.0 are included. Thus, the exposure range of the film-screen combination is up to four times that of film alone. This has proved sufficient to image from the chest wall to the nipple.

This system proved capable of meeting the image quality requirements as a mammographic receptor and was widely accepted by radiologists practicing mammography. The acceptance of this film-screen combination suggested further possible dose reductions may be possible while still maintaining adequate image quality. In 1975, Du Pont announced a faster intensifying screen, Lo-dose/2, for use with the Lo-dose film. The increase in speed was achieved by compromising screen sharpness as shown by the modulation transfer function curves in Figure 3.

According to data obtained at Albert Einstein Medical Center in Philadelphia, patient dose with the Lo-dose system was 1.2 - 1.8R with an average of 1.5R. With Lo-dose/2, it was reduced to 0.6 - 0.9R.

In 1975, Eastman Kodak announced a film-screen combination for mammography called Min-R. This combination used a single gadolinium oxysulfide intensifying screen and a single-emulsion orthochromatic film, and had system speed equivalent to that of Lo-dose/2. Other film-screen systems for mammography have been announced by other manufacturers.

FILM PROCESSING

Achieving satisfactory performance of film-screen mammography systems requires control of all variables in the radiographic imaging system, including film processing. Control of processing is especially important in mammography because maximum image receptor performance is expected.

Mammography films are generally slower in photographic speed than the medical screen films typically used in general diagnostic practice. As a result, fog levels tend to be somewhat lower and less subject to changes with processing variations. Similarly, gradients tend to be relatively insensitive to changes in temperature as shown in Figure 4 for Lo-dose film processed in CRONEX® XMD developer over the range 85° to 95° F.

Figure 5 shows that the gradient is also relatively insensitive to changes in bromide concentration. The dependence on bromide level is important because bromide in the developer functions as a restrainer which affects development rate. The bromide concentration is influenced by replenishment rates and the film size mix being processed.

These characteristics of relative insensitivity to processing changes are desirable from the standpoint of processing reproducibility and the need in mammography for films with well-controlled densities.

Perhaps one of the major processing effects is the change in film speed with processing temperature. Figure 6 shows that over an extended temperature range, the speed can vary up to a factor of 4. Around the temperature 92° F, which is recommended for XMD developer, a plus or minus variation of five degrees can change speed from approximately -28% to +38%. Obviously, smaller temperature fluctuations can be responsible for unexpected density changes.

The effect of processing temperature on speed, which is typical of most photographic products, suggests the temptation to increase system speed and reduce patient dose simply by increasing developer temperature. But, pushed processing is always accompanied by a compromise in other properties.

The speeds of the films in Figure 6 were obtained from mAs exposure values necessary to produce films of essentially matched densities. The films processed at higher temperatures were significantly more noisy than those processed at lower temperatures. Table II shows granularity data for these film samples. The data were obtained by the so-called analog method, using a rotating stage, first described by Jones. Total noise data were read using a 200um aperture to correspond to noise observed subjectively with a 2X magnifier as is often used in mammography. The total noise values include film graininess, structure noise in the phantom, and quantum mottle. The relative grain data are due to density fluctuations at 40 cycles/mm and, therefore, correspond to film graininess.

TABLE II. Effect of processing temperature on phantom image noise.
Lo-dose film processed in CRONEX® XMD, 120-second cycle

	80° F	85° F	90° F	95° F	100° F
Relative Total Noise	11.04	11.77	11.91	13.44	12.59
Relative Grain Noise	.77	.78	.80	.82	.80

*Total noise obtained with 200um aperture. Grain noise at 40 cycles/mm.

These changes in noise with processing temperature indicate that essentially all the noise increase observed on the film samples is quantum noise caused by increased film speed. Therefore, deliberate attempts to reduce patient dose by overprocessing is not recommended and should be discouraged. Processing as recommended by the manufacturer should be followed meticulously.

The industrial films commonly used for mammography prior to 1972 could not be processed in typical 90-second or 3-1/2-minute cycle medical X-ray processors. These films required much longer development times and were usually developed about five minutes by hand in a deep tank at about 70° F. By comparison, development time in a 90-second cycle is about 20 seconds at 92-95° F. Probably because these industrial films used in mammography needed hand-tank processing, some users have felt that this type of processing produces better quality and reproducibility. Attempts to improve film quality by reducing temperature and increasing time, or by using hand-tank methods on contemporary 90-second film products, are not recommended. Contemporary films are made to achieve design sensitometry under development kinetics typical of the standard 90-120-second processing cycle. These films should be processed according to the manufacturers' recommendations to obtain best results.

FASTER FILMS

Further reduction in patient dose by increasing the speed of films used in film-screen mammography systems is entirely possible. The trade-offs in image quality are predictable, but the effect on diagnostic accuracy is not.

An increase in film speed will increase quantum noise. A factor of 2 in film speed dictates that the film requires half as many X-ray photons, for a given density, and the quantum noise will increase by the square root of 2. This increase in noise will affect images of both small calcifications and soft tissue tumor edges at low density.

Some radiologists are evaluating CRONEX® MRF 31 film with the Lo-dose/2 screen for mammography. The speed of MRF 31 is nearly twice that of Lo-dose film. The contrast of MRF 31 is also higher than that of Lo-dose film. This combination is finding varying degrees of acceptability because the predictable increase in quantum noise is considered objectionable by some radiologists. Further, although the higher contrast of MRF 31 improves the visibility of some detail in the breast, it also limits the exposure range and, therefore, the ability of the film to image from the chest wall to the nipple. Further, the higher contrast increases the visibility of quantum noise. Considerable clinical experience will be necessary to determine the effect of these noise and contrast differences on diagnostic accuracy.

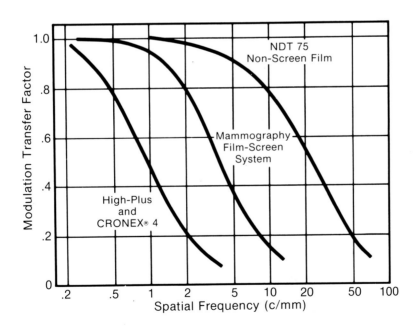

Figure 1. Modulation transfer curves comparing the mammography film-screen system with a nonscreen industrial film and a conventional medical film-screen system.

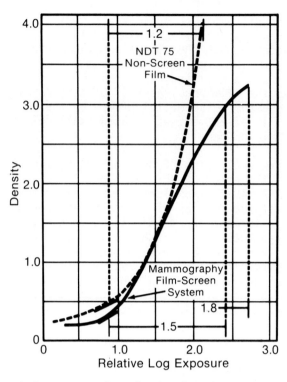

Figure 2. Sensitometric curves for the Lo-dose Mammography System and a nonscreen industrial film. Though there is a factor 7 speed difference, the curves are arbitrarily shifted to coincide at one region to emphasize differences in curve shape.

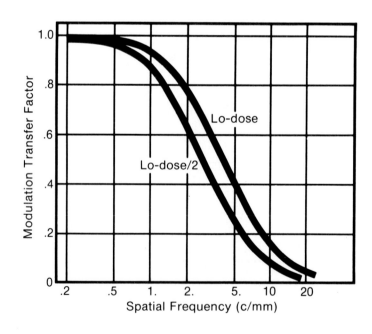

Figure 3. Modulation transfer curves comparing Lo-dose with the faster Lo-dose/2 screens.

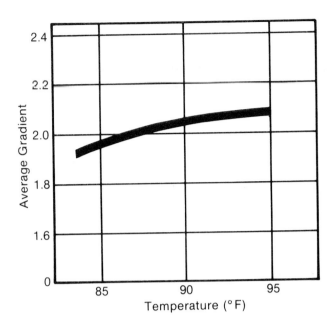

Figure 4.   Dependence of CRONEX® Lo-dose film average gradient on CRONEX® XMD developer temperature in a 120-second processing cycle. Average gradient defined as the slope between 0.25 and 2.00 net densities.

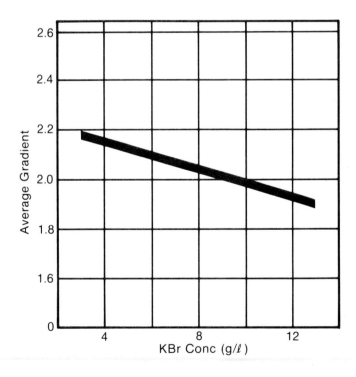

Figure 5.   Dependence of CRONEX® Lo-dose film average gradient on CRONEX® XMD developer bromide level in a 120-second processing cycle at 92° F. Normal bromide level is about 8 g/1.

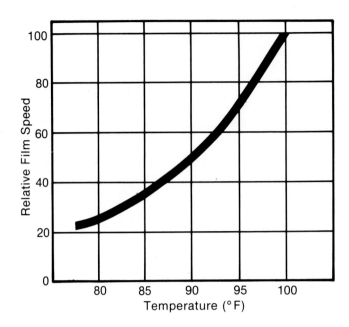

Figure 6. Change in CRONEX® Lo-dose film speed with processing temperature. Speed data obtained from mAs values required to give matched phantom film density. CRONEX® XMD developer and 120-second processing cycle.

REFERENCES

B. J. Ostrum, W. Becker, and H. J. Isard, "Low-Dose Mammography," Radiology 109: 323-326 (1973).

A. G. Haus, K. Doi, J. T. Chiles, K. Rossman, and R. A. Mintzer, "The Effect of Geometric and Recording System Unsharpness in Mammography," Investigative Radiology 10: 43-52 (1975).

J. P. Weiss and R. E. Wayrynen, "Imaging System for Low-Dose Mammography," Journal of Applied Photographic Engineering 2: 7-10 (1976).

R. S. Holland and R. E. Kellogg, "The Dependence of Quantum Noise on Screen Sharpness," Journal of Applied Photographic Engineering 3: 125-128 (1977).

R. C. Jones, "New Method of Describing and Measuring the Granularity of Photographic Materials," Journal of the Optical Society of America 45: 799-808 (1955).

FUNDAMENTAL ASPECTS OF MAMMOGRAPHIC PHOTORECEPTORS: SCREENS

Bernard Roth, MS; John F. Hamilton, Jr., PhD; and Phillip C. Bunch, PhD

Research Laboratories, Eastman Kodak Company, Rochester, New York 14650

INTRODUCTION

In screen-film mammography a single fluorescent intensifying screen in combination with a film having emulsion coated on only one side of the base support is used as the photoreceptor. The role of the screen is that of an energy converter. It provides high x-ray absorption--much higher than can be attained with a practical film emulsion--and converts the x-ray energy into light energy of a form readily absorbed by the emulsion. In addition, each x-ray quantum absorbed in the phosphor produces hundreds of light photons thus rendering a number of "emulsion grains" developable. In contrast, only one or two grains are made developable by absorption of an x-ray in the emulsion. It is these two gain factors--higher x-ray absorption and greater numbers of grains exposed--that permit the substantial reductions in the x-ray exposure required to produce a screen-film image. This exposure reduction can be used to lower patient exposure, reduce blur caused by patient motion (shorten exposure time), or permit the use of improved imaging geometry (e.g., small focal spots, long focus-film distance).

However, the light generated within the phosphor layer of the screen is emitted in all directions and thus spreads laterally as it travels to the film. Some of the factors affecting light spread--the source of image blur within a screen--are discussed and illustrated by computer simulations.

SCREEN PROPERTIES

The heart of the screen is the phosphor layer, which is an aggregate of minute phosphor crystals embedded in a plastic binder. A scanning electron micrograph of a cross-section of such a layer, enlarged 1000 times, is shown in Figure 1.

The choice of phosphor is based on several criteria:

1. high x-ray absorption
2. high conversion efficiency
3. spectral emission usable by the film
4. ability to be handled during screen preparation
5. stability when subjected to such ambient conditions as light, temperature, and moisture
6. low afterglow
7. high density

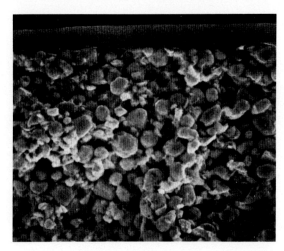

Figure 1. Photomicrograph of a cross-
section of part of an x-ray
intensifying screen. Magnification 1000X.

A schematic cross-section of a typical mammographic screen is shown in
Figure 2 to aid in identifying the various structural components of a screen.
The overcoat, usually 8 to 20 μm thick, is used to protect the screen surface
from abrasion and to facilitate cleaning. The phosphor-binder layer, typically
about 100 μm thick, is the energy converter element. The underlayer is needed
to bond the phosphor-binder to the support and may have light absorbing or
reflecting properties. The support is usually plastic, sometimes with a
cardboard laminate for increased rigidity.

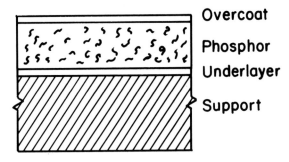

Figure 2. Schematic cross section
of an x-ray intensifying
screen.

As one would expect from the photomicrograph, the phosphor layer is a
highly turbid medium. Thus, light generated within the layer must undergo
multiple scattering events before reaching the screen surface. Also, there
is some probability that light photons will be absorbed along their path or at
the underlayer. Thus the spread of light depends on the depth within the
screen at which the light originates, the optical absorption and scattering
properties of the phosphor layer, and the optical properties of the overcoat
and underlayer.

SIMULATION OF SCREEN EMISSION

To illustrate the optical image forming properties of screens in such a manner that one and only one variable of screen design can be altered at a time, a Monte Carlo computer program (or "random walk" model) was developed to simulate the fate of light photons. Simulations were based on the choice of optical scattering and absorption parameters which yielded light-spread distributions similar to those measured for actual screens. The realism of the approach was then verified by comparison of the predicted and measured values of a series of screens differing only in thickness.

During the Conference, a movie was shown to illustrate the paths and fate of light photons within a screen as x-ray absorption and optical properties are changed. The movie was made by photographing the graphic display screen of the computer terminal used to program the Monte Carlo simulation. The purpose of the movie was to provide an appreciation of the causes of image spread within a screen and to illustrate how certain physical factors affect this property.

CONVENTIONAL MEDICAL X-RAY INTENSIFYING SCREEN

THICKNESS = 100		PHOTONS = 20
BACK REFL. = 0.90		
ORIENTATION = BACK		** HIGH keV **

SINGLE BACK SCREEN

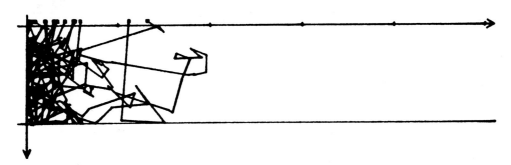

Figure 3. Simulated light photon paths. The arrowhead indicates the direction of the x-ray beam.

A sequence of three displays was used for each variable considered. Figure 3 shows the first display illustrating sequentially the path of light photons from their origin to the point at which they exited the screen surface or to the site of absorption. The diagram represents the cross-section of a 100-μm-thick hypothetical phosphor layer. A beam of x-rays is depicted on the left side by a line with an arrowhead indicating its direction. (The "back" screen designation is used when the x-ray beam is incident on the output surface of the screen. "Front" screen signifies incidence on the phosphor-base interface.) The beam of x-rays was chosen to be in the form of a line extending both into and out of the figure. Each tick mark along the screen surface is a 100-μm marker. For simplicity, only one light photon path is traced for each of the 20 x-ray absorption events shown, whereas, in reality, several hundred photons are produced by each x-ray absorption event. Where photons are absorbed in the phosphor layer, their energy is dissipated in the form of heat, and where they escape they are assumed to be incident, without further spread, on the film emulsion surface. A third simplification is in the depiction of the light distribution: light photon paths are shown in only two dimensions and on only one side of the x-ray beam.

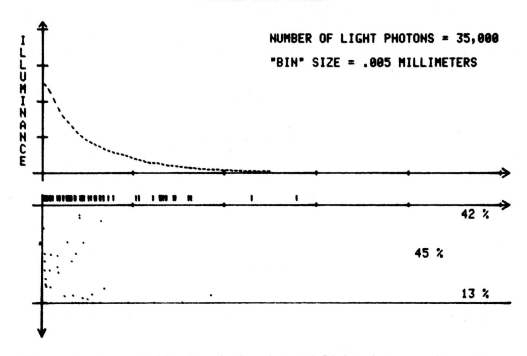

CONVENTIONAL MEDICAL X-RAY INTENSIFYING SCREEN

THICKNESS   = 100
BACK REFL.   = 0.90
ORIENTATION = BACK

PHOTONS = 100

** HIGH keV **

SINGLE BACK SCREEN

NUMBER OF LIGHT PHOTONS = 35,000

"BIN" SIZE = .005 MILLIMETERS

ILLUMINANCE

42 %

45 %

13 %

Figure 4.   Lower Half: Terminal points of light photons. Percentages
            of those escaping and absorbed are on right. Upper Half:
            Simulation of Line Spread Function.

The lower portion of Figure 4 is the second part of the three-part
sequence. Here, only the terminal points of the light photon are shown:
small dots where absorption occurred and vertical markers where photons
escaped. One hundred photons were used in this illustration to provide a
clearer illustration of the distribution of terminal point locations. To the
right are the rounded percentages for the disposition of light photons based
on following 35,000 light photons. For the conditions chosen (discussed
later) approximately 42% escape, 45% are absorbed in the phosphor layer, and
13% are absorbed in the reflecting layer between the phosphor and base.

The third part of the sequence (shown in the upper portion of Fig. 4)
shows the lateral distribution of exiting light photons arising from the
x-ray line exposure. (Since the distribution is symmetrical about the x-ray
beam, only half is shown.) Here 35,000 photons were used to increase the
precision of the distribution estimate. The number of photons was recorded
within each 5-μm interval laterally along the screen surface; had the interval
been narrower and the number of photons larger, the illuminance distribution
would have been smoother.

This distribution is called the Line Spread Function (LSF). A property
of the LSF is that it can be transformed mathematically to the Modulation
Transfer Function (MTF) which is used in Figures 7 and 8 to summarize results.
By choice, the LSFs are normalized to equal area so that, in this model, an
equal number of light photons are contained in each distribution. This method
of normalizing shows clearly both the magnitude and the direction of shifts in
distribution of light as screen parameters are changed.

In the movie the sequence of pictures just described was used to illustrate several properties of screens and their usage: high- and low-kV exposure, front and back screen orientation, and several variations of screen optical properties. Only representative examples are included herein.

LIGHT SPREAD DEPENDENCE ON X-RAY ENERGY

The hypothetical phosphor layer used in the model for Figures 3 and 4 is assumed to be used as a "back" screen, to be 100 μm thick, and to have an underlayer with a reflectance of 90%. Exposure is to an x-ray energy frequently used for general radiography ("high kV") where 15% of the x-ray beam is absorbed in a single screen. The percentages of light emitted and absorbed are shown in the lower part of Figure 4.

When the same screen is used at mammographic energies, a larger fraction of the x-ray beam is absorbed. Under low-kV mammographic exposure conditions, 80% absorption is assumed: this is reasonable for a molybdenum target tube with a molybdenum filter. An important difference can be expected between mammographic energies and those used in general radiography. For the lower energy, more of the light is emitted from the phosphor layer adjacent to the emulsion than in the higher kV case, where the distribution of light generated is more nearly uniform with depth. Thus, (1) more light escapes (although not shown, 47% escapes for the mammographic exposure case and 42% for the higher kV) and (2) the light spread is not as great since, on the average, it scatters less in reaching the film.

For comparison, the two LSFs are shown in Figure 5. For the mammographic case ("low kV"), there are more light photons closer to the x-ray line which generated the distribution: higher central peak and lower tail, therefore less spread.

EFFECT OF AN EXTREME CHANGE IN X-RAY ABSORPTION ON ILLUMINANCE DISTRIBUTION

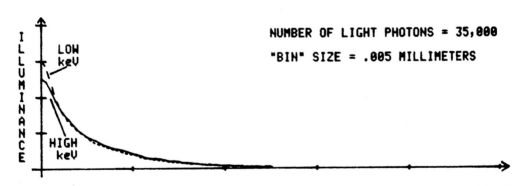

Figure 5. LSFs comparing high and low kV. Curves are area normalized.

LIGHT SPREAD DEPENDENCE ON EXPOSURE CONFIGURATION

If the hypothetical screen is inverted and used as a "front" screen instead of a "back", the effect of the distribution of light generated is even more pronounced than in the kV comparison just discussed. Where x-ray absorption is relatively high near the reflecting underlayer, less light escapes from the face of the screen than when the distribution of absorption (i.e., light generation) is highest near the screen surface: 37% versus 47%. As mentioned previously, the illuminance distributions or LSFs are normalized to the same number of emitted photons. To achieve this equal light output when used as a "front" screen, approximately 27% more x-radiation must be absorbed--27% more exposure--to offset the higher light absorption within the screen.

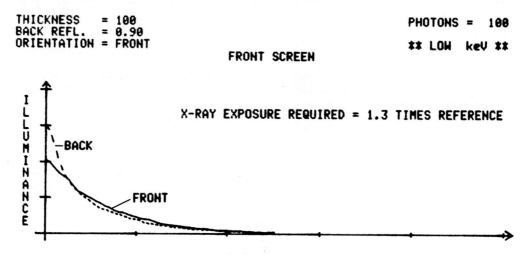

Figure 6. LSFs comparing back and front screens.

The illuminance distribution also is affected as shown in Figure 6. When the screen is used as a "back" screen, the resulting LSF is a more faithful representation of the x-ray line input than is the LSF produced in the "front" screen orientation. An alternative representation of the optical fidelity of screen performance is shown in Figure 7 where the "back" and "front" MTFs are given. Thus there are two distinct advantages to the "back" screen configuration for mammography: better MTF and lower x-ray exposure.

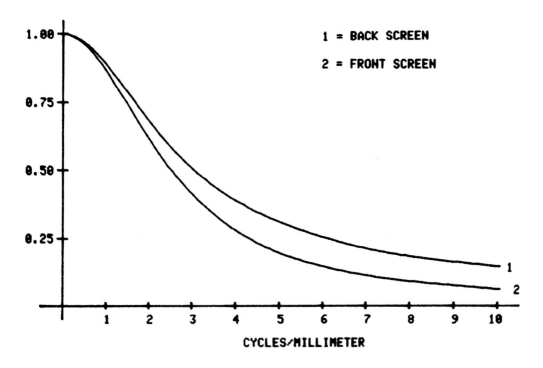

Figure 7. Modulation Transfer Functions comparing back and front screens.

LIGHT SPREAD DEPENDENCE ON SELECTED SCREEN PROPERTIES

Such dual advantages as those just described do not happen often in screen design unless there is a change in phosphor composition. Manipulating the optical properties of a screen to reduce light spread is normally accompanied by a compromise in the x-ray exposure required. In Figure 8 are MTF curves of four screen changes which improve MTF (reduce light spread) but which require greater x-ray exposure to yield equal light output.

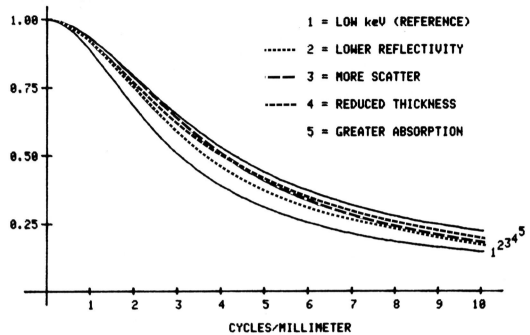

Figure 8. MTF comparisons of various screen improvements.

Curve 1. Reference screen (1X Exposure): 100 μm thick, low light absorption in the phosphor layer, highly reflecting support or underlayer.

Curve 2. Low reflecting underlayer (1.2X Exposure): Light scattered toward the support and reflected by the underlayer spreads, on the average, more than the light which is scattered in the other directions. Thus light spread is reduced by absorbing more light at the underlayer.

Curve 3. Increased light scattering in the phosphor layer (1.1X Exposure): Increased scattering increases the average path length of light photons within the phosphor layer. Photons that spread laterally travel farther and, therefore, have an increased probability of being absorbed prior to escaping through the screen surface. Thus light spread is reduced.

Curve 4. Reduced thickness (1.4X Exposure): Light spread is reduced because the average point of origin of the light is closer to the exit surface than for the reference screen.

Curve 5. <u>Greater light absorption in the phosphor layer</u> (1.6X Exposure): Light spread is reduced because photons that travel greater lateral distances must traverse longer path lengths to escape through the screen surface. With increased absorption in the phosphor layer, they have an increased chance of being absorbed.

SUMMARY

A Monte Carlo simulation of the fate of light photons generated in a turbid phosphor layer has been developed to illustrate the effects of selected optical properties of fluorescent intensifying screens on image spread and on light emission. Examples are shown which confirm the desirability of using the screen as a "back" screen, and which point out the improvement in optical image formation associated with the use of highly absorbed x-radiation (low kV) such as used in screen-film mammography. Also, examples are cited of some of the compromises in the optical characteristics of phosphor layers leading to improved MTF at the expense of radiation exposure.

FUTURE DEVELOPMENT POSSIBILITIES:
ELECTROSTATIC MAMMOGRAPHY SYSTEMS

Dr. John H. Lewis*

Techniques for imaging X radiation by predominately electronic processes are discussed in terms of the underlying mechanisms of quantum efficiency, conversion gain, system noise, and resolution. Detection processes include X-ray induced photo-conductivity in solids, liquids and gases. Recording techniques include image scanning, toning and photography. Specific examples are discussed which have potential implications for mammography.

INTRODUCTION

New and evolving radiographic imaging concepts create considerable interest within the radiology community for a variety of reasons. As has been shown by Motz and Danos[1] for example, current practice does not achieve the limits of maximum information recording at minimum patient exposure by a significant margin. Additionally, the benefits of recent innovations such as rare earth intensifying screens and CAT scanners have awakened the industry to search for other technological advances which may produce similar benefits. Electrostatic radiography in its several forms is one such area which has undergone extensive study for projection radiography.

Although assessing the potential performance and merits of imaging concepts is difficult while still in the development stage, nevertheless a fundamental evaluation based on well known and measurable standards is generally possible. Such an analysis must rely on image information theory as developed by Rose[2]. An understanding of a systems basic physical mechanisms, including stepwise and overall conversion efficiencies is required in order to utilize the techniques of image quality prediction.

X-ray photons interact with matter according to statistical probabilities producing events which are either photochemical, fluorescent, or ionizing in nature. Electrostatic imaging implies conversion of the primary X-ray photon energy into electronic charges, usually by the photoelectric process in which the energetic photoelectron produces numerous secondary ions which are subsequently utilized in image visualization. This dominant mechanism can be described symbolically by two steps:

$$h\nu + A_1 \rightarrow P\bar{e} + A_1^+$$

$$P\bar{e} + A_2 \rightarrow P\bar{e} + S\bar{e} + A_2^+$$

Where: $h\nu$ is the primary X-ray photon

   A   is an atom

   $P\bar{e}$ is a photo electron

   $S\bar{e}$ is a secondary electron

The second step above is repeated many times until the energy of the photo electron is expended. Other charge producing mechanisms also occur with lower probabilities. The Compton scattering process can be described by:

$$h\nu + A_3 \rightarrow h\nu' + C\bar{e} + A_3^+$$

*Principal Scientist, Xonics, Inc., 6849 Hayvenhurst Ave., Van Nuys, Calif. 91406.

Where: $h\nu'$ is the scattered X-ray photon

   $C\bar{e}$ is the Compton (recoil) electron

Also the photo fluorescence and Auger processes occur in conjunction with the photo electric process:

$$A_1^+ \to P_1 h\nu'' + A_1^+ \text{ or,}$$
$$A_1^+ \to P_2 A\bar{e} + A_1^{++}$$

Where: P_1 and P_2 are statistical probabilities,

   $h\nu''$ is the photo fluorescent photon

   $A\bar{e}$ is the Auger electron

It should be noted, that the photon and electron end products of the additional mechanisms $h\nu'$, $C\bar{e}$, $h\nu''$, $A\bar{e}$, have sufficient energy to continue the ionization process and produce significant numbers of secondary ion pairs as does the photo electron. All of the above processes must be analyzed in detail in evaluation of emergent radiographic imaging systems sensitivity and resolution.

For comparison of emergent electrostatic imaging concepts, three X-ray spectra representative of mammographic, extremity, and deep body procedures respectively with appropriate water targets of 5, 10, and 20 cm thickness have been chosen in a manner similar to Seelentag[3]. Each spectra is calculated assuming a tungsten anode with 3 mm of Al added filtration. The KVp and average photon energy after target filtration for each spectra is shown in Table I below:

TABLE I

REPRESENTATIVE X-RAY SPECTRA

	Spectrum	KVp	Kev
I	(mammography)	40	28
II	(extremity)	80	45
III	(deep body)	110	57

PHOTON DETECTION

Perhaps the most important single parameter in radiographic imaging is the detector X-ray photon stopping power expressed as a quantum or count efficiency. This quantum efficiency sets the statistical limits for signal to noise or quantum mottle in modern radiographic practice. Ideally the quantum efficiency would be 100% for maximum image information content. Quantum efficiency calculations for the representative X-ray spectra above for typical detector materials used in electrostatic imaging processes are presented in Table II. The detector or absorbing materials chosen are amorphous selenium, xenon, and tetramethyl-tin (TMT). Although other choices are available, these three materials are indicative of most electrostatic systems under development. All three materials despite their physical differences undergo the same X-ray photon absorption processes described in the introduction. In each case however, the probabilities of the different physical mechanisms differ and thus different techniques for optimizing imaging systems using the three mediums are required.

TABLE II

DETECTOR QUANTUM EFFICIENCY

Spectrum	Selenium (135 μ)	Xenon (10 atm-cm)	TMT (4 mm)
I	42	38	72
II	32	35	92
III	15	26	88

Recall from the discussion of X-ray interaction mechanisms that the next process in the conversion is the creation of secondary ions by collisions of the photo electron with surrounding atoms of the absorption medium. This collisional process continues until the energy of the photo electron (usually several tens of thousand electron volts) is expended. The number of secondary ions created, Ni, is determined by the total energy of the photo electron, E, and the average energy required to create a secondary ion called the W value. Not all the available energy is utilized in the creation of secondary ions. A portion of the photo electron energy is absorbed in the surrounding medium in thermalizing or non-ionizing collisions. Thus the W value can be expressed as:

$$W = \frac{E}{Ni} = \frac{Ei + Et}{Ni}$$

Where: Ei is the energy of ionizing collisions
         Et is the energy of thermalizing collisions

W values for many materials have been tabulated in numerous standard references[4] and range from 25 to 30 ev/ip for most materials.

In practice, these secondary ions are created in the bulk of the absorbing medium and must usually be collected on a charge storage surface in order to be available for the next process in the imaging chain. This collection step is accomplished by imposing a strong electric field on the absorbing medium. During the collection process a portion of the secondary ions may be lost by recombination or the number of secondary ions increased by electron amplification. Thus the usual W value as determined from atomic ionization potentials needs to be modified to include both recombination and gain in most practical systems. This modified $\overline{W}$ value expressed as electron volts per ion pair collected becomes:

$$\overline{W} = \frac{G}{C_R} \; [W]$$

Where: G is the gain coefficient
         C_R is the recombination coefficient

Ion yield measurements for the three absorbers chosen clearly demonstrate that in the case of solid or liquid absorbers, the ion recombination is a more significant factor than the electron gain, while in the case of gaseous absorbers, neither process dominates.

TABLE III

MEASURED W VALUES

Selenium	Xenon (15 KV/cm)	TMT (50 KV/cm)
50	24	50

The combination of quantum efficiency, secondary ionization efficiency, and charge collection efficiency determine an overall sensitivity of the photon detector expressed as charge collected per unit area per unit exposure. These overall detector sensitivity values (nc/cm^2-mR) are shown in Table IV below.

TABLE IV

DETECTOR SENSITIVITY
(nc/cm^2-mR)

Spectrum	Selenium	Xenon	TMT
I	.46	.56	.88
II	.61	1.7	2.3
III	.47	2.1	2.9

IMAGE RECORDING

Charge image recording techniques which utilize a wide variety of physical and chemical phenomena have been developed. Such phenomena include both direct and indirect measurement of the image charge. The most common technique is electrostatic toning, either by an aerosol or a liquid. However, much current emphasis rests on direct reading by scanning instruments. Systems under development include a scanning array of micro electrometers[5,6,7] and a laser scanner[8,9]. Small aperture PbO or Se target camera tubes have also been developed for radiography[10], but the long term degradation of the PbO has been a fundamental limitation. However, work continues in the area of electro-optic devices such as CCD arrays to record X-ray images.

Optical projection systems are also reported in literature. When deformable dielectric materials (thermo plastics, elastomers, etc.) are coated over one electrode of a typical electrostatic imaging chamber, the collected charge creates a deformation pattern which can be viewed by a schlieren projection similar to the Eidophor system developed for broadcast video viewing[10]. Such a projection system utilizing Xenon gas as the absorption medium has been demonstrated[11,12,13]. An additional, novel projection system which is an adaptation of the Wilson cloud chamber uses Xenon-alcohol vapor to create an image of condensation droplets[14].

The principles of electrophoretic displays have been applied in a radiographic system which utilizes a heavy element containing liquid such as TMT to disperse toner particles. In this system, the liquid material acts as the X-ray absorber and image charge collection medium and the toner particles act as the visualization material[15,16,17]. Electrophoretic displays can be photographed directly and a typical radiograph recorded on film is shown in Figure 1.

Numerous other systems are also being developed such as solid and liquid state ionography[18,19]. Liquid crystals and other anisotropic or birefringent materials are being considered for charge visualization devices. Other possibilities include electro/photo chromic, gas discharge, and electro luminescent effects to mention a few.

SUMMARY

Although electrostatic and electronic imaging systems have found only limited application in radiology, notably their use in mammography, interest in further development in this area remains keen. Upon reviewing the potential advantages of high quantum efficiency, and other pertinent parameters by application of image information analysis, and considering the convenience which a non-silver halide based system could bring to radiology, one can be assured that development of electrostatic imaging systems will continue.

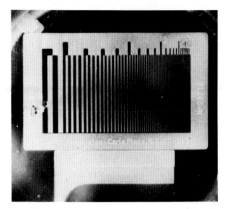

Figure 1. Electrophoretic/Liquid Absorber X-ray Display
of Resolution Target and Al Step Wedge.

REFERENCES

1. J. W. Motz and M. Danos, "Image Information Content and Patient Exposure",
Medical Physics, Vol. 5, p. 8 - 22, 1975.

2. A. Rose, Vision, Human and Electronic, Plenum Press, New York, 1974.

3. W. W. Von Seelentag, "Physikalische Grundlägen der Electroradiographie",
Rontgenpraxis, Vol. 31, Book 3, March, 1978, p. 51 - 69.

4. F. H. Attix, W. C. Roesch, E. Tochilin (editors) Radiation Dosimetry, Vol I
Fundamentals, p. 320 - 321, Academic Press, New York, 1968.

5. M. Ein-Gal, "X-Ray Imaging via Introduction Electrometry", 1978 AAPM
Annual Meeting, Abstract in Medical Physics, Vol 5, No. 4, July/August, 1978.

6. L.S. Jeromin, L.M. Klynn, "Electronic Recording of X-Ray Images", AAPM
Annual Meeting, abstract in Medical Physics, Vol 5, No. 4, July/August, 1978.

7. L.S. Jeromin, private communication.

8. A. Zermeno, et. al., "Laser Read-Out of Electrostatic Images". To be presented to the SPIE/SPSE Seminar, Application of Optical Instrumentation in
Medicine - VII. Toronto, March 25 - 27, 1979.

9. A. Zermeno, private communication.

10. B. Kazan, M. Knoll, Electronic Image Storage, p. 373 - 375, and 261 - 265,
Academic Press, New York, 1968.

11. P. W. Walton, "Optically Projected X-Ray Images from a Sealed Chamber
Ionography System", Proceedings of the SPIE, Vol 96, pp 152 - 156, 1976.

12. Pekan et al., USP 4,002,906.

13. Pekan et al., USP 4,029,960.

14. L. F. Frank, USP 4,047,031.

15. Allan, et al., USP 3,965,352.

16. Brueckner and Lewis, USP 4,079,255

17. Lewis, et al., USP 4,104,520.

18. L.A. DeWerd, P.R. Moran, "Radiographic Images by Solid State Ionography",
Proceedings of the SPIE, Vol. 96, pp 158 - 163, 1976.

19. Allan, et al., "Electron Radiography Using Liquid Absorbers", J. of Applied
Physics, Vol. 46, No. 6, June 1975.

CLOSING REMARKS

Wende W. Logan, M.D.
Consultant, Roswell Park Memorial Institute
1351 Mt. Hope Avenue, Rochester, New York 14620

So many changes have occurred since the original 1976 Reduced Dose Mammography meeting,[1] that it was not possible to include chapters on thermography, ultrasonography, and other procedures which aid in breast carcinoma diagnosis, in this second Reduced Dose Mammography meeting. Even though technically well performed mammography is the single most accurate detector of minimal breast carcinoma, no method is 100% accurate, and for this reason, these additional procedures can and should be utilized with the equivocal mammogram and/or clinical evaluation. The radiologist, who has the advantage of correlation of the mammographic appearance with breast palpation, is in an ideal position to most accurately diagnose a breast carcinoma.

In my office, a pertinent history related to the breast, is obtained on every patient. A thermogram is also performed on every patient. On all patients under the age of 35, a physical examination of the breast is performed, as well as a review of the history and thermogram results, before mammography is contemplated. A mammogram is virtually never performed under the age of 20. Between the ages of 20 and 30, mammography is performed only if a diagnosis cannot be established by means of palpation and ultrasonography. Above the age of thirty, mammography is usually performed, but often consists of only a single screen-film mammogram of each breast, rather than a routine two view study (the oblique view is the single view most commonly performed--see Logan's chapter on proper screen film technique). Since one out of every fifteen patients entering my office has breast cancer (reasons for the mammograms are multiple, varying from a palpable mass (60%), unilateral nipple discharge, positive family history, prior mastectomy, baseline mammogram at age fifty, etc.), considerable care must be paid to any suspicious radiographic or palpable abnormalities. Coned down magnified views are performed of any possible radiographic evidence of calcification, or asymmetrically positioned or unusually dense glandular tissue, as well as palpable masses in patients without discernable radiographic abnormality on a routine mammogram. These magnified coned down views, (with the RSI microfocus unit) are performed with the asymmetric or dense glandular tissue, or palpable mass, positioned tangential to the remaining breast tissue, in an attempt to isolate this region from overlapping glandular tissue elsewhere in the breast. The tangential view is not always possible, with centrally located lesions (with central lesions, the craniocaudad view, or a slight oblique from craniocaudad, is usually the best position to visualize the density separate from surrounding glandular tissue). The magnified view enables much greater accuracy of diagnosis of suspicious lesions[2,3] (see figure 9 in Logan's chapter on Grid vs Magnification).

Ultrasonography has proven to be an extremely valuable aid for evaluation of smoothly outlined densities.[4] Magnification views of these smoothly outlined densities occasionally show no evidence of an irregular border, in which case intracystic carcinomas or medullary carcinomas cannot be ruled out. If fluid is demonstrated via ultrasonography in a clinically worrisome palpable density, aspiration is usually performed, in order to assure the referring clinician, that the lesion is indeed a cyst. Pneumocystography (injection of air into the cyst), is not routinely performed in this office, since intracystic filling defects can be detected by ultrasonagraphy). Figures 1 - 3 demonstrate the important role of ultrasonagraphy in breast cancer diagnosis.

Ductography is performed whenever a unilateral nipple discharge occurs, irrespective of the type of discharge. Ductography frequently detects small carcinomas and/or papillomas that cannot be seen on routine mammography.[5,6]

Needle aspiration cytology is often performed, using a 21 gauge thin walled biopsy needle, which has been specially designed by Universal Medical Instruments* (catalogue number 4526-42-2721). More cellular material has been able to be obtained with these needles, because the thin walls provide more of a cutting edge than a thick walled needle, and the lumen is larger than that of an average 20 or 21 gauge needle. Needle aspiration cytology should not be performed unless the pathologist has had experience with breast needle aspirations, since interpretation is more difficult than that of paraffin tissue sections. At Strong Memorial Hospital, needle aspirations were performed on all surgical breast biopsy specimens, with interpretation of results compared to paraffin tissue interpretations, for an entire year. At that point, the cytology department felt that enough experience had been obtained, and in vivo needle aspiration of breast lesions was begun. Although the preliminary results of the needle cytology interpretations have been encouraging, not enough material has been accumulated at this point to predict what role this will play in breast cancer diagnosis. I predict that in the indeterminate lesion, needle aspiration will prove to be highly valuable in determining whether or not to biopsy.[7]

When a biopsy is recommended, copies of the mammograms are performed on a Delcomat Copier** (on 100 mm x 100 mm duplicating film), to assist the surgeon. If the radiographic lesion is non-palpable (as occurs in 1/4 of the carcinomas), a 1:1 copy of the calcifications is performed in addition, to assist in preoperative localization, and also to assist in radiographic verification of the calcification on tissue specimen radiography, post biopsy. The film copies are sent in preference to the original mammograms, since 20% of original mammograms that are mailed to surgeons are subsequently lost, thus interfering with proper interpretation of the mammogram of the remaining breast, subsequently. (The Delcomat Copier also can be utilized to minify mammograms small enough to directly mount on 35 mm slides for teaching purposes.)

Magnification and ultrasonography, and the other described procedures, have enabled radiographic diagnosis of great specificity. In the past three years, of 3000 patients, 270 breast carcinomas were suspected radiographically. Two hundred of these 270 biopsies proved to be breast carcinoma. Many of the seventy nonmalignant biopsies were "pre-malignant" lesions such as severe focal atypia, and multiple papillomatosis. An analysis of the first 1000 patients evaluated in 1976, by the above described methods, showed that fifty of fifty-five carcinomas were diagnosed correctly via mammography[8] for a radiographic accuracy of 91%. The five missed carcinomas were detected within one year of the radiographic "negative" examination. (At this point, it might be well to point out that many reported articles of mammographic accuracy of diagnosis do not include a one year follow up of the patients, to determine which carcinomas were missed radiographically--the one year interval "miss" rate of radiographic diagnosis is, and should be, an important measure of the efficacy of mammographic diagnosis, and should not be excluded from any evaluation of efficacy of the particular method being evaluated.) While further radiographic image improvements have occurred since the initial evaluation in this office (i.e. improved detector systems, grid use), a one year observation

* also comes in longer lengths for lung and other skinny needle biopsies.
** Old Delft.

necessary before a true accurate analysis of the results can be presented. These are in progress in this office at this time, and will be subsequently reported.

THE FUTURE

The future of mammography has never looked better. In the H.I.P. study in the 1960's, for every breast carcinoma found in women under the age of fifty, solely via mammography, three carcinomas were found solely by physical examination.[9] In sharp contrast, the mammograms have improved so dramatically since the 1960's, that in the B.C.D.D. projects in the 1970's, in women under the age of fifty, for every breast carcinoma detected solely by physical examination, six breast carcinomas were detected solely by mammography--an 18-fold relative increase in detection rate by mammography (Fig 4), as compared physical examination. Technically poor mammography images, however, are more harmful than no mammographic examination at all--a sense of false complacency can be induced by a falsely negative mammogram, which may dissuade the referring physician from obtaining a surgical consult until metastases have occurred. For this reason, proper x-ray equipment and detector systems must be utilized, with strict attention paid to the technical factors of breast positioning and compression. Specialized x-ray equipment solely for the purpose of mammography is not absolutely necessary when xeromammography is performed. However when screen-film mammography is performed, specialized x-ray equipment should be utilized, in order to provide proper compression, and the specialized soft x-ray beam necessary for adequate contrast. Specialized x-ray equipment is supplied with the XERG method.

While considerable sophistication in the art and science of imaging has developed since the 1976 meeting, a state of confusion now exists with respect to breast glandular x-ray dose. This is understandable however, since the Northeast Physics Center depth dose data results have not had ample time to be assimilated before this meeting. At the next Reduced Dose Mammography Meeting (tentatively planned for 1980) it will obviously be of extreme importance to be as accurate and specific as possible when discussing dosage. One should describe the methods utilized for measurement of average glandular dose, including x-ray beam half value layers, average breast thickness, and entrance exposure (including back scatter). Also, when average glandular doses are computed, it should be stated whether an adipose-skin shield (and if so, the thickness), has been used. The method of measurement of the exposure should also be included, since thermoluminescent dosimetry measurements tend to be slightly less than those obtained with the Garrett-Holt ionization chamber, when very low energy levels are being measured (such as with the screen film method). Breast entrance exposures, and mid-plane breast doses are both inadequate indicators of average glandular dose, and therefore cannot and should not be utilized in comparison of the dose of one method to another.

The excellent screen film mammography screening program described in Tabar's chapter, with age matched control group, will undoubtedly prove to lower mortality rates due to breast carcinoma, including women between the ages of 40 and 50, since detection rates of carcinoma are excellent in this age group. Because of the hysteria induced by the former higher x-ray doses, in the United States, coupled with statistical evaluation of outmoded mammography methods, it is doubtful that mammography screening will be reintroduced in the United States in the near future. It is also doubtful, because of the controversy, that a similar controlled study could ever be performed in the United States, and it is indeed fortunate that a screening program can be performed elsewhere, to remove all doubts of the efficacy of reduced dose mammography to detect carcinoma. I predict that the screening results in Sweden will subsequently prove that the decision to delete asymptomatic women between the ages of 40 and 50 from mammography screening in the B.C.D.D. project, was an error in judgement.

70,000,000 chest films were performed in the United States last year. Over 1/3 of the chest films included a lateral view. Since the average glandular dose to the breast in a lateral chest film, is only slightly less than the average glandular breast dose described in Tabar's chapter, if lateral views were not performed on asymptomatic women under the age of 30 obtaining routine chest films, the same average glandular dose could be "stored", for a future occasional screening mammogram in the future, far more efficaciously in terms of diagnostic yield.

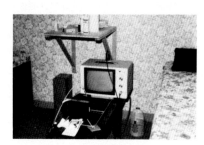 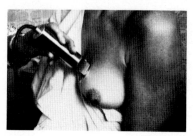

Figure 1.   A- A Bronson-B Ophthalmic Ultrasound Scanner. The unit is small, inexpensive, and extremely valuable in the evaluation of indeterminate lesions. In the diagnostic situation, about 20% of patients benefit from this additional evaluation, following equivocal mammogram results. B- Virtually every mass 1 cm., or larger is able to be evaluated. The transducer is simply placed over the mass, (with a water soluble gel interface), and a poloroid recording of the oscilloscope appearance is obtained.

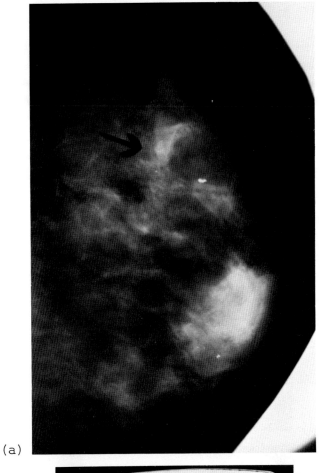

(a)

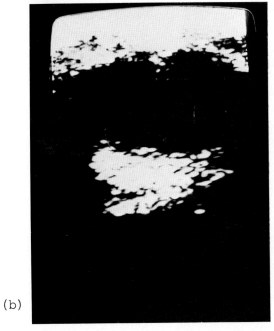

(b)

Figure 2.   A is a lateral mammogram (the arrow points to a palpable firm
density, the border of which is obscured by surrounding glandular
tissue). B is a poloroid image of the Bronson-B Ultrasound
scan, revealing a classical cyst.   This was aspirated, with dis-
appearance of the mass.   Surgery was cancelled.

547

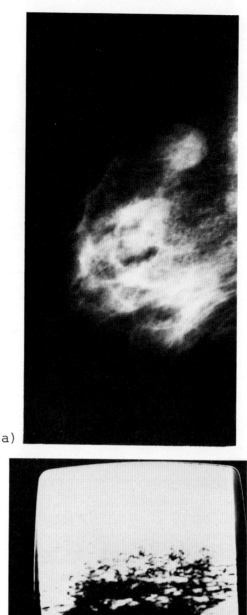

(a)

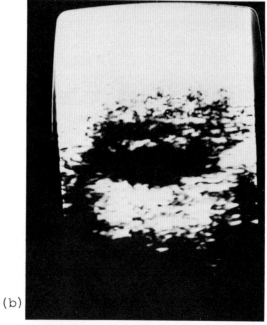

(b)

Figure 3. A is a lateral mammogram on a patient with a smoothly outlined
easily movable density, thought to represent a cyst, both
clinically and radiographically. The Bronson-B scan (B),
revealed a slightly irregular outline to the density, as well
as internal echoes, indicative of a soft tissue density. The
radiologist's opinion was revised, biopsy was recommended, and
this proved to be a medullary carcinoma.

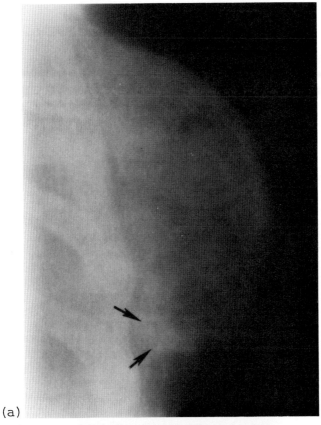

(a)

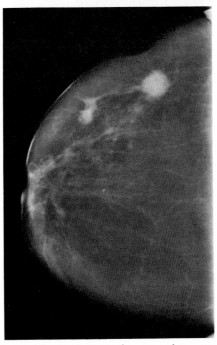

(b)

Figure 4. A demonstrates a breast carcinoma, detected in 1969, as seen
on Kodak Industrial AA hand-processed film, without specialized
x-ray equipment, and without compression, at 2000 mR av. gl. dose.
B shows a Kodak NMB film-Min-R screen mammogram, performed on
the GE Mammex unit, using vigorous compression, at 150 mR av. gl.
dose. The carcinoma outline is well delineated, with slightly
irregular borders.

REFERENCES

1. Logan, WW, Breast Carcinoma-The Radiologist's Expanded Role, John Wiley and Sons, Ed., NYC, NY, 1977.

2. Logan, WW: Overview of the radiologist's role in breast cancer detection. In, Breast Carcinoma: The Radiologist's Expanded Role, Logan, WW, Ed., Wiley and Sons, Publ., NYC, NY, 1977, pp 344-352

3. Muntz, EP, Logan, WW: Focal spot size and scatter supression in magnification mammography. A.J.R.. 1979 (in press).

4. Cole-Beuglet, C.,Beique, RA.;975. Continuous ultrasound B-scanning of palpable breast masses. Radiology 125-128, 1975.

5. Sartorious OW: "Contrast ductography for recognition and localization of benign and malignant breast lesions: an improved technique," Breast Carcinoma: The Radiologist's Expanded Role, pp 281-300, Logan, WW(Ed.), John Wiley and Sons, Publ., NYC, NY, 1977.

6. Logan, WW: Overview of the radiologist's role in breast cancer detection. In, Breast Carcinoma: The Radiologist's Expanded Role, Ed., Logan, WW, Wiley and Sons, Publ., NYC, NY, 1977, pp 353-356.

7. Zajicek, J:"Fine-needle aspiration biopsy of palpable breast lesions", Breast Carcinoma: The Radiologist's Expanded Role, Logan, WW, Ed., John Wiley and Sons, Publ., NYC, NY, pp 319-324.

8. Logan, WW, "Breast carcinoma: the radiologist's role in a non-screening situation. Presented at the RSNA, Dec, 1977.

9. Shapiro, SP, Strax, P, Venet W: Changes in 5-year breast cancer mortality in a breast cancer screening program. Seventh National Cancer Conference Proceeding: 663-673. American Cancer Society, New York, 1973.

INDEX